# Muscle Revolution

Marco Toigo PhD

# Muscle Revolution

## Concepts and Recipes for Building Muscle Mass and Force

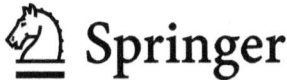

Marco Toigo PhD
Zürich, Switzerland

ISBN 978-3-662-68047-6        ISBN 978-3-662-68048-3   (eBook)
https://doi.org/10.1007/978-3-662-68048-3

This book is a translation of the original German edition „MuskelRevolution" by Toigo, Marco, published by Springer-Verlag GmbH, DE in 2019. The translation was done with the help of artificial intelligence (machine translation by the service DeepL.com). A subsequent human revision was done primarily in terms of content, so that the book will read stylistically differently from a conventional translation. Springer Nature works continuously to further the development of tools for the production of books and on the related technologies to support the authors.

Translation from the German language edition: "MuskelRevolution" by Marco Toigo, © Springer-Verlag GmbH Deutschland, ein Teil von Springer Nature 2019. Published by Springer Berlin Heidelberg. All Rights Reserved.

© The Editor(s) (if applicable) and The Author(s), under exclusive license to Springer-Verlag GmbH, DE, part of Springer Nature 2023
This work is subject to copyright. All rights are solely and exclusively licensed by the Publisher, whether the whole or part of the material is concerned, specifically the rights of translation, reprinting, reuse of illustrations, recitation, broadcasting, reproduction on microfilms or in any other physical way, and transmission or information storage and retrieval, electronic adaptation, computer software, or by similar or dissimilar methodology now known or hereafter developed.
The use of general descriptive names, registered names, trademarks, service marks, etc. in this publication does not imply, even in the absence of a specific statement, that such names are exempt from the relevant protective laws and regulations and therefore free for general use.
The publisher, the authors, and the editors are safe to assume that the advice and information in this book are believed to be true and accurate at the date of publication. Neither the publisher nor the authors or the editors give a warranty, expressed or implied, with respect to the material contained herein or for any errors or omissions that may have been made. The publisher remains neutral with regard to jurisdictional claims in published maps and institutional affiliations.

This Springer imprint is published by the registered company Springer-Verlag GmbH, DE, part of Springer Nature.
The registered company address is: Heidelberger Platz 3, 14197 Berlin, Germany

Paper in this product is recyclable.

# Foreword

In practically every magazine you will find tips and recommendations from "experts" on how to train effectively and efficiently and on optimal nutrition. In bookstores, books on strength and fitness training fill entire shelves and departments. Television is also teeming with relevant messages and the Internet represents a veritable jungle of information in this regard. How is a normal person who wants to find out about training and nutrition supposed to find his way through this swamp of opinions? Because this much is clear: There are not nearly as many scientifically proven facts on the subject of training and nutrition as there are training recommendations and so-called training systems.

To find your way through the jungle of training and nutrition opinions and to sharpen your eye for the essentials, there is only one thing to do: acquire the necessary expertise. All you need is understandable, quality-controlled information. The source of quality-controlled expert information is all *peer-reviewed published* literature (literature that has been peer-reviewed by independent experts prior to publication) from a wide variety of disciplines in the natural sciences of muscle research, such as muscle physiology, molecular and cell biology, genetics, neuroscience, nutritional science, and biomechanics. Only by integrating the different scientific perspectives and findings and comparing them with training practice does an overall picture emerge from which conclusions can be drawn as to what is sensible or proportionate in terms of training and nutrition.

In this book, I try to build a logical and robust bridge between this scientific knowledge and training and nutrition practice. I know at this point there would normally come a point where the author subtly signals his expert status to you so that you believe what is in the book. This is usually done by communicating status symbols, that is, a list of scientific awards, athletic accomplishments, years of experience, or simply muscular looks. You won't find that bling-bling here. I prefer to let hard facts speak for themselves.

MarcYigo PhD

# Instructions for Use of This Book

The book consists of the following five elements: Main Text, Summaries, Info Boxes ("Knowledge Drops"), Illustrations, and Bibliography. The boxes, which are distributed throughout the book, aim to answer widely asked questions briefly and clearly. The bibliography provides the precise details of any academic papers, books, or websites cited in the text. The illustrations and diagrams are intended to help illustrate textual content and thereby make it more understandable, or to provide another approach. The main text is divided into 24 chapters, all of which provide a very deep, yet practical insight into the nature (science) of skeletal muscle and its malleability through Resistance Training.

In this book you have several access modes and content difficulty levels at your disposal. This allows you to approach the content according to your previous knowledge and interests. For example, in the boxes you will quickly get well-founded answers to your questions without first having to rummage through countless pages. Starting from these boxes, you can go into more detail in the relevant chapters, or you can jump in at any chapter and explore the rest of the content from there, thanks to the cross-references. The summaries reflect the presented contents in a concise form and sometimes show the practical relevance with concrete tips. Finally, you can also use the book as a classic textbook and reference work.

The first third (Chaps. 1, 2, 3, 4, 5, 6, 7, and 8) of the book deals mainly with basic muscle physiology. This can seem a bit dry at times, but is no less important. Hang in there! You will be rewarded with enlightening and unexpected insights. We then turn to the peculiarities and laws of voluntary muscle (fiber) use in Resistance Training and explore how you can specifically influence skeletal muscle development and strength through training and nutrition. The focus is always on the transfer of scientific findings into everyday training.

I hope that you will benefit from this book by understanding, first and foremost, how Resistance Training, nutrition, and muscle adaptation interact based on individual prerequisites, and what the practical consequences are for your training and nutritional habits. I wish you an interesting and satisfying journey into the wonderful world of muscle training!

# Acknowledgments

I thank the physicist Raphael Barengo for the artistic graphic realization of my raw illustration templates. Many thanks to Marko Cevid and Jan Zierold who skillfully edited the text of the 1st edition. I thank my former PhD and master's students for their critical discussions and contributions to the visual material. I thank the editors of Springer-Verlag Marion Krämer and Martina Mechler for their support in realizing this book project. A special thanks goes to Jonathan von Oppen, who fully committed himself to this project during his internship at Springer and made an optimal cooperation possible. Furthermore, I am very grateful to Dr. Sandro Müller, my long-time colleague, for his extremely valuable support in the realization of the 2nd edition. I would also like to thank Dr. Andrea Scherer, Bradley Turner, and Daniel Fitze for their help in checking the proofs and the translation. Finally, I thank the many readers of this book. They not only make the 2nd edition possible but also contribute to the further development of the book with their constructive feedback.

# Contents

1 **What Are We Talking About? Clear Thinking Through Clear Terminology and Vice Versa**    1
   1.1 Muscles Contract: Not (Only)!    1
   1.2 Mice Under the Skin    3
   1.3 Why Skeletal Muscles Do Not Have Eccentric Airs and Graces    4
   1.4 Do Not Be Deceived by Appearances    5
   1.5 The "Trinity" of Force Production    6
   1.6 The Relationship Between the Rate of Change of Length and the Force of a Muscle    7
   1.7 What Does "Exercise" Actually Mean and How Is It Quantified?    9
   1.8 If You Want to Lose Weight, Fly to the Moon!    10
   1.9 Muscles Only Want One Thing: To Rotate Loads Around Joints    10
   1.10 Why Your Muscles (Have to) Work Even Though You Are Not Performing Any Work    12
   1.11 What Do Human Muscles Have to Do with Horses?    13
   1.12 Force Always Tastes Like Newtons    14
   1.13 Why You Should Not Confuse Your Training Resistance with a Projectile    15
   1.14 Jogging on the Leg Press    15
   1.15 Summary: Why Muscle Force Does Not Always Lead to Visible Movement    16

## 2  All that Glitters Is Not Gold — 19
2.1  Surrogates for Internal Muscle Force — 19
2.2  How Strong Is "Strong"? — 20
2.3  Maximum Force Is Not Equal to Peak Force — 20
2.4  Decoding Muscle Force — 21
2.5  Muscles in the Zebra Skin — 25
2.6  Spoilt for Choice When Selecting the Best Training Tool? — 26
2.7  Not All Machines Are Created Equal, or Are They? — 26
2.8  The Ominous Force Curve — 28
2.9  Summary: Don't Blindly Follow the Squat Trend — 31

## 3  Thick and/or Long? A Never Ending Question — 33
3.1  The Functional Role of Muscle Length — 33
3.2  The Functional Role of Muscle Thickness (Muscle Cross-Sectional Area) — 36
3.3  Summary — 38

## 4  The Neuromuscular Origin of Muscle Force — 41
4.1  The Muscles in the Brain — 41
4.2  How Is Muscle Force "Coded"? — 42
4.3  Muscle Fibers, as Part of the Motor Unit, Always Work as a Team — 44
4.4  Why Are Neuromuscular Connections Dotted? — 44
4.5  Not All Muscle Fibers Run from Tendon to Tendon — 45
4.6  Neuromuscular Catchment Areas — 47
4.7  How Motor Units Can Differ — 48
4.8  Summary — 50

## 5  A Bouquet of Cellular Diversity — 51
5.1  The Colorful World of Muscle Fibers — 51
5.2  Molecular Motors of the Muscle — 52
5.3  Fiber Type-Specific Motor Classes — 53
5.4  Distribution of Muscle Fiber Types in Humans: What Determines It? — 56
5.5  Changes in the Distribution of Muscle Fiber Types Due to Training or Inactivity — 59
5.6  Why You Can Produce More Force Pliometrically than Miometrically — 60

|   |   |   |
|---|---|---|
| 5.7 | Summary: Does "Fast" Training Make Your Muscle Motors Faster? | 62 |

## 6 Muscular Energy Bundles — 63
- 6.1 The Dynamics of Muscular Energy Consumption — 63
- 6.2 Matching Supply and Demand — 64
- 6.3 Muscle Fibers Have Several Resources for Regenerating Energy — 64
- 6.4 The Phosphagen System: A Firework of Energy — 65
- 6.5 The Glycolytic System: Sugar-Sweet ATP Regeneration — 67
- 6.6 Mitochondrial Respiration: Why We Need Oxygen — 72
- 6.7 Mitochondria: Small but Mighty! — 73
- 6.8 Integration of the Three Systems for the Regeneration of ATP — 74
- 6.9 Summary: ATP Molecules Resemble Rechargeable Batteries — 75

## 7 Why You Fatigue During Exercise — 77
- 7.1 The Different Components of Neuromuscular Fatigue — 77
- 7.2 Metabolites as Fatigue Mediators — 77
- 7.3 Microtraumata as Fatigue Mediators — 78
- 7.4 From Muscle Mice to Sore Muscles — 79
- 7.5 Summary: The Lore of Being Sore — 80

## 8 The Molecular and Cellular Muscle Universe — 81
- 8.1 Muscle Regeneration: A Balancing Act — 81
- 8.2 DNA: The Mother Molecule of All (Muscle) Proteins — 82
- 8.3 All Muscle Fibers Are Muscle Cells, But Not All Muscle Cells Are Muscle Fibers — 85
- 8.4 When Satellite Cells Are Awakened — 86
- 8.5 The Gift of Self-Renewal — 87
- 8.6 Muscle Spindles Also Contain Muscle Fibers — 92
- 8.7 Characterisation of Human Muscle Tissue — 92
- 8.8 Summary — 94

## 9 How You Can Influence Which Muscle Fibers Are Used in Training — 97
- 9.1 Back to the Motor Units — 97
- 9.2 How Is the Force of a Muscle Modulated During Voluntary Force Production? — 98

| | | |
|---|---|---|
| 9.3 | Muscle War Zone: Recruit and Fire! | 98 |
| 9.4 | How Do Recruitment and Increase in Firing Frequency Encode the Level of Force? | 99 |
| 9.5 | What Do Autonomous Reserves Have to Do with Hibernation? | 100 |
| 9.6 | The Tonic Recruitment Threshold | 101 |
| 9.7 | The Regular Recruitment of Motor Units | 102 |
| 9.8 | Mechanism of Recruitment of Motor Units | 102 |
| 9.9 | Where Brain Meets Muscle | 105 |
| 9.10 | How Is the Rate of Force Development Encoded by Recruitment and Frequency? | 107 |
| 9.11 | Practical Relevance: Force Magnitude and Rate of Force Development | 110 |
| 9.12 | Do You Want Big and Strong Muscles? Weaken Them! | 112 |
| 9.13 | Can Type 2 Fibers Be Selectively Activated? | 115 |
| 9.14 | Neuroanatomical Muscle Cartography | 116 |
| 9.15 | Force Transmission Between Neighbours | 121 |
| 9.16 | Tensional Integrity and Mechanotransduction: To What Extent Do Muscle Fibers Have Integrity? | 122 |
| 9.17 | Can a Muscle Be Specifically "Sculpt"? | 123 |
| 9.18 | Summary | 125 |

## 10 When Resistance Training Meets Muscle Plasticity — 129

| | | |
|---|---|---|
| 10.1 | How Do Muscles Adapt To Resistance Training? | 129 |
| 10.2 | Length Adaptation (Longitudinal Hypertrophy or Atrophy) in Animals and Humans | 130 |
| 10.3 | Radial Growth of Muscle (Radial Hypertrophy or Atrophy) in Humans | 144 |
| 10.4 | Summary | 145 |

## 11 How Is Skeletal Muscle Protein Synthesized and Broken Down? — 147

| | | |
|---|---|---|
| 11.1 | Building Muscle Protein Mass | 147 |
| 11.2 | The Relationship Between MPS and MPB | 148 |
| 11.3 | How Your Muscles Hypertrophy and Atrophy Hourly | 149 |
| 11.4 | Summary | 150 |

## 12  Dietary Protein as an Anabolic Stimulus — 153
- 12.1 Whole-Body Protein Metabolism Is Not Equal to Muscle Protein Metabolism — 153
- 12.2 The Anabolic Effect of Dietary Protein on Muscle Metabolism — 154
- 12.3 Protein Quality Counts! — 158
- 12.4 The Protein Quantity Counts as Well! — 165
- 12.5 Why Eating Alone Isn't Sufficient to Bulk Up Muscles — 168
- 12.6 The Concept of Full Muscle — 169
- 12.7 Amino Acids, Protein Shakes or Meals? — 171
- 12.8 Are Carbohydrates Necessary in a Protein Shake? — 172
- 12.9 Why Not Take Isolated Amino Acids? — 174
- 12.10 Summary — 174

## 13  Resistance Exercise as an Anabolic Stimulus — 177
- 13.1 The Acute Anabolic Muscle Response to Resistance Exercise — 177
- 13.2 Bridging the Gap Between Muscle Protein Synthesis and Motor Unit Recruitment — 178
- 13.3 How Does Training Intensity Affect Muscle Protein Synthesis? — 179
- 13.4 The Dose-Response Relationship Between Training Load and the Acute Increase in Muscle Protein Synthesis — 180
- 13.5 What Influence Does the Muscular Time Under Tension Have on the Anabolism of the Muscle? — 182
- 13.6 Which Is More Effective: Single-Set or Multi-set Training? A Pointless Question — 183
- 13.7 The Key to Muscle Growth — 184
- 13.8 The Difference Between Time Under Tension, Effective Time Under Tension and Number of Repetitions — 193
- 13.9 Is Pliometric (Eccentric) More Effective than Miometric (Concentric)? — 195
- 13.10 Skeletal Muscles Also Have a "Feeling of Satiety" — 195
- 13.11 What Is the Optimum Time Interval with Which to Train a Particular Muscle? — 196
- 13.12 Misconception of Supercompensation — 197
- 13.13 Summary — 198

## 14 The Synergistic Relationship Between Resistance Exercise and Dietary Protein Intake — 201
- 14.1 The Synergistic Effect Between Resistance Exercise and Dietary Protein — 201
- 14.2 Protein Intake: Best Before, During or After Resistance Exercise? — 205
- 14.3 Does Resistance Exercise Affect Protein Digestion? — 208
- 14.4 Is Carbohydrate Intake Necessary Immediately After Resistance Exercise to Maximize MPS or Minimize MPB? — 209
- 14.5 Is the Anabolic Response of the Muscle Weaker if You Train with Relatively Empty Muscle Glycogen Stores? — 210
- 14.6 Transfer from Acute to Long-Term Effects? — 211
- 14.7 When Does Protein Supplementation Make Sense? — 213
- 14.8 Summary — 220

## 15 Does Endurance Training Inhibit Muscle Growth? — 225
- 15.1 Who Bites Whom: The Resistance Training the Endurance Training or Vice Versa? — 225
- 15.2 Why Muscle Protein Synthesis Is Not a Priority in the Presence of Energy Stress — 226
- 15.3 Misconception of Periodization — 227
- 15.4 Does Resistance Training Make Sense for Endurance Athletes? — 230
- 15.5 Why Resistance Training Hardly Makes Your Heart Fitter — 231
- 15.6 Summary — 233

## 16 The Hunt for Hormonal Ghosts — 237
- 16.1 Whole Body or Split Training? — 237
- 16.2 Why Testosterone Is Overrated as an Anabolic Hormone — 238
- 16.3 How Does Resistance Exercise Affect the Blood Concentration of Anabolic Hormones? — 239
- 16.4 Summary — 243

## 17 Men Are Not Martians and Women Are Not Venusians — 245
- 17.1 What Does Planetary Science Have to Do with Gender-Specific Muscle Development? — 245
- 17.2 How the Contraceptive Pill Can Affect Your Muscle Mass — 247
- 17.3 XXY — 248

|  |  |  |
|---|---|---|
| | 17.4 Summary | 248 |

## 18 Specificity of Adaptation to Training — 251
- 18.1 Does Your Right Arm Benefit When You Exercise Your Left? — 251
- 18.2 Initially with the Shotgun, Later with the Precision Rifle — 251
- 18.3 Exerceuticals — 252
- 18.4 Summary — 253

## 19 Why Muscle Training Is Not Optional — 255
- 19.1 The Hidden Sides of the Skeletal Muscles — 255
- 19.2 The Muscle-Bone Unit — 258
- 19.3 The Bone-Building Potential of Training and Exercise Purely from the Perspective of the Bone Deformation Achieved: Practical Tips — 260
- 19.4 Training During Pregnancy — 262
- 19.5 "From the Age of 25, Muscle Force and Mass Go Downhill": If You Believe So! — 262
- 19.6 Anabolic Resistance — 263
- 19.7 The Anti-aging Effect of Resistance Training — 266
- 19.8 Summary — 269

## 20 At the End of the Day, What Makes You Aesthetic? — 271
- 20.1 The Difference Between Muscle Mass and Body Mass — 271
- 20.2 If Measuring, Then Correctly — 272
- 20.3 Fat Loss — 274
- 20.4 Why You Do Not Continue to Lose Weight Despite Even More Exercise — 275
- 20.5 About Problem Zones and Cellulite — 279
- 20.6 Is There an Optimal Time of Day for Muscle Training? — 282
- 20.7 The Path from Training Stimulus to Muscle Adaptation — 285
- 20.8 Summary — 285

## 21 Nature's Whim: The Extent of Adaptation to Training Is Individual — 287
- 21.1 Interindividual Variability of Adaptation to Training: The New Mantra? — 287
- 21.2 Twice as Much Muscle Mass: Without Training! — 290

|  |  |  |
|---|---|---|
| | 21.3 What Can Be Expected in Terms of Average Muscle Growth? | 292 |
| | 21.4 Why We Sometimes Confuse Cause and Effect in Training Too | 293 |
| | 21.5 Summary | 295 |
| **22** | **Neural Aspects of Resistance Training** | **297** |
| | 22.1 Force Versus Exercise Competence | 297 |
| | 22.2 Is a Bigger Muscle Also a Stronger Muscle? | 299 |
| | 22.3 Are 100 Newtons Equal to 100 Newtons? | 301 |
| | 22.4 Core Training | 302 |
| | 22.5 Rate of Force Development | 306 |
| | 22.6 Summary | 309 |
| **23** | **Anabolic Enhancers** | **311** |
| | 23.1 Vitamin D | 311 |
| | 23.2 β-Hydroxy-β-Methylbutyrate (HMB): Top or Flop? | 314 |
| | 23.3 Fish Oil as an Anabolic Enhancer | 316 |
| | 23.4 Creatine Supplementation: Why? What for? | 317 |
| | 23.5 Summary | 319 |
| **24** | **Go for It!** | **321** |
| **References** | | **323** |
| **Index** | | **337** |

# 1

# What Are We Talking About? Clear Thinking Through Clear Terminology and Vice Versa

## 1.1 Muscles Contract: Not (Only)!

What is the first thing that comes to mind when you hear the commonly known term "muscle contraction"? Well, I don't have to be psychic to guess that you automatically think of the contraction or shortening of the muscle. This is not surprising at all. Even the definition in the *Duden foreign dictionary* is "(Med.) the contracting (esp. of muscles)". Unfortunately, this definition is woefully inadequate to describe muscle function and misleads us into misconceptions. Why?

Imagine you are standing upright, your arms are hanging by your sides and you are holding a dumbbell in your right hand. Experience shows that you can move the selected dumbbell mass up and down several times without difficulty. Now bring the dumbbell to your chin, just as you would bring an apple to your mouth. What happens during this bending movement? When lifting (pulling) the dumbbell, the arm flexor muscles, among others, produce force while the forearm bones, to which the muscles are attached by tendons, approach the humerus and shoulder blade. From the outside, the muscles shorten and the angle between the upper and lower arm becomes smaller. So how does the dumbbell get back to the starting position? In this case, you can do this by deliberately reducing the force applied. This reduces the muscular torque compared to the external torque – the dumbbell moves back to the starting position as a result. When lowering (braking), the arm flexor muscles therefore also generate force, but they become longer on the outside and the angle between the upper and lower arm increases. If you pause briefly at the

© The Author(s), under exclusive license to Springer-Verlag GmbH, DE, part of Springer Nature 2023
M. Toigo, *Muscle Revolution*, https://doi.org/10.1007/978-3-662-68048-3_1

reversal points between flexion and extension (or *vice versa*) while holding against the dumbbell, no movement is visible from the outside, but your muscles are still generating force continuously.

But there is a second way, how you can bring the dumbbell to the starting position (stretched arms to the side of the body, hands to the side of the hips). To do this, imagine that you – attached by your feet – hang upside down on a horizontal bar, still holding the dumbbell with a bent forearm to the chin. In this case, you get to the starting position by having the opposite muscles (the so-called antagonists) of the arm flexors, the arm extensor muscles, move the dumbbell back by extending at the elbow joint. In the process, mainly the arm extensor muscles produce force, and shorten (external view). As a result, the angle between the upper and lower arm increases. The intended effect of some muscles, for example the arm flexors, is therefore to reduce the angle between the upper and lower arm (angle of the elbow joint). For other muscles, such as the arm extensors, this is exactly the opposite.

What do we learn from these observations? The muscles *try to* shorten, but the shortening is not necessarily the result. Depending on the amount of force produced and the amount of force to be overcome, the result can also be a relative lengthening or no change in length (always viewed from the outside, of course). Equating muscle contraction with muscle shortening therefore falls far short of the mark. If you concentrate exclusively on the muscle-shortening movement phase when training your muscles, because you think or have been told that your muscles only work in this movement phase, you neglect the other forms of use that are just as important for training success. Furthermore, you are ignoring the fact that it is precisely the aspect of neural activation and force production (regardless of the direction of length change) that is central to training adaptations. And if muscle contraction is supposed to equal muscle shortening, how please should the commonly used term combination "isometric muscle contraction" be understood? Exactly. Not at all, because "isometric" – "iso-" (gr. ísos for similar, corresponding, equal) and "-metric" (referring to the meter as a unit of length) – means something like "equal length", which contradicts muscle contraction if it is understood as muscle shortening.

> **Box 1.1: Quintessence: What Is "Functional Training" Really?**
> Skeletal muscles are essential for the function of our organism and thus for our health. They fulfil several important tasks. In the context of human movement, the actual function of skeletal muscles is to produce force (see Sect. 1.15). In doing so, the muscle tries to shorten itself, which it often does in everyday life. For example, when you bring an apple to your mouth, your biceps muscle

shortens. However, muscle shortening is not always the result of force production. In other words, externally visible limb movement is not necessarily the result of muscle force generation. You will become aware of this fact as soon as you try to lift a tank with maximum effort. It will not budge even though your muscles are generating a lot of force. Similarly, when holding or carrying shopping bags, your shoulder and neck muscles produce force even though the shopping bags remain more or less at the same height. Finally, in everyday life it often happens that you have to slow down movement, for example when walking or going down stairs. After you put your foot down, the knee bends and the thigh muscles produce force to prevent you from buckling. In this case, the muscles produce force while they are stretched a bit. From these observations, it is clear what "functional" really means for a muscle: it is stimulated voluntarily or reflexively by nerve impulses and produces force. Whether a movement is externally visible and how fast this movement is, depends primarily on the amount of muscle force produced relative to the force imposed by the external load and the lever arm. Muscle force characteristics in turn depend on neural and muscular factors, namely the recruitment and firing frequency of motor units and the structural and metabolic properties of their muscle fibers. In this sense, your training is automatically "functional" once your muscles are neurally stimulated and producing force. However, the target of a muscle's force production (shortening) can vary because a single muscle can normally perform multiple movement tasks. For example, the biceps muscle not only has the task of flexing the elbow, but also of rotating the wrist outward or lifting the arm forward when the elbow is flexed. From this perspective, training becomes more functional when you train a specific muscle in all of its movement tasks. In resistance training, this means that you should work the different anatomical-neuromuscular compartments of a muscle, *nota bene* if they exist, with several, functionally different exercises. This increases the chance that the training effects will also be effective in your sport or during everyday activities. In other words, it increases the transfer effect of resistance training. One thing is clear: there is no convincing scientific basis for claims that single-joint exercises are less functional than multi-joint exercises.

## 1.2 Mice Under the Skin

Incidentally, etymologically the term "muscle" can be derived from the Latin word *musculus* (little mouse), because the image of shortening muscles resembles the idea of mice running under the skin. Historically, the first attempts to explain how muscles work date to the Greek physician Hippocrates (460–377 BC). However, it was Galen (129–216 AD), a physician from Pergamon (now Bergama, Turkey), who attempted to explain muscle function mechanistically. Among other things, he postulated that there was a substance in the brain (lat. *spiritus animalis*) that was able to flow through the nerves, which were imagined to be hollow, into the muscles and expand them. This, according to his conception, would activate the muscles. This theory was so pervasive that it lasted into the seventeenth century. It was not until 1663 that Swammerdam showed, by means of an elegant neurophysiological experiment, that an isolated muscle does not increase its volume when stimulated. This experimentally disproved Galen's theory. Apparently, however, the equally clear result was overlooked that stimulation also does not lead to a reduction in volume (i.e. volume contraction) of the isolated muscle. Nevertheless, to this day the inappropriate expression of muscle contraction can stubbornly persist. But you know better now: instead of "contraction", just use "force production"!

## 1.3 Why Skeletal Muscles Do Not Have Eccentric Airs and Graces

Besides "isometric", the two adjectives "concentric" and "eccentric" are also very often combined with the noun "muscle contraction", only these two adjectives are even more meaningless in the context of skeletal muscle activity than the aforementioned "muscle contraction". "Concentric" means something like "having a common center" (referring to circles) while "eccentric" can be translated as "lying outside the center (of circles)." While these two geometric terms are compatible with the physiological or pathological adaptations of the heart muscle, or ventricles, they do not make sense in the context of heart muscle and skeletal muscle function. Even if a cardiac enlargement is eccentric in nature (e.g., a left ventricular only cardiac enlargement) and the cardiac muscle then produces force under eccentric conditions, in the process the muscle fibers become progressively shorter, remain the same length, or are stretched under special circumstances. The further meaning of "eccentric" as "unusual in an exaggerated way", then makes the term combination "eccentric contraction" finally a curiosity.

You may wonder why I keep emphasizing the outside view. The answer is: because quite different processes can be going on inside. The many muscle fibers (i.e., the multinucleated muscle cells) are organized in bundles (fascicles) and embedded in a network of connective tissue, commonly called the extracellular matrix. Externally, the muscle is surrounded by a layer of coarse connective tissue (muscle fascia). Muscle fibers and extracellular matrix are connected to tendons via the muscle-tendon junction, which in turn is the link to bone. In this context, one speaks of the muscle-tendon unit (Fig. 1.1).

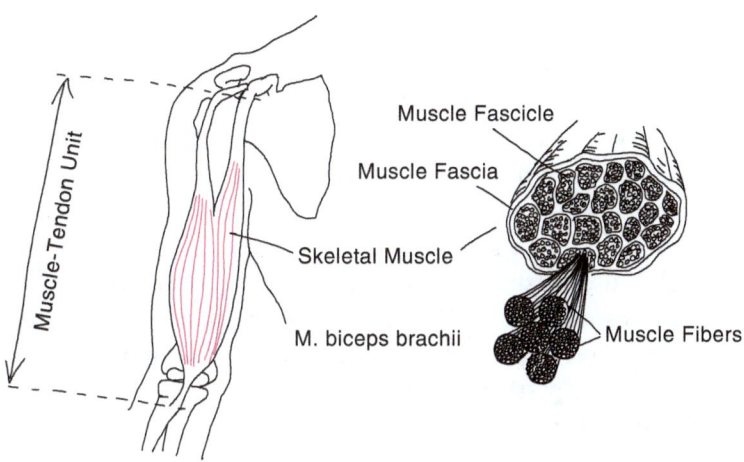

**Fig. 1.1** Muscle-tendon unit and structure of skeletal muscle. Note that under given circumstances the length of the muscle-tendon unit may increase with simultaneous muscle shortening. Therefore, the length of the muscle-tendon unit is not the same as the muscle length. A skeletal muscle consists of many bundles of individual muscle fibers (fascicles)

## 1.4 Do Not Be Deceived by Appearances

When viewed from the outside, for example in the case of the arm flexor muscles, the joint angle between the upper and lower arm becomes smaller, one speaks of the muscle shortening. Strictly speaking, however, it is the muscle-tendon unit that shortens and not necessarily the muscle or the muscle fascicles in all cases. How so? Think of the two-legged jump. You can initiate this jump from a standing position. In doing so, you swing your arms and simultaneously bend your knees (squatting motion), and then immediately shoot up into the air. This is called a *countermovement jump*. By definition, such countermovements involve a stretch-shortening cycle, in this case for the knee extensor muscles. It is typical for stretch-shortening cycles that, due to the higher preload at the beginning of the shortening of the muscle-tendon unit (*i.e.* at the end of the lowering movement in the squat), the tendon stretch is greater than the fascicle stretch. This means that the fascicles of the knee extensor muscles shorten before any movement occurs in the knee joint (*i.e.*, the muscle-tendon unit does not change length during this phase). During the jump, the fascicle length then remains relatively constant while the tendons snap back at high speed (the muscle-tendon unit becomes shorter). If the muscles had to shorten at high speed in order to perform the jumping movement, muscle force would be low (see Sect. 1.6).

The rapid shortening of the muscle-tendon unit therefore depends primarily on the shortening of the tendon during stretch-shortening cycles. In contrast, the shortening of the muscle-tendon unit of the knee extensor muscles in movements without a stretch-shortening cycle, for example in a two-legged jump without a countermovement (i.e. starting in a squat position), is primarily due to the shortening of the muscle fascicles (more or less constant tendon length; Cormie et al. 2011). At the same time, during this type of jump, the calf muscles (specifically the medial head of the twin calf muscle, M. gastrocnemius medialis) behave like the thigh muscles during the jump with stretch-shortening cycle. The Achilles tendon plays an important role in connection with energy storage and release.

As I have just explained to you, the term "muscle contraction" as well as the adjectives "concentric" and "eccentric" used with it are inadequate or incorrect to describe muscle function. What is needed is an unambiguous and correct nomenclature. In English, the problem has been solved by simply using the adjectives shortening, lengthening or *isometric* before muscle *action*. This way you are describing the result of muscle function. The function of the muscle is, as mentioned before, to produce force. In doing so, it attempts to shorten.

## 1.5 The "Trinity" of Force Production

As early as 1938, Hubbard and Stetson recognized that muscles can perform their function under three conditions. They called these three conditions "miometric", "isometric" and "pliometric" (Hubbard and Stetson 1938). These adjectives are composed of the Greek prefixes "mio-" (shorter), "iso-" (equal), and "plio-" (longer) and the word "-metric" and accurately sum up the result of force action or force application on the length of the muscle-tendon unit. For the rest of the book, therefore, instead of "concentric, isometric, eccentric contraction," I will speak of "miometric, isometric, pliometric force production."

How can you remember which change in length "miometric" and "pliometric" stand for ("isometric" is already established in linguistic usage)? Quite simply, in the word "pliometric" the letter "l" occurs for "longer" or "long". Always be aware when reading that the adjectives are primarily describing the change in length of the muscle-tendon unit. The book will also frequently refer to muscle fibers. Consequently, in the context of individual muscle fibers or muscle fiber bundles, the adjectives refer to the length of these structures. Finally, note that the adjective "pliometric" used here should not be confused with "plyometric training". The latter is colloquially used to describe jump training.

## 1.6 The Relationship Between the Rate of Change of Length and the Force of a Muscle

On the one hand, the force-velocity relationship (Hill 1922; Katz 1939; Fig. 1.2) describes the fact that a muscle produces less force with increasing shortening velocity. Conversely, this means that a muscle can only produce a large force when shortened if the shortening velocity is low. You know this from your daily experience: a pencil (low load, little muscle force) can be moved faster than a tree trunk (high load, much muscle force), even if in both cases you try to move the resistance as fast as possible. On the other hand, the force-velocity relationship describes that at negative shortening velocity, i.e. stretching, increasingly more force is produced as the stretching velocity increases until it reaches a plateau, and more than isometrically possible. You are also familiar with this phenomenon from practice. When you lower the dumbbell each time in training (braking part of the movement or negative shortening speed), the load feels lighter because the muscle is stronger in this force production mode. The amount of muscle force generated therefore

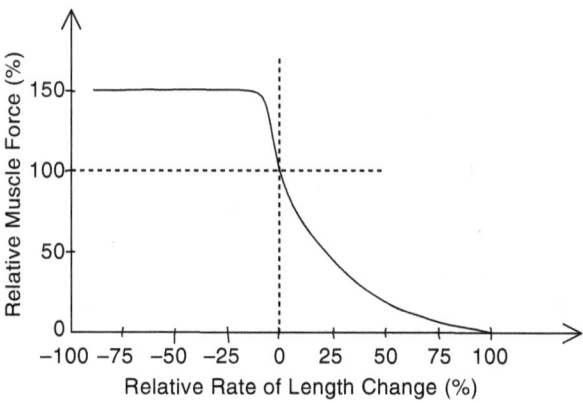

**Fig. 1.2** Force-velocity relationship for a skeletal muscle. Note that when the rate of length change is negative (i.e., pliometric activity), muscle force increases rapidly at first, then does not change as it progresses, and decreases sharply as the rate of shortening increases (positive) (i.e., miometric activity). Muscle force production with a shortening speed of zero is referred to as isometric muscle activity

depends on the speed of the change in length of the muscle, but this in two respects: direction and amount.

## Direction

By convention, during force production with muscle shortening, the velocity is positive, while during force production with muscle stretching, it is negative. Incidentally, terms such as "positive or negative phase of movement" and "negative training" are derived from this. When the rate of change in length is zero, force production takes place isometrically.

## Amount

During miometric force production, you can move the physical body being moved faster if its weight force is small relative to the instantaneously available peak voluntary force. During pliometric force production, the rate of change in length (in this case, elongation) is greater when the object's weight force is large relative to the instantaneously available peak voluntary force. In other words, the heavier the dumbbell for a given muscle force, or the more fatigued your muscle is for a given external load, the faster the braking phase.

> **Box 1.2: What Can You Deduce for Your Training from the Described Force-Velocity Relationship?**
>
> You can deduce two things: First, when miometric force production is fast, the muscle force produced is relatively small. Conversely, the slower the rate of shortening, the more force the muscle can produce. Assuming that high internal forces can be beneficial for muscle strengthening during training, the training load should be moved slowly during muscle shortening. Second, muscle force is always greater at maximal activation during pliometric force production (regardless of stretch speed) than during isometric or miometric force production. Try to move slowly at all times during training, even if that is not always the visible result.
>
> As an example, I describe here the performance of negative pull-ups (negative training). If you can do less than four anatomically perfect and slowly executed pull-ups, a pull-up bar and a small staircase are completely sufficient for this experiment. Climb the stairs and hold onto the bar with an underhand grip so that your chin is higher than the bar when your neck is straight, and your forearm, upper arm, and shoulder are in the same plane on each side. Now angle your lower legs and cross your feet while still holding firmly in the starting position. You are now literally hanging in the air. Now try to slow down the downward movement of your body evenly and slowly (in about 10 s). Do not let go of the bar when you reach the bottom and immediately and quickly climb back up

> the stairs to the starting position. Repeat the braking process. You will notice that as you brake more and more (i.e., repetitions), the downward motion becomes faster and faster, even though you are using maximum voluntary effort to try to slow your body down. After a few repetitions you will virtually free-fall, i.e. in less than 1 s – this point in time then corresponds to the end of the exercise.

## 1.7 What Does "Exercise" Actually Mean and How Is It Quantified?

Now that we have clarified the movement function of muscles, we are in a better position to examine the meaning of the term "exercise". *Exercise* is the potential disruption of homeostasis by muscle activity that is either exclusively or in combination miometric, isometric or pliometric in nature. This definition takes into account that, on the one hand, disruption of metabolic processes is likely, but that, on the other hand, movement may not necessarily be a result. Moreover, the definition can be applied to all situations and all muscles (cardiac muscles, smooth muscles and skeletal muscles). Incidentally, this definition is also applicable to the term "physical activity". The difference between exercise and physical activity is therefore the different context of muscle activity and the related different interpretation of the motivation or intention of the individual.

The next question is how to quantify training. The answer to this question can be found in the International System of Units (*Système International d'Unités*, SI). The SI was introduced in 1960 as the twelfth resolution of the eleventh General Assembly on weights and measures. It is administered by the *International Bureau of Weights and Measures* (http://www.bipm.org), which publishes the SI reference booklet every few years. This sets out the internationally recognised quantities, units and symbols that apply to all measurements. In science, following the SI is mandatory, because it is the only way to compare measurement results from different (laboratory) corners of the world. In training practice, one should at least be able to distinguish which terms are SI-compliant and which do not make sense.

## 1.8 If You Want to Lose Weight, Fly to the Moon!

As I said, one important function of muscles is to exert force. Of course, muscles also perform other fundamental functions for our survival, which I will discuss later. But what is force anyway? In 1687 Isaac Newton published his work *Philosophia Naturalis Principia Mathematica* (Mathematical Principles of Natural Philosophy). In it, he formulated three principles or laws of motion. The concept of force comes from the first of Newton's three laws, the law of inertia. It states, in simple terms, the following: Force is that which acts to change the state of rest or the uniform rectilinear state of motion (*i.e.*, motion with constant velocity and no change in direction). The SI unit of force is the newton (N). Thus, in the case of linear motion, that is, motion along a straight line, a force applied to a stationary or moving object tends to accelerate the object. The "reluctance" or inertia of the object to change its state is due to its mass.

The SI unit for mass is the kilogram (kg). Due to the effect of gravity, mass exerts a force and this force corresponds to the weight of the object. The two quantities "weight" and "mass" are often not distinguished from each other, especially when it comes to our body properties. Body weight is a force and should therefore be expressed in newtons, whereas body mass should be expressed in kilograms. If your body mass is 80 kg, then your body weight on earth is approximately 800 N. If you want to lose body weight, fly to the moon. There you will weigh about six times less than on Earth. Joking aside, it is more likely that you want to lose fat mass and gain muscle mass, and I hope the contents of my book can help you do that.

## 1.9 Muscles Only Want One Thing: To Rotate Loads Around Joints

However, especially in the context of training, we are not primarily interested in the linear effects of force, but rather the angular effects. If you bring an apple to your mouth with one hand, the hand rotates around the elbow joint, i.e. the apple moves circularly and not linearly around the elbow joint. Even if you move an object more or less along a line (for example, when pressing a dumbbell up), the straight-line motion of the dumbbell comes only from simultaneous rotation of the humerus at the shoulder joint and the forearm bones at the elbow joint. Consequently, the action of a muscle manifests itself as a torque around the corresponding joint rather than as a linear force. The reluctance of the body to change its angular motion is called the moment of inertia. The moment of inertia, in turn, depends on the mass of the physical body and the distribution of that mass about the axis of rotation. The muscular torque is calculated from the vector cross product between the moment arm and the acting force. The moment arm, in turn, represents the magnitude of the muscle force component perpendicular to the joint's center of rotation, while the lever arm corresponds to the distance between the joint's center and the point of force application on the bone being moved (in the example of the biceps brachii muscle, the two-headed arm muscle, this corresponds to the tendon attachment point on the forearm bone). Simply put, the moment arm is the distance perpendicular to the line of action of the muscle force from the line of action to the pivot point (joint).

The SI unit of torque is the newton metre (Nm). Muscular torque opposes the torque generated by the external force (Fig. 1.3). Thus, if you are holding a dumbbell in your hand, the external torque is equal to the product of the magnitude of the weight force component of the dumbbell acting *perpendicular to* the forearm and the distance of the dumbbell from the center of the elbow joint. Roughly speaking, this distance is equal to the length of your

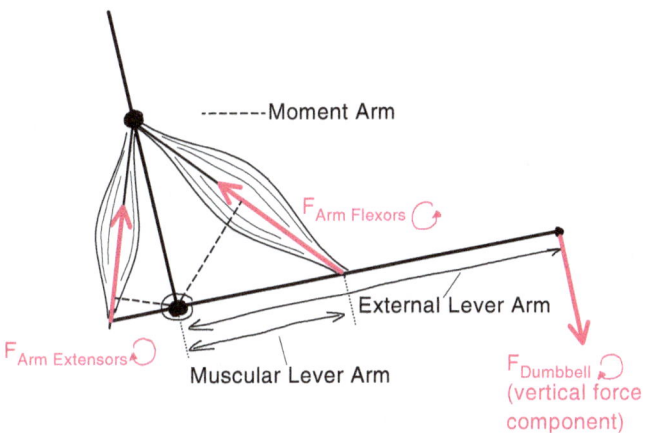

**Fig. 1.3** Forces acting during a biceps curl with a dumbbell. The muscle-tendon unit of the arm flexors shortens (miometric force production) only if the muscular torque (product of the magnitude of the moment arm and the muscular lever arm) of the arm flexors is greater than the sum of the torques caused by the training resistance (dumbbell) as well as the arm extensor muscles. The external torque is equal to the product of the amount of the weight force component of the dumbbell perpendicular to the forearm and the external lever arm

forearm bone. From these considerations it becomes clear why you feel the most resistance during the lifting of a dumbbell (bending at the elbow joint) in that joint position where the forearm bone is horizontal to the surface of the earth: At that position, the weight force of the dumbbell acts exclusively perpendicular to the forearm bone. If the muscular torque of a muscle (e.g. the arm flexor muscle, M. brachialis) is greater than the external torque and also greater than the torque of the antagonist muscle (in this case the arm extensor, M. triceps brachii), the resulting muscle action is miometric in nature. In the opposite case, the muscle action is pliometric. If the opposing torques are in balance, there is no externally visible movement (isometric case).

## 1.10 Why Your Muscles (Have to) Work Even Though You Are Not Performing Any Work

If the point of application of a force moves in such a way that the direction of movement is wholly or partially in line with the direction of the force, mechanical work is performed. Consequently, mechanical work is calculated from the product of force times distance (displacement). But beware! Mechanical work is only done (i.e. the sign of the work is positive) if the distance travelled is opposite to the direction of the force. The SI unit for distance is the metre (m). Mechanical work is thus given by the product newton times meter (Nm), which corresponds to the SI unit joule (J). In the context of exercise, however, the concept of mechanical work should be taken with a grain of salt. Think of isometric muscle force production. For example, if you are standing upright holding a heavy bag steady, your trapezius muscles are producing a lot of force, but the external mechanical work done is zero because your hands are not moving.

In principle, therefore, exercise must not be equated with the performance of external mechanical work. In addition, when using the term mechanical work, the energetic or thermodynamic system must always be specified. Indeed, in the case of a movement, the whole body or only individual limbs or segments can be considered as a system. The mechanical work performed then corresponds to the net change in the energy of the defined system. In the context of exercise, one therefore distinguishes internal and external work. Consider the following case. There is a very heavy dumbbell on your desk and you try to lift it with maximum effort. However, you do not even begin to succeed – the use of the muscle-tendon unit is consequently isometric. What happens inside the muscle? The muscle fibers shorten, while the elastic components of the extracellular matrix and the tendons stretch to their limit. Strictly speaking, the muscle (or the muscle fibers) is doing mechanical work. This can be called internal work. Nevertheless, the external mechanical work remains zero. The term "internal" can also be used to refer to the mechanical work that must be done simply to move one or more parts of the body, regardless of whether external work is being done. Think of leg movements while riding a bicycle and now imagine that you are mimicking them on a stationary bike without pedals. The external mechanical work is zero in this case. But you do have to do (internal) mechanical work to move your legs at all.

## 1.11 What Do Human Muscles Have to Do with Horses?

The rate at which mechanical work is performed is called power. Power is also a construct from classical mechanics. Historically, the use of this mechanical quantity can be traced back to the Scottish inventor James Watt (1736–1819). Based on the design of Thomas Newcomen (1663–1729), Watt further developed the steam engine by improving its efficiency. At the time (the beginning of the Industrial Revolution), industrial processes were powered by horses. Watt therefore proposed to quantify the effectiveness of steam engines relative to that of horses. Hence the term *horsepower* coined by Watt. The SI unit of power is the watt (W). One watt is equal to one joule per second ($Js^{-1}$). So what is energy? Energy manifests itself in different forms, for example in heat, light, electricity, chemical reactions, sound and, of course, motion. In the case of motion, we speak of kinetic energy. Forms of energy can be converted into each other. For example, ingested food is digested, including converting complex insoluble material into simple soluble substances. These soluble substances can then be transported in the body and absorbed by body cells.

Conversely, metabolic intermediates (metabolites) can also be transported from the cells by the blood and taken up by other cells or excreted via respiration or urine. When an enzyme (a molecule, usually a protein, which has a catalytic effect) interacts with a substance, the substance is called a "substrate". During the interaction between substrate and enzyme, energy can be released, but often energy is invested. The energy currency in our cells is adenosine triphosphate (ATP). During exercise, ATP provides the chemical energy for muscle fibers to produce force, – and when movement occurs in the process, to convert chemical energy into kinetic energy. A change in energy means that external and/or internal work has been done. When chemical energy is converted into mechanical energy, heat is also released.

Exercise is therefore accompanied by heat production (thermogenesis). If the energy release is aerobic, the conversion of the substrates requires the supply of oxygen. In anaerobic reactions, energy release occurs without oxygen consumption, even if the oxygen supply is good. In endurance sports in particular, it is a major challenge to match external power or speed so that energy availability (supply) is matched to energy requirement (demand). Conventionally, energy is said to be the capacity to do mechanical work. However, in the context of exercise, this definition can be misleading. As we have seen previously, the conversion of chemical or metabolic energy is not necessarily expressed as external mechanical work (as the example of isometric force production shows), but results in other forms of energy exchange (heat production). In the context of exercise, it is therefore more appropriate if we understand energy as that which must be "spent" in order to exercise.

## 1.12 Force Always Tastes Like Newtons

Well, muscles are not steam engines. Nevertheless, the concept of external (internal is often ignored) mechanical work and power can be applied to steady state cyclic activities, for example cycling, with certain limitations. Unfortunately, however, the concept of mechanical power is often misused in training or sport. As described earlier, the concept of external mechanical work is not at all useful to describe, let alone quantify, the training stimulus during an isometric muscle engagement. The situation is similar in "explosive" sports such as sprinting, shot put, hammer and discus throwing, or vertical or horizontal jumping disciplines. There, athletes are mistakenly said to have great power, or worse, great speed-strength or explosive-strength. Strike the last two terms from your vocabulary, because these entities do not exist in the SI system. Force has only one SI unit: the newton! I will explain immediately why you should replace these terms with "impulse" or *"rate of force development"*.

"Impulse" is a term from classical mechanics that is fundamental to training and sports, especially when a projectile is involved. This projectile can be a ball (shot put), a hammer (hammer throw), a discus (discus throw) or the athletes' body (in vertical or horizontal jump). In the case of linear motion, Newton's second law states that the increase or decrease in momentum of a physical body depends on the impulse, that is, the magnitude and direction of the applied force and the duration of the force application. This principle also applies to angular motion. For jumps and throws, the take-off or throw velocity represents the directed quantity, which is more decisive for athletic performance than the mechanical power.

## 1.13 Why You Should Not Confuse Your Training Resistance with a Projectile

Speed, understood as directionless velocity, is the distance travelled per unit of time. The SI unit of time is the second (s), so that the SI unit for speed is $ms^{-1}$. Speed is calculated by dividing the amount of momentum by the mass of the physical body. Consequently, to achieve a high take-off or throw speed, the athlete must maximize the impulse. This is accomplished by either increasing the peak force, the rate of force development or the duration of the force application. The greater the force you can generate in a given time interval, the greater the impulse. It is therefore not surprising that the ability to develop force quickly (especially in the first 40 ms) helps to maximize the impulse. Rate of force development is therefore more strongly associated with jump and sprint acceleration than mechanical power. Thus, the characteristics of "movement speed" or "explosiveness" go back to the ability to generate a large impulse. In the first instance, therefore, we should ask ourselves what neural and muscular factors determine this. Once these factors have been identified, we can investigate whether they can be trained, and if so, what the training should best look like.

What relevance do these considerations of mechanical impulse have for your training in the gym? If you want to build force and mass at the muscle tissue level, do not consider the training load to be moved (e.g. dumbbell, weight block, etc.) as a projectile! If you give the dumbbell a very high impulse, the dumbbell will continue to move "by itself" afterwards, and you will then automatically have to use less muscle force. As you will see later, this is the opposite of what is beneficial for muscle building.

## 1.14 Jogging on the Leg Press

And what about "strength endurance"? Endurance athletes in particular and their coaches often (still) think they need good "strength endurance" and that they can train it by moving low loads countless times in the gym. Unfortunately, when we look at the SI, this conceptual construct is also meaningless. The construct is also wholly inadequate to describe the ability to perform, sustain, and/or tolerate a particular movement task (*e.g.*, cycling, running). In the case of cycling, "strength endurance" is more likely to mean the ability to maintain as high an external mechanical output on the bicycle as possible for as long as possible. In other words, the duration to voluntary exhaustion (the point at which the exercise task can no longer be performed) should be as long as possible for a given power output that is as high as possible. Analogous considerations apply to runners in terms of running speed (rather than external mechanical power). So, even in the case of "strength endurance", one must first ask on what neural and muscular factors the desired ability is based, whether these factors can be trained at all, and if so, how this can best be done. The mechanisms that lead to increased power on the bike or running speed are not necessarily the same as those that increase the length of time it takes to reach exhaustion. It should therefore be obvious that it is hardly purposeful for endurance movements to be performed on a strength machine for the purpose of increasing "strength endurance".

## 1.15 Summary: Why Muscle Force Does Not Always Lead to Visible Movement

When your muscles generate force and shorten in the process, it is correctly referred to as miometric force generation. Colloquially, however, the term "concentric contraction" is even more common. During miometric force production, the training load is overcome, for example when lifting a dumbbell. A more typical example from everyday life is climbing a flight of stairs. In doing so, your thigh and glute muscles are generating force miometrically. Conversely, we speak of pliometric force generation (colloquially: "eccentric contraction") when your muscles become longer or are actively stretched during force generation. This happens during braking movements, such as going down stairs. The third possible effect of force generation is isometric force generation (colloquially: "isometric contraction"). In this case, your muscles generate force, but this does not result in any outwardly visible movement. Just think of carrying a heavy shopping bag, where several muscles (including shoulder, neck, forearm muscles) generate force isometrically, while the shopping bag, in relation to your body segments, practically does not move from the spot. Finally, in connection with the external effect of force generation, one often encounters the two proper nouns "positive" and "negative" (e.g. "negative training", see Sect. 1.6). These property words have nothing to do with "good" and "bad" in the context of training, but they refer to the sign (plus for positive or minus for negative) of the external mechanical work done during the movement (the energy expended by the body), which can be calculated as follows: Work = Force times Displacement. In the example of climbing stairs, the force is equal to your body weight and the distance is equal to the height of the stairs traveled (height of one step times number of steps). When climbing the stairs (overcoming phase), the work done is positive by definition, i.e. it carries a positive mathematical sign, when descending the stairs the sign is negative. "Negative training" therefore describes the same thing as "eccentric training" or indeed pliometric force generation. Very important for understanding is the following: The function of a muscle is to generate force. In doing so, it always *tries to* shorten. However, muscle shortening is not always the result of your effort. Whether a movement is externally visible (and how fast this movement is) depends not only on the force exerted by your muscles, but also on the amount of external load. In other words, the muscle always *tries to* generate force miometrically, but depending on the relationship between your muscle force (or effort) and the external force (load), the result will be miometric, isometric or pliometric.

# 2

# All that Glitters Is Not Gold

## 2.1 Surrogates for Internal Muscle Force

From our considerations it is clear that the term "strength training" is meaningless or confusing. Yet intuitively it would be so logical: Whoever does "strength training", trains his strength, what else? But what exactly is meant by "strength training"? Does it mean increasing your weight? You now know that you can achieve this goal more easily if you travel to the North Pole. Gravity is stronger there than at the equator. But perhaps you mean the internal force of your muscles. Or is it rather the force you can exert externally? Or by force, do you in fact mean torque, or perhaps just "the muscles"? Unfortunately, actual muscle force cannot be measured directly in living humans. This would require cutting at least one end of a tendon, connecting it linearly to a force sensor, and activating the muscle. Instead of internal muscle force, two surrogates are usually used in humans.

We have already learned about the first type of surrogate. These are the external torques and forces (e.g. ground reaction force, pedal force, etc.). From these external quantities, the internal forces and torques can be estimated using inverse dynamics under many assumptions, for example about the lever ratios. A second surrogate that is often, but not necessarily usefully, used for muscle force is muscle size. This is measured as muscle volume, muscle (fiber) cross-section, lean mass, or the muscle mass calculated from these. In fact, the correlation between muscle size and external torque or external force is not as good as one would expect. Studies in humans have shown that leg muscle size only explains about 25–50% of the variability in torque or force. Thus, more muscle size or mass is not necessarily associated with an improvement in muscle function that is physiologically relevant in the context of exercise (Anliker and Toigo 2012). I will discuss this important aspect in more detail later (see Sect. 22.2).

## 2.2 How Strong Is "Strong"?

In very few fitness centres or sports clubs is your training success for the trained muscles systematically and scientifically correct or justifiable recorded, for example as external force in newtons or as external torque in newtons times meter. In order to capture the training success in its entirety, it would also be necessary to determine the peak torque value as well as the times reached to voluntary exhaustion (static or dynamic) at fixed percentages of the peak value and standardized exercise execution. In practice, you can usually only fall back on two SI quantities: the mass of the resistance (*e.g.* the dumbbell) in kilograms and the time in seconds. These are also the two quantities you can use to modulate the training stimulus. If you always perform an exercise in exactly the same way in terms of anatomical execution, *range of motion* (ROM), etc., you will become "stronger" in that movement task or exercise if you can move a higher load (mass of external resistance) and/or move the load longer. If anything, instead of "strength training", it should be called load training. Then you would also be more aware that the ability to move (accelerate and decelerate) and/or hold a load describes more of a skill than a muscle property.

## 2.3 Maximum Force Is Not Equal to Peak Force

There is an important difference between the peak force that can be produced at will during a functional or movement maneuver and the maximum voluntary force. In a two-legged *countermovement jump*, the typical peak ground reaction force acting on a forefoot is approximately 1.2 times the body weight. During multiple hops on one leg with the knee extended and no heel contact, the typical peak force is approximately 3 to 3.5 times the body weight, approximately 2.5 to 3 times higher than during the *countermovement jump* (Anliker and Toigo 2012). Note that the internal (muscle) forces are always greater than those you can generate externally as a result. This has to do with the fact that the muscular moment arms are practically always smaller than the lever arms. As a very rough estimate, you need about 20 N of muscular force to move 10 N of body weight. If you stand upright on one leg and lift your heel minimally off the ground with your knees extended, the ratio of the distance from the forefoot to the joint (lever arm) and from the joint to the Achilles tendon (moment arm) is in the range of 2.5:1. The calf muscles must therefore exert 2.5 times your weight force to maintain this position. At approximately 800 N body weight (80 kg body mass), this corresponds approximately to a muscle force of 2000 N. Applied to the previous example, this means the following: If a ground reaction force equivalent to 3.5 times your body weight force acts on your forefoot during a one-legged hop, your calf muscles produce approximately 8.75 times your body weight force. If your body mass is 80 kg, this corresponds to a muscle force of approximately 7000 N. For comparison: The weight force of a small car is about 8000 N!

Accordingly, in order to determine the maximum voluntary force, the functional or movement manoeuvre with the highest typical peak force must be selected. An often neglected aspect of determining maximum force is the fact that for any given level of muscle activation, maximum force occurs during pliometric force production. Human muscle fibers produce 1.4 to 2.1 times more tension (force per cross-sectional area) during active stretching (i.e. the muscle fiber is stretched while it is producing force, i.e. it is active) than during active shortening, depending on the type of fiber (see Sect. 5.6). You will also be familiar with this phenomenon from practical experience: When a load is lowered, it feels lighter than when it is lifted. From these considerations it follows – in order to speak of a maximum voluntary force – that the force must firstly be acquired with a movement manoeuvre that produces the highest typical peak force, and that secondly it must also be measured with the maximum possible muscle activation during a pliometric effort.

> **Box 2.1: The Terms "Peak Force" and "Maximum Force" Are Not Synonyms**
> The force measured during a movement test at maximum voluntary effort corresponds to the peak voluntary force. The peak force measured during pliometric force production at maximum voluntary effort corresponds to the maximum force, provided it is the movement manoeuvre that produces or can produce the highest force.

## 2.4 Decoding Muscle Force

The term "muscle activation" is understood to mean that an action potential is triggered at the muscle fiber (Fig. 2.1) due to a depolarization of the cell membrane (sarcolemma), which propagates simultaneously in both directions along the length of the muscle fiber (Fig. 2.2). Molecular sensors in the

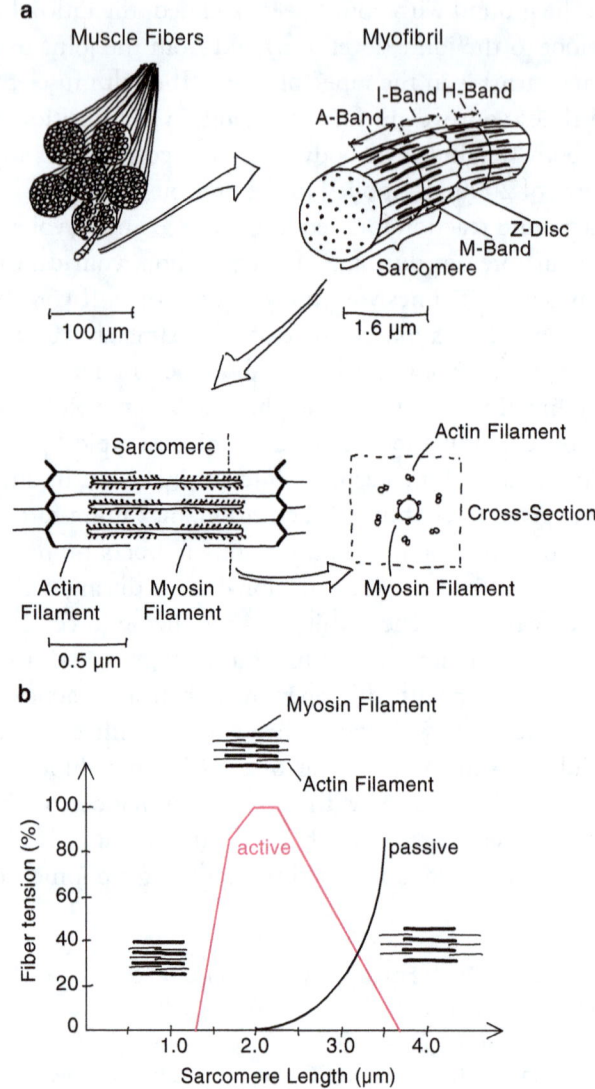

**Fig. 2.1** Structure of a muscle. (**a**) Structure of muscle fibers. (**b**) Force-length relationship of a single sarcomere. Note that muscle fibers are composed of parallel myofibrils and myofibrils are composed of serially arranged sarcomeres. Sarcomeres can produce different amounts of force depending on the length or degree of overlap of actin and myosin filaments (active force production, red line). With increasing sarcomere length (elongation), the passive force (black line) in the sarcomere also increases, which in turn counteracts elongation

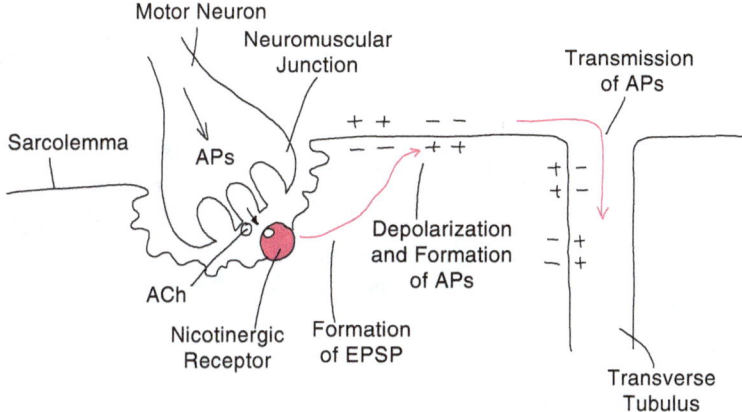

**Fig. 2.2** Stimulus transmission from motoneuron to muscle fiber. The incoming action potentials (APs) in the motor neuron cause acetylcholine (ACh) to be released at the synapse (contact point between motor neuron and muscle fiber), which binds to a nicotinic receptor of the postsynaptic membrane (i.e. the muscle fiber membrane, the sarcolemma). This membrane generates an excitatory postsynaptic potential (EPSP, cf. also Sect. 9.9 regarding the EPSP in the axon hillock of the motor neuron cell body), which above a certain threshold leads to a sequence of APs. The APs run along the sarcolemma and are conducted into the T-tubules. AP, action potential; EPSP, excitatory postsynaptic potential (see Sect. 9.9 and Fig. 9.3). (According to Clauss and Clauss 2009)

sarcolemma detect the electrical voltage generated by the action potential and trigger the opening of calcium channels in the terminal cisternae of the sarcoplasmic reticulum inside the muscle fiber (Fig. 2.3). The increase in calcium concentration results in increased binding of calcium ions to troponin C (Fig. 5.1). Troponin C, together with the other two troponin subunits (I and T), regulates the spatial arrangement of tropomyosin. At low calcium concentrations, tropomyosin blocks the binding sites between actin and myosin, also known as thin and thick filaments. Only the increased binding of calcium ions to troponin C and the subsequent rearrangement of troponin I and T allow the tropomyosin to be pushed away and thus an interaction, i.e. the formation of a bridge, between actin and myosin.

The consequence of this interaction is the initiation of a cross-bridge cycle (see Sect. 5.2) with accompanying cleavage of ATP, whereby force (and, depending on this, movement) is produced (see Fig. 5.1). As long as action potentials are triggered at the sarcolemma and the calcium concentration in the region of the myofilaments actin and myosin remains elevated, force production takes place. As soon as impulses and calcium concentration decrease,

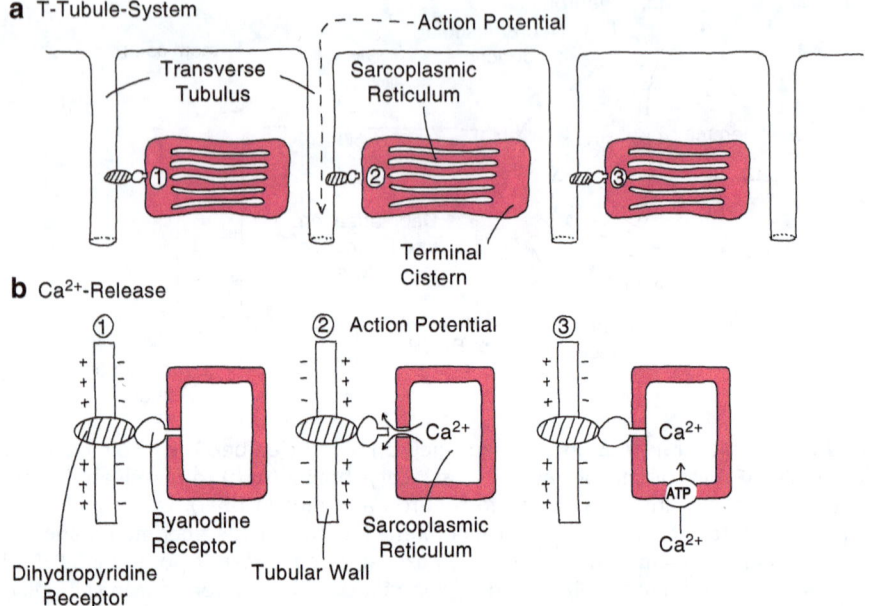

**Fig. 2.3** Coupling between depolarization at the sarcolemma and calcium release in the sarcoplasm. (**a**) Conduction of a muscle action potential via the T-tubule system and coupling of the electrical signal via the receptors to Ca$^{2+}$ release from the terminal cisternae of the sarcoplasmic reticulum. (**b**) Mechanism of Ca$^{2+}$ ion release. In the initial state, Ca$^{2+}$-ions are located in the lumen of the sarcoplasmic reticulum ①. When the membrane of the T-tubules is depolarized ②, the conformation of the dihydropyridine receptor (DHPR) changes. This opens the ryanodine receptor and Ca$^{2+}$ ions flow from the sarcoplasmic reticulum into the cytosol of the muscle cell, the sarcoplasm. The Ca$^{2+}$ ions are transported back into the sarcoplasmic reticulum, consuming energy ③. (According to Clauss and Clauss 2009)

force decreases. This is due to the fact that the calcium ions inside the muscle fiber are actively pumped back into the sarcoplasmic reticulum, i.e. with energy expenditure (cleavage of ATP) (Fig. 2.3). This is done by means of molecular pumps located in the membrane of the sarcoplasmic reticulum. As soon as the calcium concentration falls below a critical value, the inhibition of tropomyosin resumes. This is referred to as relaxation. The faster a muscle can pump back the calcium, the faster the relaxation. The ATP concentration must be regenerated during tension and relaxation, which occurs through the breakdown and conversion of food components (e.g. glucose, fatty acids, etc.) and/or their mobilisation from dynamic body stores (e.g. glycogen in muscle and liver, triglycerides from white fat cells, etc.).

The more parallel cross-bridge cycles that can take place (directly dependent on the calcium concentration around the myofilaments), the greater the resulting muscle (fiber) force. Thus, while the number of parallel cross-bridge cycles affects muscle fiber force, the number of serial cross-bridge cycles affects the maximum unloaded (i.e., occurring without external resistance) shortening velocity of a muscle fiber. The greater the number of serial cross-bridges, the higher the maximum unloaded shortening velocity. Actin and myosin filaments interlock and together form hexagonal lattices (six actin filaments surround one myosin filament) and several such lattices form a myofibril (Fig. 2.1a). A muscle fiber contains quite a few such myofibrils. The interlocking of myofilaments actin and myosin is responsible for force production and movement. Myofibrils can in turn be divided into functional contractile subunits called sarcomeres (Fig. 2.1a). The total number of sarcomeres within a muscle fiber therefore depends on the fiber length (number of sarcomeres in series or serial cross-bridge cycles) and the fiber cross-section (number of parallel sarcomeres or parallel cross-bridge cycles).

Within a muscle fiber, at a given calcium concentration, the possible number of parallel-connected cross-bridges depends, on the one hand, on the degree of overlap of the actin and myosin filaments and, on the other hand, on the number of myofilaments (i.e. actin and myosin filaments). The degree of overlap depends on the instantaneous length of the corresponding sarcomere. The relationship between sarcomere length and force is described by the so-called force-length relationship (Fig. 2.1b): For a very short or a very long sarcomere, the degree of overlap is smaller (i.e. force production is less) than for an intermediate length (force production is greater). This is one of the reasons why you cannot produce the same amount of muscle force at every joint angle position. In turn, the number of actin and myosin filaments is proportional to the cross-sectional area of the muscle fiber. If the cross-sectional area of a muscle fiber changes, so does the potential of the fiber to produce force. If the cross-sectional area becomes smaller or larger, the fiber force potentially becomes smaller or larger accordingly.

## 2.5 Muscles in the Zebra Skin

The interlocking pattern of actin and myosin arrangement is also responsible for the transverse striation visible under the light microscope in longitudinal fiber section. This is why skeletal muscle is often called striated muscle. One should simply not forget that the cardiac musculature is also transversely striated.

A myofibril can be divided into at least five regions based on its optical properties: The regions that contain only myosin filaments are called the

A(nisotropic) band. The regions which contain only actin filaments are called the I(sotropic) band. Where actin and myosin filaments overlap are called H zones, where the H stands for light ("hell" in German). The black dark line, which is in the middle of the I-stripes, is called a Z-disk (Z for between, or "zwischen" in German). The distance between two Z-disks corresponds to the length of a sarcomere. Finally, in the middle of the A band is a relatively dense zone called the M line (Fig. 2.1a).

## 2.6 Spoilt for Choice When Selecting the Best Training Tool?

There are now a number of training aids available to help build muscle force and mass. There are roughly two classes: Free weights and machines. The exercises in which the training aids are used can also be roughly divided into two classes: those in which the movement being trained only involves one joint (e.g. seated leg extensions), and those in which movement takes place in several joints at the same time (e.g. leg press or squat). The former are often called isolation or single-joint exercises and the latter compound or multi-joint exercises. In English, the terms *open kinetic chain exercise* and *closed kinetic chain exercise* are also used. A kinetic chain is open in the sense that hand or foot are free to move, as in the "biceps curl" or "seated leg extension" exercises. Handstands and squats, on the other hand, would be closed kinetic chain exercises.

## 2.7 Not All Machines Are Created Equal, or Are They?

In the case of machines, which in the broadest sense can also include cable hoists and the like, a distinction must again be made according to design and functional principle. It is beyond the scope and intention of this book to discuss all conceivable variations. I would therefore like to explain only the most important differences. Irrespective of the nature of the resistance (weight of the metal discs, electric motor, compressed air, muscle force, etc.), the resistance can vary (or not) depending on the design of the device, namely

- within the *range of motion* (ROM) for machines with eccentric *cam* and/or
- between miometric and pliometric use (e.g. machines where the load is selectively higher during the pliometric phase) and/or

- from repetition to repetition (adaptive machines, i.e. the resistance decreases with increasing fatigue).

Furthermore, there are individual equipment manufacturers who produce machines with direct resistance. By "direct" is meant that the resistance is applied to *the* bone that is to be moved by muscle force (isolation exercise, see above). Take for example the exercise "pullover".

"Direct" here means that the resistance attaches to the upper arm and that the upper arm is moved or held against this resistance primarily by the force of your large back muscle. Finally, unlike free weights, machines provide rotational resistance. The weight force of a free weight is always directed toward the center of the earth, while movements in a joint (such as flexion or extension) are rotational movements. Even if the resistance, such as the barbell in the bench press, moves linearly, the upper arm bones rotate in the shoulder joint and the lower arm bones rotate in the elbow joint. Single-joint machines for performing isolation exercises can now be designed so that the resistance acts as far as possible against the direction of rotation.

Finally, it should be mentioned that there are also machines where not the resistance but the movement speed is specified, i.e. you always push or pull with maximum effort – the movement speed remains constant. However, the supposed strongest horse in the argumentative racing stable of the equipment producers is the variable rotation resistance within the ROM, also called "adaptive resistance". The idea behind adaptive resistance is that the external torque generated by the training resistance and the lever arm is varied, according to the angle-torque relationship of the muscle, i.e. the internal torque: in the joint positions where the muscular torque is greatest (where you are "strongest"), the external torque should be greatest and *vice versa*. This is supposed to make the workout particularly effective or superior relative to free weight training. Incorrectly, people always talk about the force curve in this context.

> **Box 2.2: Machine or Free Weight Training?**
> The question of which workout – machine *or* free weight training – is *fundamentally* better for building muscle makes no sense. You don't get big muscles because you train with free weights instead of machines. Conversely, you don't have small muscles because you train with machines instead of free weights. The choice of training tool (whether machine, free weight, your own body, etc.) is secondary. If you train properly and have good (epi-)genetics (see Chap. 21), you can achieve good results with both free weights and machines or your own body

weight as training resistance. Machines, free weights, pulleys, body weight, etc. are not mutually exclusive. What is more important is *how* you perform the exercises (see Chap. 9) and that a gradual increase in resistance is possible (progressive training). If the execution of the exercise is poor (and yes, unfortunately this is the case in many training facilities), the best training tools are of no use. The focus should be on the execution of the movement instead of the training equipment. High quality training is the be-all and end-all of injury-free and quantitatively successful muscle and force building. I therefore advise a pragmatic approach. Depending on the exercise, choose the training tool that makes you feel the muscles you want to train the most, i.e. the one that "hurts" the most.

## 2.8 The Ominous Force Curve

It is now claimed that there is a natural, ideal force curve (often referred to as the "strength curve") of the muscle and that the resistance of the training equipment must be adapted to this as far as possible, firstly to train effectively and secondly to avoid dysbalances. The selling point is that imbalances in the force curve, defined as a deviation of the muscle's force curve from the natural ideal curve, causally lead to musculoskeletal problems such as back pain. Unfortunately, however, most claims related to the force curve are nonsense. The big problem, in fact, is that the course of muscle force during joint rotation does not necessarily correspond to the course of muscular torque, because the moment arm can also vary during joint rotation. Muscular force and muscular torque must therefore not be used as synonyms. Furthermore, the force curves (more precisely the length-force relationships) of human muscles are unknown.

**Lessons from the Frog Muscle**
The relationship between sarcomere length, joint angle, moment arm, internal muscle force and muscular torque has so far only been determined for the frog semitendinosus muscle. This double-jointed muscle of the ischiocrural musculature is attached to the pelvis and lower leg and contributes to leg flexion.

In corresponding experiments on the frog, the above measures were recorded over a ROM of 180° (from full knee joint extension at 0° to full flexion at 180°, with the hip joint always flexed 90°) (Lieber and Boakes 1988a, b). Muscular torque was highest at approximately 110° of flexion, whereas muscle force peaked at slightly less than 160° of flexion. The moment arm was greatest at approximately 90° of flexion. Here, the measurement points for the moment arm described a parabolic arc (increasing with knee flexion up to 90° and decreasing thereafter) and those for the force described a straight line (i.e., increasing linearly with flexion up to 160°). Thus, even in this isolated musculoskeletal system, torque resulted from the interaction between muscle and joint properties and not merely from one or the other (Fig. 2.4). Claims that machines with adaptive resistance are *fundamentally* more effective therefore have no scientific basis.

In addition, the length-force relationship of a muscle is dependent on the angular positions of the joints it affects (in the example of the frog muscle, the hip joint angle). For example, it can be assumed that the length-force relationship of the biceps muscle varies depending on the shoulder joint position in which a biceps curl is performed (i.e. depending on the position of the humerus in relation to the shoulder joint or torso).

### The Vagaries of the Force Curve

There is a second problem associated with the optimal force curve. In the frog experiment described above, the average sarcomere length decreased from 3.6 to 2 μm during knee flexion, meaning that each sarcomere had to shorten by 1.6 μm. Now, this number doesn't necessarily have to be that large because the more sarcomeres there are in series, meaning the longer the muscle fibers, the less each sarcomere has to shorten for the same change in muscle length. If there had been twice as many sarcomeres in series, each sarcomere would have

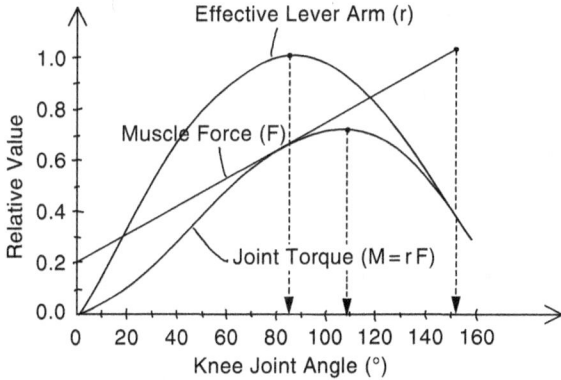

**Fig. 2.4** Interaction between muscle and joint properties. The joint angle at which the highest muscle force can be produced does not necessarily have to be the same as the joint angle at which the highest muscular torque can be generated. The reason for this is that not only the force, but also the effective moment arm can vary depending on the joint angle. In the example of the frog muscle shown, you can see that the highest muscular force occurs at a much larger joint angle (between 150 and 160°) than the highest torque (about 110°). (Adapted from Lieber and Boakes 1988b)

had to shorten by only 0.8 µm. The change in the length of individual sarcomeres, which varies depending on the number of sarcomeres in series, therefore results in a change in the degree of overlap between actin and myosin, or in the number of crossbridges, and thus in the muscle fiber force, which depends on the muscle length and varies in magnitude.

Suppose a muscle-joint system were set up so that the muscle is shortest at 40° of extension and longest at 80° of extension. The functional joint ROM in this case would be 40°. Now assume further that the number of sarcomeres in series, or the length of the muscle fibers, increases significantly. What happens to the joint ROM? On the one hand, the joint ROM increases with the increase in the number of serial sarcomeres (see Sects. 3.1 and 10.2), say from 40° to 75°. On the other hand, however, the angle-muscle force relationship also shifts in the direction of larger joint angles: at minimum length, the joint angle now assumed is 70° (instead of the original 40°), at maximum length it is now 145° (instead of the original 80°).

This example shows that the relationship between muscle fiber length (number of sarcomeres in series) and moment arm length determines how much the sarcomeres will shorten during joint rotation and therefore how much the internal muscle force will vary during joint rotation: If the length of the fibers is large relative to that of the moment arm, the change in sarcomere length and thus fiber force during joint rotation will be small. However, if the length of the fibers is small relative to that of the moment arm, the sarcomere length and fiber force will vary greatly during joint rotation.

The ratio between fiber and moment arm length was estimated in humans for different muscles of the lower body. The gluteus maximus muscle (large gluteal muscle) had the highest ratio of 79.5, followed by the gluteus minimus muscle (small gluteal muscle) with 13.9 and the sartorius muscle (sartorius) with 10.8. The soleus muscle had the lowest ratio (0.9). The anterior and posterior thigh muscles were only slightly above this at 1.8 and the gastrocnemius (twin calf) muscle also had a low value of 1.5. For the other leg muscles (adductors, pronators, etc.) the values are somewhere between 1 and 8. These figures mean that the internal muscle fiber force varies much more in the gluteus maximus muscle during joint rotation than in the soleus muscle, where it remains virtually constant. So even if the exact internal force curve during joint rotation were known (which it is not), there would be little additional benefit to be expected from the use of specially designed machines with eccentric cam for muscles with a low to moderate muscle fiber to lever arm length ratio.

### Why Dysbalances Are Natural

The exciting thing is that the number of sarcomeres in series or the muscle fiber length is not a constant value, but is regulated depending on the (dis-) use or training of the muscle, i.e. the number of sarcomeres in series increases or decreases. I will explain the exact mechanisms and the consequences for practice in detail in Sect. 10.2. This much in advance: muscle (fiber) length adapts to strain such that its sarcomeres operate at optimal length, that is, at or near the plateau of the length-force relationship (Fig. 2.1b). At this length, the filament overlap is optimal and the resulting force is maximal. This automatically means that the force curve (i.e., the length-force relationship) of the muscle is the result of typical muscle loading. "Optimal" should therefore be understood relative to the muscle's current pattern of use. In other words, for an elite athlete who uses a particular muscle in athletic movement primarily at a shortened length, training on a machine with a matched force curve may be suboptimal or, in the worst case, inhibit performance. Why?

If muscle fibers are adapted to specific everyday use at short muscle length, meaning they have relatively fewer sarcomeres in series, and then are used in resistance exercises (whether free weights or machines) over an unusually long muscle fiber length, a relative increase in length is triggered. Specifically, this means that more sarcomeres are incorporated in series to accommodate the new functional use at greater muscle length – the force curve shifts towards greater muscle length (see example above). One consequence of this is that for the same joint angle, there is now a different muscle force and possibly a different torque acting. If we now assume that, for example in a javelin thrower, the muscular torques are tuned depending on the angular position within and between the muscles so that the javelin can be thrown as far as possible, it becomes clear that a shift in the force curve can influence (negatively or positively) the athletic task of throwing the javelin.

## 2.9 Summary: Don't Blindly Follow the Squat Trend

Some swear by resistance training with free weights. Others preach resistance training on machines. Not to forget the followers of training with body weight. As different as these three schools of thought may be, they all have at least one thing in common: All of them claim that their means of training is the most effective. This is despite the fact that there are people in each camp who are very muscular and strong. You guessed it: the choice of training equipment, be it a barbell, a machine or your own body, can hardly be *the* decisive factor for training success. If you want to use resistance training to exploit your individual genetic potential in terms of muscle force and mass gain, you should rather focus on temporarily weakening your muscles during training. Yes, weaken! Thus, the goal of training is to trigger adaptive processes in muscle and nerve cells that result in them becoming more muscular and stronger. In that respect, it's not so much about showing others what feats you can do with a loaded barbell. If the exercise execution is poor, the best training tools are of no use.

The same applies to the so-called "basic exercises" such as the squat, deadlift and bench press, which are (once again) in fashion. In the fitness centers you can see more and more young customers, but also older people, who struggle endlessly with such exercises, often, as it seems, more badly than well. This supposed "boom" is triggered, among other things, by claims and promises from coach gurus and the like, according to which the execution of such "basic exercises" is mandatory for increasing muscle mass (and force), that only through such "golden exercises" can you achieve a firm buttocks or that these exercises are even more "functional" than others.

You can believe anything, of course, but there is still no hard scientific data to back up the above claims without ifs and buts. Rather, it can be assumed that there is fundamentally not one exercise that is the best exercise for all people. The exercises with which you can best "reach" the muscles to be trained depend on your anatomical conditions, your motor skills and abilities (e.g. with regard to muscle interplay), the mobility of the joints involved, etc. The activation of the target muscles in the training process is not always the same. While activation of the target muscles in training is an important prerequisite for the desired training adaptations to occur over time, it is not a guarantee. Rather, a suitable mechanical and metabolic stress on the target muscles is required to ensure that the muscle-building processes are stimulated over a long period of time (see Chap. 13). This is why the quality of training is probably more decisive than the means of training: the supposedly "best" exercise is of no use if you *cannot* perform this exercise correctly, for whatever reason. My basic advice is to train each muscle in its complete range of motion (see Sects. 9.14 and 9.18) and to select those exercises and training aids that will allow you to fatigue the target muscles most safely and efficiently. For each exercise, start by choosing the means of exercise that makes you feel the muscles you want to train the most, i.e. that "hurts" the most during the exercise, in a good sense.

# 3

# Thick and/or Long? A Never Ending Question

## 3.1 The Functional Role of Muscle Length

The shortening of a muscle fiber results from the shortening of the individual sarcomeres. Therefore, a muscle can shorten by several centimeters, although a single sarcomere can only shorten by about 1 μm (micrometer; one millionth of a meter). As mentioned earlier, the number of sarcomeres, both parallel (i.e., side by side) and serial (i.e., one behind the other), can be altered depending on the training stimulus. A detailed discussion of this follows in Chap. 10. For now, I would like to outline the functional relevance of the number of parallel and serial sarcomeres.

First, let's compare two muscle fibers that have different numbers of sarcomeres in series for the same cross-sectional area (i.e., the same number of sarcomeres arranged in parallel). For the same muscle fiber length, the average sarcomere length is shorter for the fiber with more sarcomeres in series, or for the same average sarcomere length, the muscle fiber with more sarcomeres in series is longer. Based on the same fiber length, the potential length excursion is greater for the fiber with more sarcomeres in series, meaning it can produce force over a further distance (Fig. 3.1a). Although the maximum fiber force is the same due to the same cross-sectional area, for the muscle fiber with the higher number of sarcomeres in series, the maximum fiber force occurs at a greater fiber length. Now, for which of these two fibers is the maximum unloaded shortening velocity higher? The answer is: for the fibers with more sarcomeres in series. Why? Velocity, as a vector quantity, is characterized by the direction (e.g., shortening or lengthening) and the amount of distance

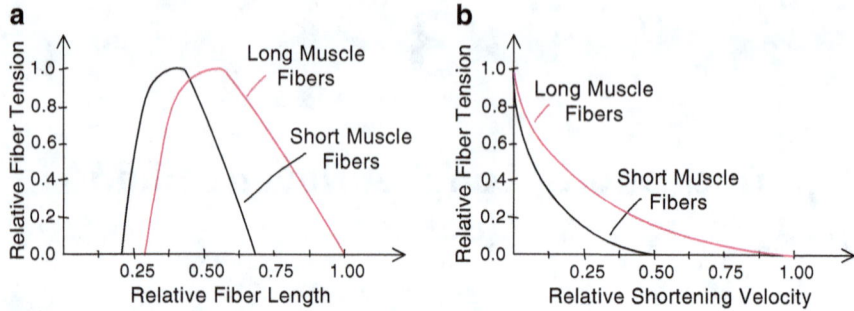

**Fig. 3.1** Length-tension and velocity-tension relationships of short and long muscle fibers. (**a**) Length-tension relationship. (**b**) Velocity-tension relationship. Note that the relative fiber tension is the fiber force normalized to the cross-sectional area of the muscle fiber (tension = force per area)

traveled – in our case, the distance of fiber length change. Now, the individual sarcomeres in a muscle fiber can all shorten at the same rate, that is, they shorten by the same distance per unit time. Consequently, if there are more sarcomeres in series, the muscle fiber can shorten by a greater distance per unit time than it would if there were fewer sarcomeres, which corresponds to a higher rate of shortening. In other words, a muscle fiber with more sarcomeres in series (a longer fiber) can shorten by a greater distance in the same time interval than a shorter fiber (Fig. 3.1b).

If we now transfer these considerations to all fibers in an isolated muscle, this means for the same number of muscle fibers in the muscles that

- a longer muscle compared to a shorter muscle is not *a priori* longer because its sarcomeres are longer at rest, but because there are more sarcomeres in series,
- a longer muscle is more stretchable compared to a shorter one,
- the peak force is generated after an increase in the length of the muscle with greater muscle length than was previously possible with smaller length,
- the theoretical maximum internal muscle force is the same for both muscles,
- the maximum shortening speed is greater in the long muscle relative to the short muscle, and
- the longer muscle can develop more force relative to its maximum force at the same relative shortening speed as the shorter muscle.

You may wonder why the latter is the case? The longer muscle is known to have more sarcomeres in series. Therefore, for the same rate of muscle shortening, the rate of shortening of each sarcomere in the longer muscle is less than that of the sarcomeres in the shorter muscle. Because of the force-velocity relationship, this means that each sarcomere in the longer muscle can generate more force under these circumstances (Fig. 3.1b).

> **Box 3.1: Does Resistance Training Make You Slow?**
>
> Yes and no. Yes, in terms of intrinsic force production. As an untrained person, you will slow down when you start resistance training (regardless of how fast you perform the movements!). Incidentally, the same is true for all other forms of training (see Sect. 5.5 for a detailed discussion).
>
> Resistance training doesn't make you slower in terms of movement speed, though. Your peak voluntary movement speed generally tends to increase over time (unless you become so extremely muscular that your muscles get in each other's way). This may sound confusing, but it's not. Let's say that before and after a resistance training period of several months, we measure the speed with which you can move your forearm to your upper arm. Let's further assume that training allows you to double your biceps muscle force. Now, after the training period, can you move your forearm to your upper arm faster or slower? The answer is faster, because the weight of the forearm is unlikely to have doubled in the same period of time. You know from the force-velocity relationship (see Sect. 1.6) that the lower the force, the higher the possible shortening velocity. If the force in the biceps muscle increases relative to the weight of the forearm, this means nothing other than that the forearm has become "lighter" and can therefore be moved faster.
>
> Increasing muscle cross-section and force therefore tends to make your movements faster, not slower. Despite this, you often come across athletes claiming that resistance training makes them slow. Is there any truth to this? In javelin throwing, the speed at which the javelin is thrown certainly plays a central role, and it can be assumed that in order to achieve the highest possible throwing speed, all the muscles involved must produce the correct torque in the correct joint position, which in turn depends on the correct muscle length. If this interaction of the angle-torque-relationships is disturbed by asymmetric length adaptations in an untargeted (or unknowing) way, the result can be a lower movement speed and thus a lower release speed. However, as you know by now, a muscle also changes the number of sarcomeres in series depending on the type of activity. Lenghtening resistance training is very suitable for this (see Sect. 10.2).
>
> Mistakenly, such a (temporary) possible decrease in movement speed is typically interpreted as resistance training or muscle growth making a movement slow. You now know better: resistance training or muscle thickness growth do *not a priori* make a movement slower, but the length adaptation possibly triggered by the changed length stress (whether this is due to resistance training or other possible everyday activities) can have a negative or positive effect on the speed of the movement due to the change in the angle-torque curves.

## 3.2 The Functional Role of Muscle Thickness (Muscle Cross-Sectional Area)

Let us now compare two fibers which have the same length (i.e. the same number of serially arranged sarcomeres) but have a different cross-sectional area (i.e. a different number of parallel sarcomeres). Both fibers can produce force over the same distance (length), but at each fiber length, the force of the thinner fiber is smaller relative to the thicker fiber (Fig. 3.2a, due to different numbers of parallel sarcomeres). However, the fiber length at which the maximum fiber force occurs is the same for both fibers, as is the maximum unloaded shortening velocity (Fig. 3.2b, due to the same number of serially located sarcomeres). However, the isometrically measured force (shortening velocity equal to zero) is greater for the thicker fiber compared to the thinner fiber (Fig. 3.2b, greater number of parallel sarcomeres). Analogous to the relationships for different muscle fiber lengths, the observations on muscle fibers with different cross-sectional areas can also be transferred to whole muscles with different cross-sectional areas (but the same number of muscle fibers). However, there are two things to keep in mind. First, we assume in the considerations that the muscle density (in mammals 1.056 g cm$^{-3}$) is constant. Second, muscle architecture may vary from muscle to muscle. What is meant by the term "muscle architecture"? The fibers of a muscle can be oriented differently relative to the axis along which the muscle generates force (which corresponds to the line connecting the two ends of the tendon). This means that the muscle fibers can be oriented at one or more angles to the tendon axis, depending on the muscle architecture. There are basically three types of muscle architecture. In a muscle with a spindle-shaped architecture (e.g. biceps brachii muscle, two-headed arm muscle), the muscle fibers run parallel

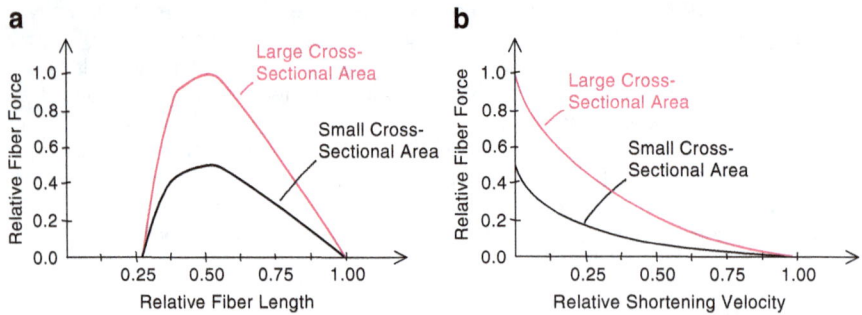

**Fig. 3.2** Length-force and force-velocity relationship of muscle fibers with small and large cross-sectional area. (**a**) Length-force relationship. (**b**) Force-velocity relationship

to the axis along which the force is transmitted to tendons and bones (Fig. 3.3a). In unipennate muscles (e.g. vastus lateralis, outer thigh muscle), the muscle fibers are at a defined angle (the pennation angle) to the said axis (Fig. 3.3b). Finally, in multipennate muscles (e.g., gluteus medius, gluteus medius), the fibers are at multiple angles to the axis. This different muscle architecture leads to several functional peculiarities. In a spindle-shaped muscle, muscle fibers oriented parallel to the tendon direction transmit all their force toward the tendons. In contrast, a unipennate muscle, in which the muscle fibers are, say, at an angle of 30° to the force-generating axis, transmits only 87% of its force along this axis. On the other hand, a pennated muscle can accommodate more muscle fibers in a given volume, resulting in a larger *physiological cross-sectional area* (pCSA).

From these considerations, it is clear that there is an important difference between the anatomical or geometric muscle cross-sectional area (i.e. the cross-sectional area at one or more points along the length of the muscle and perpendicular to it) and the pCSA. The pCSA (in mm²) for a muscle is calculated as follows:

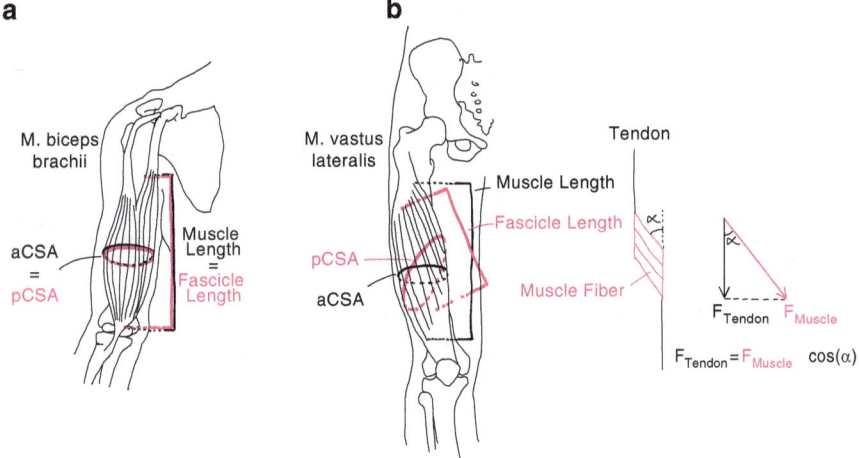

**Fig. 3.3** Muscles with different architecture. (**a**) In the case of the spindle-shaped biceps brachii muscle, the muscle length corresponds to the fascicle length and the anatomical muscle cross-sectional area (aCSA) corresponds to the physiological muscle cross-sectional area (pCSA), shown here using the example of a biceps head. (**b**) In the case of the unipennate vastus lateralis muscle (outer thigh muscle), both the muscle length and the fascicle length as well as the aCSA and the pCSA can differ. The muscle force ($F_{Muscle}$) that can be transmitted to the tendons ($F_{Sehne}$) depends on the pennation angle α. The greater the pennation angle, the smaller the force that can be transmitted from the muscle to the tendons and vice versa (while the cross-sectional area of the muscle fibers remains constant)

$$\mathrm{pCSA}\left(\mathrm{mm}^{2}\right) = \frac{\text{Muscle mass}(\mathrm{g}) \times \cos(\text{pennation angle} \alpha)}{\text{Muscle density}\left(=1.056 \times 10^{-3} \mathrm{g\ mm}^{-3}\right) \times \text{Fibre length}(\mathrm{mm})}$$

This formula makes it easy to understand why, for a spindle-shaped muscle, the anatomical cross-sectional area is equal to the pCSA (Fig. 3.3a, in contrast to Fig. 3.3b): The pennation angle is 0. The cosine of 0 is 1. The muscle mass divided by the muscle density gives the muscle volume. Dividing the muscle volume by the fiber length gives the cross-sectional area, which in the example of the spindle-shaped muscle corresponds to the pCSA.

The more pronounced the muscle pennation, the shorter the fiber length relative to the muscle length, i.e. the smaller the quotient between the two quantities. In spindle-shaped muscles, the quotient is larger (tends more towards 1), which in turn means that the fibers are similar in length to the muscles. In the human body, therefore, there are muscles whose architecture is better suited to the production of high forces – such as the pennated muscles of the quadriceps femoris (four-headed thigh extensor) and the triceps surae (three-headed calf muscle) – than others that are better suited to faster and greater changes in length – such as the spindle-shaped muscles of the ischiocrural musculature or the dorsiflexors of the foot.

> **Box 3.2: Not All Muscle Cross Sections Are Created Equal**
>
> For two muscles with the same geometric muscle cross-section, the maximum muscle tension (force per cross-sectional area) is greater for the muscle with the larger physiological cross-sectional area. A training-induced change in the pennation angle (e.g. by changing the fiber length, i.e. addition or subtraction of sarcomeres in series) leads to a change in the muscle force that you can develop in the tendon direction.

## 3.3 Summary

The volume and, for a given chemical composition and thus density, the mass of a muscle fiber is determined by the length of the fiber and the cross-sectional area of the fiber along the length of the fiber. If the fiber gains length while the cross-sectional area remains the same, the fiber mass increases. If the cross-sectional area increases while the length remains the same, the fiber mass also increases. The same applies, of course, to any combination of increase in length and increase in cross-sectional area.

While the increase in length is due to an increase in the number of sarcomeres in series (with more or less constant average sarcomere length), the increase in cross-sectional area is due to an increase in the number of sarcomeres lying side by side (i.e. parallel). Depending on the degree and type of usage, these two quantities can be positively or negatively affected (see Chap. 10). The totality of the changes in the number of serially and parallel arranged sarcomeres within a muscle fiber thus determines its instantaneous mass, geometric shape and force generation properties (length-force relationship and force-velocity relationship).

Consequently, the totality of fiber changes within a skeletal muscle affects its force generation properties. In addition, for pennate muscles, such as the outer thigh muscle, changes in fiber cross-sectional area and length can affect the pennation angle. This in turn affects how much of the muscle force generated can actually be transferred to the tendons and therefore bone. If your thigh muscle gains x% in mass, that does not automatically mean you are getting x% "stronger" outward. In fact, it depends on where the extra mass (i.e. in this context, the extra sarcomeres) are incorporated and how this changes the pennation angle.

# 4

# The Neuromuscular Origin of Muscle Force

## 4.1 The Muscles in the Brain

In connection with the sequence of events from muscle (fiber) activation to force production described above, we speak of *excitation-contraction coupling*. Now, how does activation occur, that is, what triggers action potentials in the sarcolemma? Activation occurs in voluntary movements by a signal (movement command) from nerve cells (neurons) in the brain. This signal travels to the spinal cord where it is transmitted to the motor neurons (motoneurons), that is, an action potential is triggered in the axon hillock of the motoneurons (the trigger zone). This propagates along the axon (a myelinated, long tube-like nerve cell extension, also called a neurite) via the neuromuscular synapse (the motor end plate, the connecting link between the nerve and muscle fibers) to the muscle fiber (Fig. 4.1). The term "nerve" refers to many motoneuron axons that are surrounded by a connective tissue sheath. In reflexive muscle use, the muscle-activating signal does not originate from neurons in the brain, but from sensory neurons (e.g. in the skin or in the muscle itself).

Just think of the case when you touch a hot stove top out of carelessness – you will reflexively pull back your hand. This quick reaction is only possible because the signal from the sensory neurons does not have to be conducted via the brain to the spinal cord, but reaches the spinal cord directly. Of course, the brain does receive sensory feedback during the reflex. Action potentials in the muscle can also be triggered involuntarily in other ways, for example by electrostimulation of the nerve fibers or the muscle. The method of functional electrostimulation is used by therapists in the clinic and is used when patients

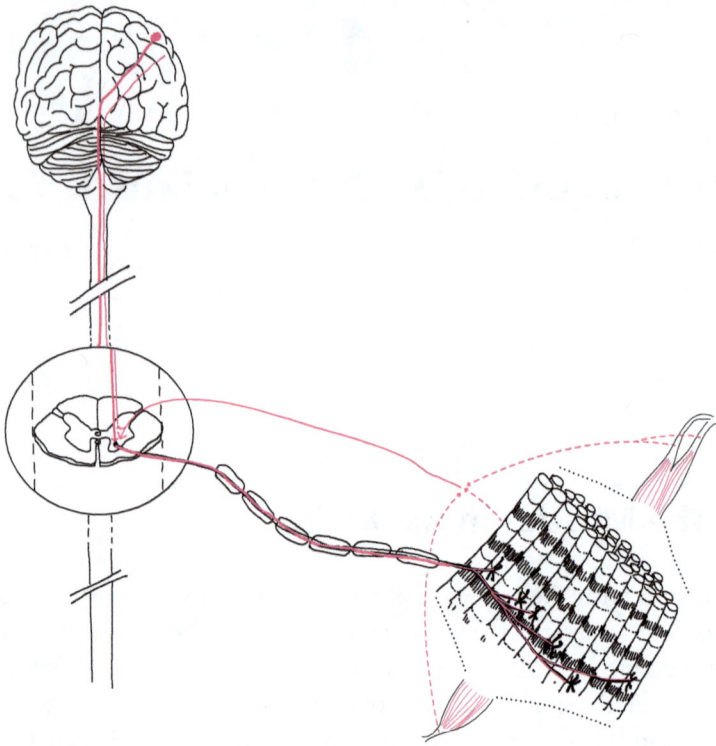

**Fig. 4.1** The neural axis. Voluntary movements require coordination between the various components of the motor system. The main components of the motor system are the motor cortex, the basal ganglia, the thalamus, the midbrain and cerebellum (collectively shown as the brain in the upper left), and the spinal cord (center, left) and the motoneurons recruited there that innervate the muscle fibers (right). Note that starting from the muscle and tendons (and the skin, for that matter), feedback signals travel to the spinal cord and brain. These signals, in turn, can influence motor output. The thicker solid red line symbolizes the descending neuronal signal pathway, while the ascending signal pathway (feedback signal) is shown with thin (solid and dashed) red lines

can no longer activate their muscles independently. This can be the case with nerve and/or spinal cord injuries or also after operations.

## 4.2 How Is Muscle Force "Coded"?

How can the force level of a single muscle fiber be influenced at will? In other words, how is it possible that you can influence whether a single muscle fiber produces much or little force? We have seen that the force production of a muscle fiber is normally coupled to a neural signal. The excitation of the muscle fiber, including the release of intracellular calcium ions, occurs relatively quickly (about 5 ms). In contrast, the processes of subsequent force production and relaxation are relatively slow (about 100 ms). The result of force production, the twitch, therefore lags behind activation. If the muscle fiber now receives a second nerve impulse (impulse here understood as a synonym for impulse or drive), calcium is again released. If the second impulse arrives before the muscle fiber is relaxed, that is, before the 100 ms has elapsed, then there is a summation of calcium concentration around the myofilaments and thus a summation of force. In other words, the two impulses partially superimpose. The superposition concerns the part of the calcium ions that could not yet be pumped back into the sarcoplasmic reticulum because of the insufficient time interval. This is referred to as temporal summation. For a given fiber cross-sectional area (number of parallel sarcomeres), the fiber force therefore depends on both the number and the temporal sequence of impulses from the motoneuron. A higher fiber force results if the neuronal impulses occur at high frequency, because then there is less time for relaxation. However, if the time interval between two impulses is too short, then the second impulse has no effect. This effect is due to the fact that the sarcolemma is refractory, i.e. insensitive, to renewed depolarization for a certain time.

The refractory period – which in skeletal muscle fibers, unlike in cardiac muscle fibers, is only a few milliseconds – is therefore the time span in which no further action potential can be triggered after a preceding action potential at the sarcolemma. The frequency at which a single motor neuron transmits impulses to muscle fibers is called the firing frequency or firing rate. This corresponds to the inverse time interval between two impulses – the SI unit is $s^{-1}$. Here, a pulse frequency of 1 $s^{-1}$ corresponds to one pulse per second or 1 Hz (Hertz). At high firing frequencies (approx. 100 $s^{-1}$), complete tetanic force production occurs, i.e. the individual twitches are no longer apparent in the temporal recording of the fiber force, and the fiber force appears as a smooth curve.

**Frequency Coding**
The strategy of grading muscle fiber force by changing the neural impulse frequency is called frequency coding. Frequency coding represents one of two basic ways in which the central nervous system can adjust muscle force. If high or low muscle forces are required, then high or low frequency impulses can be administered by the central nervous system. On its own, however, frequency coding is not particularly effective in terms of force gradation. There are two reasons for this: From electrical stimulation experiments on the

rabbit tibialis anterior muscle (anterior tibial muscle), it is known that muscle force increases by a maximum of 4 to 5 times when the stimulation frequency is increased from 5 to 100 Hz. This dynamic range is much smaller than the typical dynamic range of muscle force. Thus, the force measured at the fingertip during a grasping movement can vary by a factor of 1000!

This wide range is necessary to master a wide variety of movement tasks in everyday life, from holding a pencil to typing on a keyboard to carrying a shopping bag to holding onto a pull-up bar. A second reason why frequency coding alone is not the ultimate coding strategy is that the steadiness of force production decreases dramatically at very low stimulation frequencies. This means that the fluctuation in force level increases. However, this is exactly the opposite of what is desired for fingers or hand dexterity. Fortunately, muscle force control is more sophisticated via the central nervous system. To be clear again, muscle force has a neural component and a muscular component. Accordingly, muscle force is a neuromuscular product.

## 4.3 Muscle Fibers, as Part of the Motor Unit, Always Work as a Team

While at the level of muscle tissue the sarcomere or, due to the symmetrical sarcomere structure, half the sarcomere represents the functional unit of force production, the functional unit of the neuromuscular system and thus of movement is the motor unit. A motor unit includes an α-motoneuron and all muscle fibers innervated (excited) by that motoneuron. As mentioned previously, the cell bodies of motoneurons are located in the anterior horn of the spinal cord. One axon emanates from each cell body of a motoneuron. Many axons from different cell bodies run in bundles in peripheral nerves to the muscles and innervate them (Fig. 4.1). A peripheral nerve therefore contains a large number of axons, one end of which is formed by the individual cell bodies of the motoneurons in the spinal cord and the other end of which leads to the muscle.

## 4.4 Why Are Neuromuscular Connections Dotted?

The existence of task-specific subsets of motor units within the same muscle (in the above example of the biceps brachii muscle) brings me to the question of how muscles and muscle fibers are innervated, i.e. supplied with nerves or motoneurons. As mentioned earlier (Sect. 4.1), a peripheral nerve contains many motoneuron axons. Bundled in the nerve, the axons reach the muscle. There the nerve branches into smaller branches as appropriate, and in adult humans each individual axon innervates exactly one muscle fiber, approximately in the middle of its fiber length. One can visualize these zones of innervation histochemically in the muscles of human cadavers. Each individual motor endplate (i.e., neuromuscular synapse) then appears as a single point and, when viewed from a distance, a dark stripe, called the endplate stripe, is seen in the center of the muscle.

This innervation site makes sense because the signal strength of the action potential triggered on the cell membrane of the muscle fibers decreases as it propagates with increasing distance from the end plate. If the muscle fiber were now innervated at one end, the action potential would not be able to reach the other end of the fiber at all due to signal attenuation. The consequence would be that force would only be produced in one fiber region (the other would remain relaxed). Due to the then pronounced force and length inhomogeneity of the sarcomeres, the fiber would become very susceptible to microtrauma (see Sect. 7.3).

## 4.5 Not All Muscle Fibers Run from Tendon to Tendon

In fact, it can be observed that with increasing fascicle length, the number of neuromuscular synapses generally also increases, i.e. the longer the muscle, the more endplate strips can be observed. Muscles with multiple endplate strips are referred to as multiply innervated muscles. In non-primates (mice, guinea pigs, rabbits), the fascicles of muscles with only one endplate stripe are always shorter than 35 mm. Thus, in singly innervated muscles, a single neuromuscular synapse supplies an average 35 mm long muscle fiber in these mammals. Muscles with longer fascicles have multiple endplate strips that are regularly spaced. With each additional endplate strip, the average fascicle length supplied by an endplate strip also increases, by approximately 10–12 mm.

Since a single muscle fiber is basically innervated by only one motoneuron, this means that multiply innervated muscles have intrafascicular-ending muscle fibers. Intrafascicular-ending muscle fibers are muscle fibers that do not run the entire length of the muscle (i.e., from tendon to tendon) but end somewhere in the muscle. In order for longitudinal and transverse force transmission to still be possible, these fibers are coupled to other muscle fibers via myomyonal connections (connections between two fiber ends, where one fiber end is laterally attached to the end of another fiber; the fibers are laterally connected). The existence of multiple innervated muscles, or muscle fibers terminating intrafascicularly, naturally raises the question of how this complex organization is controlled motorly by the central nervous system, or what a motor unit is composed of. Does a motor unit include all intrafascicular fibers linked longitudinally by myomyonal junctions, or those arranged in parallel at a particular level of the fiber, or does a motoneuron even supply randomly (i.e., unevenly distributed) intrafascicularly terminating muscle fibers? Unfortunately, there are no answers to these questions yet.

In adult primates, unlike non-primates, most muscles of the extremities are singly innervated, meaning that the muscles have exactly one endplate stripe and the muscle fibers run continuously from tendon to tendon. In primates, lengths of up to 14 cm have been measured for singly innervated muscle fibers, meaning that the section of muscle fiber supplied by a neuromuscular synapse is much longer than for the smaller, non-primates mentioned above. However, there are also multiply innervated muscles in humans. For example, in large humans, the sartorius muscle (sartorius) can be up to 60 cm(!) long. Significantly, it contains five to seven neurovascular compartments, each of which is traversed by an endplate strip. This muscle is thus clearly multiply innervated. The gracilis muscle (slender muscle) and the latissimus dorsi muscle (broad back muscle) are also multiply innervated muscles and have multiple endplate strips. The semitendinosus muscle (semitendinous muscle) is divided by a tendon strip into two compartments, each of which is singly innervated. Similarly, the human rectus abdominis (straight abdominal muscle) has multiple tendon plates (these, along with the muscle, give rise to the image of the infamous six-pack). The shorter fascicles in the headward muscle bellies are typically single innervated, while the longer fascicles (footward) are multiple innervated. These facts are relevant for two reasons. First, together with the aspect of neuroanatomical organization in the spinal cord (see Sect. 9.14), they form the physiological basis for understanding differences in shape of the same muscle from individual to individual. Secondly, they reinforce the view that, anatomically/functionally speaking, a muscle should be worked in as many ways as possible if you want to maximise hypertrophy or increase the chance of a positive transfer to the sport. For example, whether you need your straight ab muscles to move the pelvis towards the rib cage when the rib cage is fixed, or to move the rib cage towards the pelvis when the pelvis is fixed, the demands on each muscle belly will not be the same.

## 4.6  Neuromuscular Catchment Areas

In muscle, the axons or motoneurons branch to varying degrees into a few to several hundred terminal branches. Normally, each terminal axon branch innervates exactly one muscle fiber. Motor units can vary in size with respect to the number of innervated muscle fibers. Thus, the size of the motor unit is defined by its innervation number (number of innervated muscle fibers). Large motor units have a large number of innervations; they thus consist of a motor neuron and many muscle fibers. In contrast, smaller motor units have a lower innervation number. The innervation number is also characteristic for the average increase in force that results from the activation of the motoneuron. The lower the innervation number, the more finely graded the muscle force can be. The size of motor units can vary greatly between different muscles but also within the same muscle. In the case of the interosseus dorsalis I muscle (a hand muscle), the range of innervation numbers extends from approx. 21–1770. The "strongest" motor unit of this muscle (in terms of the number of fibers) is therefore about as strong as an average-sized motor unit of the gastrocnemius medialis muscle (the medial part of the twin calf muscle).

The muscle fibers belonging to a motor unit are not evenly distributed or scattered over the entire cross-sectional area of the muscle. They usually cover a partial area, which at the same time is also interspersed with muscle fibers from other motor units. The functional purpose of this arrangement is that the force of a motor unit can be distributed over a larger tissue area. This minimizes mechanical stress in focal muscle regions. Many of the classic animal experiments on the motor unit were conducted in the late 1960s and early 1970s around Robert Burke and colleagues (e.g., Burke et al. 1973). The researchers isolated individual motor units of the hind paw of a cat and measured both the electrophysiological properties of the motor neurons and the mechanical properties of the motor units within the whole muscle. They did this by directly electrically stimulating the cell bodies of the isolated motoneurons via a microelectrode. You may recall: If the stimulation is strong enough for the individual cell body, an action potential is triggered in the axon hillock of the motoneuron (in the trigger zone) according to the all-or-nothing principle (i.e. either there is an action potential or there is not). This spreads via the terminal axon branches to all muscle fibers belonging to this motor unit and activates them.

## 4.7 How Motor Units Can Differ

It was found that the motor units of the cat's paw could generally be distinguished on the basis of three physiological characteristics (Burke et al. 1973),

- the twitch behavior of the motor unit,
- the fatigue behaviour with a defined stimulation pattern and
- the appearance of the tetanic voltage curve at medium stimulation frequency.

Regarding the first point, it was demonstrated that some motor units developed a high twitch force after a single electrical impulse, while others, relatively speaking, showed medium and low twitch forces. Moreover, it became apparent that force increase and decrease occurred at different rates during the single twitch. This gradation of rapidity (fast, medium fast, slow) was consistent with the gradation of twitch force (high, medium, low).

The "stronger" motor units can therefore also produce force more quickly. The second distinguishing feature concerns the fatigue index, i.e. how great the loss of force is after repeated stimulation (one 40 Hz pulse per second over several minutes). In this regard, it was shown that the majority of motor units had either a fatigue index less than 0.25 or greater than 0.75 (i.e., could produce less than 25% or more than 75% of the initial force after 2 min of stimulation). The third and final criterion for classifying motor units concerns the progression of force as a function of time during incomplete tetanic force production. The physiological significance of this criterion is unclear. Be that as it may, there were motor units in which force increased on average with time, and others in which force first increased but then decreased slightly.

Based on these three criteria, three main types of motor units can be distinguished: First, there are those that can develop force quickly, have a low fatigue index (i.e., are quickly *fatigable*), and for which the force drops sharply over time (abbreviated FF, Fig. 4.2a). Then there are the motor units that can develop force quickly, have a high fatigue index (i.e. are relatively fatigue

---

**Fig. 4.2** (continued) less force, and take longer to reach peak force during a single twitch. In return, they are more resistant to fatigue compared to FF-type units. (c) S-type motor units consist of α-motoneurons with small cell bodies and axons. They innervate few muscle fibers. Compared with those of the FF and FR types, these units can produce less force during a single twitch and, relatively speaking, take a long time to reach peak force. On the other hand, they practically do not fatigue. TwTp (twitch time to peak), time taken for the force generated by the motor unit during a single twitch to reach the peak value. (According to Burke et al. 1973)

# 4 The Neuromuscular Origin of Muscle Force

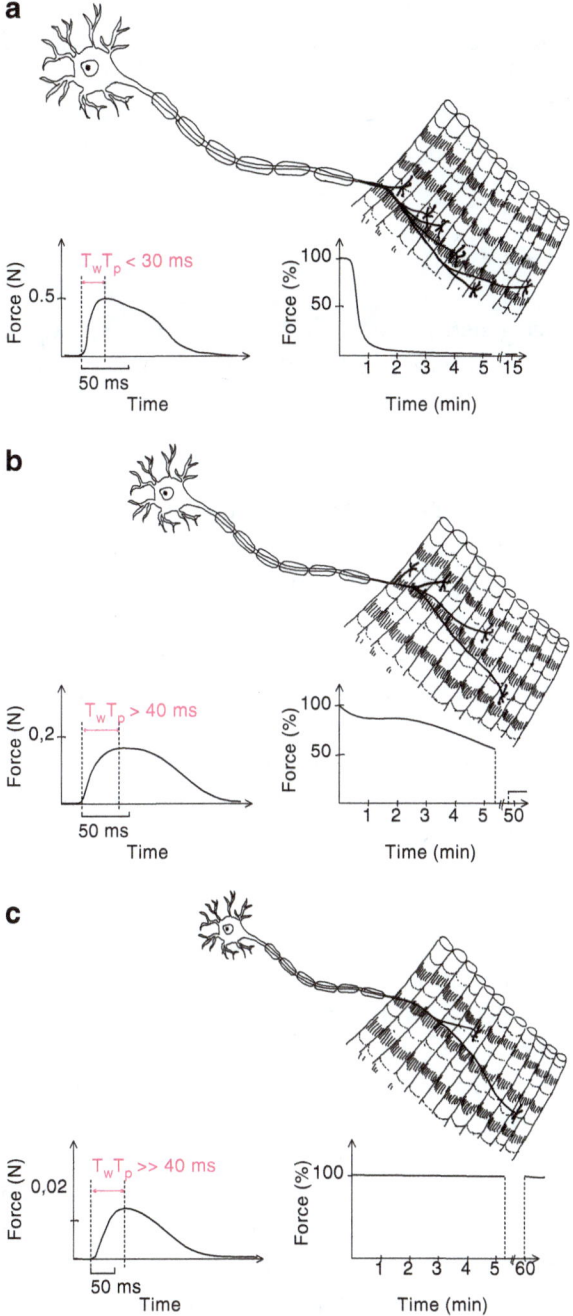

**Fig. 4.2** Anatomical and physiological characteristics of the three types of motor units. (**a**) FF-type motor units consist of α-motoneurons with large cell bodies and axons. They innervate many muscle fibers. They can generate a lot of force in a short time, but tire quickly. (**b**) FR-type motor units are smaller than FF-type units, generate

*resistant*) and are characterized by a smaller drop in force (abbreviated FR for *fast fatigue resistant*, Fig. 4.2b). Finally, there are the motor units that can only produce force slowly, have a high fatigue index and whose force trace practically does not drop under the conditions described above (abbreviated S for slow, Fig. 4.2c).

## 4.8 Summary

Based on the force generation and fatigue properties, 3 groups of motor units can be distinguished experimentally: FF (*fast fatigable*) type motor units consist of α-motoneurons with large cell bodies and axons. They innervate many muscle fibers. FF motor units can generate a lot of force in a short time, but they fatigue quickly. FR (*fast fatigue resistant*) motor units are smaller than FF motor units (i.e. they contain fewer muscle fibers), generate less force and take longer to reach peak force during a single twitch. In return, they are more fatigue resistant compared to FF motor units. Finally, S-type motor units consist of α-motoneurons with small cell bodies and axons. They innervate few muscle fibers. Compared to FF and FR motor units, S motor units can produce less force during a single twitch and take a relatively long time to reach peak force. On the other hand, they practically do not fatigue.

Please do not understand this classification as an exact demarcation between the different groups of motor units, but much more as a rough guide. Motor units are not DIN-normed. Generally speaking, it is therefore more appropriate to speak of motor units with low or high recruitment thresholds and to see this recruitment threshold as a continuum between two extreme values (very low to very high). For didactic reasons, I will continue to speak of the 3 groups FF, FR, and S in this book.

The force of a muscle can in principle be graded by the recruitment and frequency of motor units. For this purpose, imagine a theater stage that can be illuminated with many dimmable lamps of varying light intensity. Each lamp can be controlled separately from the control room. The brightness on the stage now depends on how many lamps are switched on and at what light intensity they burn. In this analogy, the brightness corresponds to muscle force, the lamps to the sum of the muscle fibers belonging to a motor unit, the control room to the spinal cord, and the dimmable light switches to the cell bodies of the motor units. The switching on or off of lamps to increase or decrease brightness thus symbolizes the strategy of recruiting motor units, while the frequency of motor units corresponds to the process of dimming.

# 5

# A Bouquet of Cellular Diversity

## 5.1 The Colorful World of Muscle Fibers

What determines the described physiological properties of the motor units? As an attentive reader, you already guessed it: by the innervated muscle fiber type. Indeed, the physiological properties of the muscle fibers belonging to a motor unit roughly correspond to those of the motor unit. That muscle fibers are heterogeneous was first observed in the early eighteenth century. Even at that time, it was noted that the color could vary from bright white to deep red depending on the muscle. Muscles were therefore classified as red or white on the basis of their color. The color gradation, by the way, comes from the varying content of myoglobin. Myoglobin is a muscle protein that, like hemoglobin in the blood, can bind oxygen. Oxygen-loaded myoglobin gives muscle tissue a reddish color, similar to how oxygen-loaded hemoglobin makes arterial, oxygen-rich blood appear red. With the development of new measurement methods, many characteristics were discovered by which fibers can be distinguished. These characteristics can be broadly classified into four key physiological categories:

- Metabolism (ATP production and energy supply)
- Rate of force development ("molecular motors", energy conversion)
- Excitability of the sarcolemma (triggering of an action potential)
- Excitation-contraction coupling (control of intracellular calcium concentration)

Basically, the classification of muscle fibers is problematic because the different schemes only work or apply to the particular property under investigation. In other words, the correlation between the classification schemes is poor to non-existent. This can be seen just by the example of the two features "muscle color" and "shortening speed". Contrary to the common belief that "red" equals "slow", certain fibers can be very red and still be fast. It is therefore extremely important to remember that muscle fibers have a wide and almost continuous spectrum of morphological, metabolic and force production related properties. Classification schemes should therefore be understood as templates that we place on this continuum for convenience.

## 5.2 Molecular Motors of the Muscle

Let us now turn to the physiological properties of the different types of fibers, starting with energy metabolism. Like all other cells in the human body, muscle fibers require energy to "finance" their basic functioning, which includes maintaining resting membrane potential. Unlike other cells, which need energy "only" to maintain normal physiological processes, muscle fibers need to generate additional energy for force production and movement. The actin-myosin cross-bridge cycle of muscle contraction, which involves the cleavage of ATP, represents the determinant of energy consumption and thus the energy demand side. So let us first turn to this energy demand.

In the many cross-bridge cycles, which occur simultaneously but asynchronously during muscle use, one ATP is cleaved per cross-bridge cycle to form adenosine diphosphate (ADP) and inorganic phosphate ($P_i$). In brief, a cross-bridge cycle comprises the following steps:

1. A molecule of ATP binds to the myosin head with subsequent detachment of the myosin head from actin.
2. ATP is cleaved to ADP and $P_i$, with ADP and $P_i$ still remaining at the myosin head. This cleavage has two effects: the lever arm of the myosin folds forward and the affinity between myosin and actin increases.
3. $P_i$ is split off and a so-called power stroke occurs, i.e. a lever arm rotation with a step movement of the actin filaments of approx. 5–10 nm in the direction of the M-line. This produces a force of about 4 pN (i.e. 4 × $10^{-12}$ N).
4. With the subsequent detachment of ADP, the initial state is reached, i.e. the cross-bridge cycle has been run through once (Fig. 5.1).

# 5  A Bouquet of Cellular Diversity   53

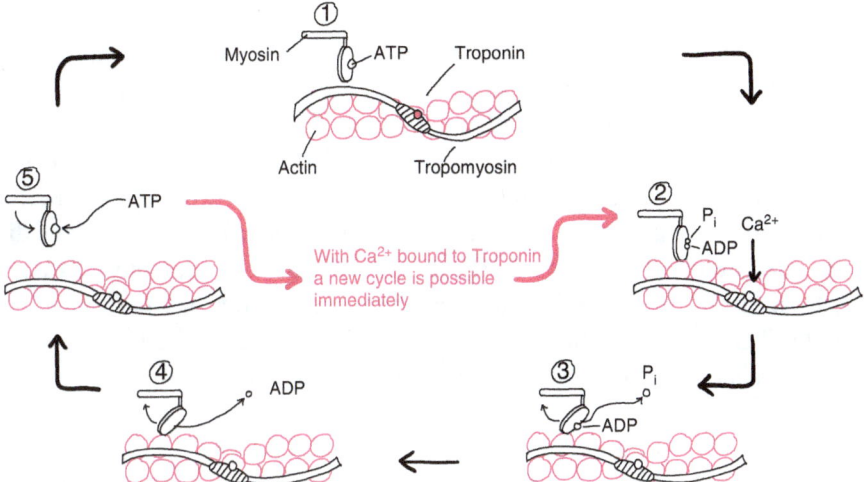

**Fig. 5.1** Sequence of the cross-bridge cycle. ① At rest, without Ca²⁺ bound to troponin, tropomyosin blocks the binding site for the myosin head at actin. ② When Ca²⁺ is released from the sarcoplasmic reticulum and binds to troponin, the binding sites for the myosin heads on actin become free. ATP is cleaved in the myosin head into ADP and phosphate ($P_i$). ③ When the phosphate is cleaved, the myosin heads angle 45°. ④ If ADP is also cleaved from myosin, the myosin heads angle at 50°. ⑤ The myosin heads do not detach from the binding site until ATP attaches to the head. (According to Clauss and Clauss 2009)

As the cross-bridges perform this microscopic rowing movement in the mio- or pliometric case many times in succession at ever new locations along the actin filament, the macroscopic movement occurs. In the isometric case, the myosin head always attaches to the actin filament at the same point.

> **Box 5.1: Why Do Dead People Become Rigid?**
>
> With the onset of death, the ATP concentration in the muscle fibers drops to zero. The bound cross-bridges can therefore no longer be released, but remain in the so-called rigor complex. This rigid anchoring of actin and myosin, which lasts until the dissolution of the myofibrillar proteins, manifests itself in stiff muscles (latin *rigor mortis*). Since ATP prevents this rigidity or dissolves the bond, one often speaks of the softening effect of ATP.

## 5.3  Fiber Type-Specific Motor Classes

The myosins of the sarcomere are hexamers consisting of two *myosin heavy chains* (MyHC) and two pairs of *myosin light chains* (MyLC). ATP cleavage takes place in the catalytic center of the MyHC, so that their ATPase activity (the amount of ATP cleaved per unit time by the ATPase enzyme) determines how many cross-bridge cycles can be repeated per second. The higher the ATPase activity of the MyHC, the more often the same cross-bridge is active per second and the greater the unloaded shortening rate. Therefore, the shortening rate of a (half-)sarcomere or fiber is coupled to the average rate of ATP cleavage in the MyHC. Different MyHC isoforms are expressed in skeletal muscle (isoforms are different forms of the same protein). These isoforms differ in the rate of ATP cleavage – it can vary at least six-fold, from 22 to 131 $s^{-1}$. In addition, the more crossbridges there are in series, i.e. the longer the muscle fiber, the faster the unloaded shortening speed of the fiber, and the more parallel crossbridges there are, the higher the force generated (see Sect. 2.4).

In mammals as a whole, at least eleven sarcomeric MyHC isoforms encoded by eleven *MYH genes* can be distinguished. However, not all isoforms are expressed (produced) in every species and the predominantly expressed isoform may also differ from muscle to muscle. For example, the predominant MyHC isoform in atypical muscles such as the extraocular muscles (muscles that allow the very rapid, saccadic eye movements) or the masseter muscles is different from that in typical skeletal muscles such as the thigh muscles.

As far as typical skeletal muscles are concerned, three primary MyHC isoforms are distinguished in adult healthy humans: Type 1, Type 2A, and Type 2X. MyHC type 1 fibers have low ATPase activity relative to the other isoforms, and are therefore slow in terms of the rate of ATP cleavage. MyHC type 2 (2A/2X) have relatively high ATPase activity and are faster relative to MyHC type 1. MyHC type 2X are again faster than MyHC type 2A. MyHC type 1 are innervated by S-type motor units, and MyHC type 2A and MyHC type 2X are innervated by FR- and FF-type motor units, respectively. In addition, in skeletal muscle fibers of rodents such as mice and rats, but not humans, the MyHC-2B isoform is also expressed. Its rate of ATP cleavage is even higher than that of MyHC type 2X. A single human skeletal muscle fiber usually expresses predominantly one of the three MyHC isoforms mentioned above (1, 2A, 2X). However, there are also so-called hybrid fibers, i.e. muscle fibers that simultaneously express several isoforms in similar amounts. It is obvious that muscle fibers can be classified on the basis of the expression of the MyHC isoform (i.e. its molecular motor). Accordingly, we distinguish at least five types of MyHC fibers in adult humans (1, 1/2A, 2A, 2A/2X, and 2X), with 1/2A and 2A/2X fibers being hybrid fibers. For simplicity, we limit ourselves here to the three "pure" fiber types 1, 2A, and 2X.

**Box 5.2: What Is Meant by the Distribution of Muscle Fiber Types?**

The distribution of the fiber types of a muscle can basically be understood in two ways. In the first case, the fibers of a muscle are typed and the number of fibers of all existing fiber types is determined in the histological cross-section of a muscle sample (Fig. Diversity of muscle fiber types). The distribution of fiber types is calculated from the number of individual muscle fiber types relative to the total number of fibers (expressed as a percentage). In the second case, all muscle fibers are also typed, but their respective cross-sectional area is determined at the same time. From this, one then calculates the distribution of the fiber area, i.e. how much of the total fiber area is taken up by one fiber type. From a functional point of view, the cross-sectional area of the fiber types in a muscle seems to be more important than the numerical proportion of the fiber types.

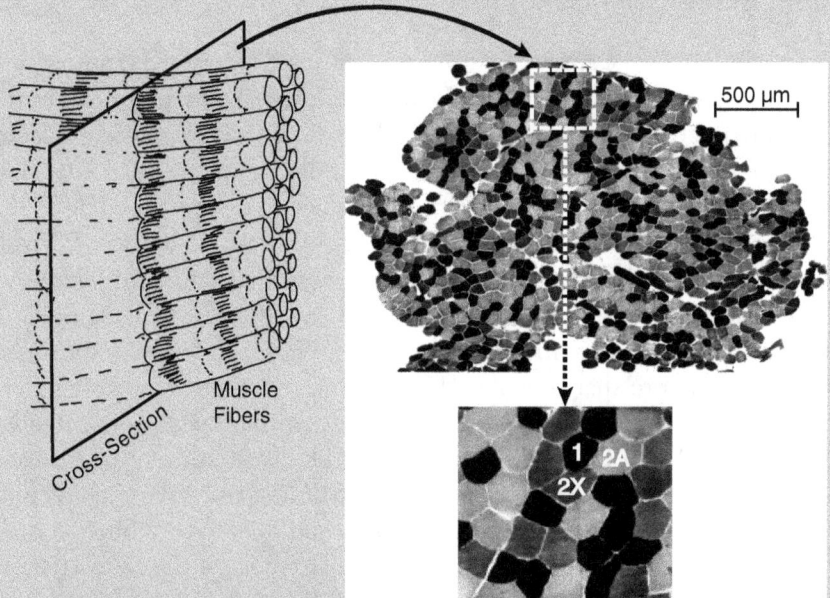

**Diversity of muscle fiber types**

In humans, according to the classification pattern of MyHC (myosin heavy chains), three "pure" muscle fiber types are distinguished: Type 1, Type 2A, and Type 2X. *On the left,* a group of muscle fibers is shown. *On the right* is shown the result of histological staining of the section through the muscle fibers. This is a sample from the vastus lateralis muscle (outer thigh muscle) of an untrained male in young adulthood, obtained as part of one of our studies. The muscle sample was cut perpendicular to the direction of the muscle fibers into slices of a thickness of 8 µm. The slices were then placed on slides and stained using histochemical methods. The myofibrillar ATPase reaction with acidic pre-incubation (pH 4.6) reveals the individual muscle fiber types. Above, several hundred muscle fibers can be seen in cross-section. The staining intensity of the individual muscle fibers reflects the MyHC isoform predominant in the fiber. As the section below shows, type 1 MyHC fibers appear very dark in this staining method, type 2A fibers appear light, and type 2X fibers are in the middle. Note the size scale to get an idea of the diameter of individual muscle fibers.

In general, the distribution of fiber types in humans is very heterogeneous. This applies both to an interindividual comparison – the same muscle is considered in different people – and to an intraindividual comparison, which is either between different muscle groups such as upper body *vs.* lower body muscles or side-specific (in top athletes e.g. playing leg *vs.* standing leg).

## 5.4 Distribution of Muscle Fiber Types in Humans: What Determines It?

As part of a large-scale study of 270 untrained and 148 trained (endurance or resistance training), light-skinned North American women and men (average age approximately 24 years, range: 16–33 years) of average body size and mass, 418 muscle samples were obtained from the vastus lateralis (outer thigh muscle). Analysis of these muscle samples revealed that approximately 25% of the subjects had either less than 35% or greater than 65% type 1 MyHC fibers in the vastus lateralis muscle (Simoneau and Bouchard 1989). However, the variability found was high in both males and females. For example, the percentage of type 1 fibers in females was 18–85%, which tended to be slightly higher compared to that in males (15–79%). On average, females had 51% type-1, 37% type-2A, and 12% type-2X fibers, with corresponding standard deviations (SD) of 13, 10, and 9. In males, the distribution of fibers was as follows: 46% type-1 (SD 15), 39% type-2A (SD 12), and 15% type-2X fibers (SD 9). Similar – approximately 50% type 1 and 50% type 2 fibers – is also estimated to be the distribution of muscle fiber types for the rectus femoris, gastrocnemius, deltoid and biceps brachii muscles. In the soleus muscle, however, the distribution is 75–90% type 1 and 10–25% type 2 fibers, so it contains predominantly type 1 fibers. The triceps brachii muscle is different: It has only 20–40% type-1 and 60–80% type-2 fibers in humans.

Simoneau and Bouchard's (1989) study of the vastus lateralis muscle also showed a wide variability in fiber cross-sectional areas. Thus, in females, they found an average cross-sectional area of 4044 µm$^2$ (SD 846), 3594 µm$^2$ (SD 818), and 2837 µm$^2$ (SD 884) for type 1, type 2A, and type 2X fibers, respectively. Males were found to have a larger average fiber cross-sectional area, especially for type-2 fibers: 4591 µm$^2$ (SD 1058), 4958 µm$^2$ (SD 1177), and 4439 µm$^2$ (SD 1254), respectively, for the respective fiber type (Simoneau and Bouchard 1989). The greater average fiber area in males relative to that in females is accompanied by the greater average muscle mass in males relative to females. This fundamental difference in muscle mass develops during puberty. During this phase of increased hormone production, the testosterone concentration in men rises to a markedly higher level, which increases muscle mass at this stage of development (possibly with a selective effect on type 2 fibers). The fact that young women on average have a lower muscle mass than young men therefore has to do with the gender-specific hormone release during puberty. But be careful: this in no way means that adult women have a lower adaptive potential for resistance training compared to men (see Sect. 17.1)!

Studies of monozygotic and dizygotic twins were then conducted to determine what accounts for the variance (i.e., scatter of data points) in the percentage of type 1 fibers. It was possible to attribute approximately 45% of the total variance to genetic factors, approximately 15% to experimental conditions (sample collection and processing), and approximately 40% to environmental factors (training, diet, geographic environment, etc.) (Simoneau and Bouchard 1995). However, it is unclear at what stage of development the environmental influences can have any effect at all. It is true that the muscles of athletes in sprint sports tend to have a higher number of type 2 fibers (about 75%) than untrained athletes (about 45%), and the muscles of endurance athletes tend to have a higher proportion of type 1 fibers (about 75%) than untrained athletes. However, it is also true that the data points for the proportion of type 1 fibers in untrained individuals scatter so much around the mean value that the scatter range also contains the values of all sprinters (total scatter range) and almost all endurance athletes.

It is therefore not clear whether the proportion of type 1 fibers in these extreme examples of elite athletes is the result of their training, and if so, at what stage of their physical development the interaction between training and genes took place, or whether these individuals simply "ended up" in the sports for which they are suited by their muscular make-up (see also Chap. 21).

In any case, for athletic performance, the cross-sectional area of the individual fiber types seems to be more important than their numerical proportion. Take the example of two men, Jim and Joe. The numerical proportion of each muscle fiber type in their vastus lateralis (outer thigh muscle) is identical, say 46% type 1, 39% type 2A, and 15% type 2X fibers. If the proportion of cross-sectional area for the three fiber types is the same on average for both (see above data for cross-sectional area), then the area distribution for both is approximately 45% type 1, 41% type 2A, and 14% type 2X fibers. However, if Jim's type-2A fibers have a cross-sectional area twice that of Joe's (no difference in the other fiber types), the area distribution of the fibers in Jim's muscle is 32% type-1, 58% type-2A, and 10% type-2X fibers. The situation becomes even more complicated when you take into account that, of course, it is not only the relative distribution of fiber type that affects performance, but also the absolute muscle mass. So if Joe has a much larger thigh muscle mass relative to body mass compared to Jim, in absolute terms, it is no longer clear whether there will be differences in performance and which components of performance they will affect (e.g. force, speed, etc.).

A real, scientific case study is intended to illustrate this fact. The distribution of fiber types in terms of number and area in the vastus lateralis muscle (outer thigh muscle) of a world champion and Olympic medalist in shot put and his long-time training partner in a highly trained state at the end of his career were examined. The first thing that stood out was that the muscle samples from both athletes contained virtually no type 2X fibers (see below). The different type 2 fibers were therefore combined in the evaluation.

What is your estimate of how fiber types were distributed numerically for the two? Based on the above averages for athletes in sprint sports, your estimate for both athletes should be about 25% type 1 and 75% type 2 fibers. Well, for the training partner this was approximately true (33% to 67%), but not for the world champion. For him, the type 1 fibers were clearly in the majority (60% to 40%). However, if we look at the average fiber cross-sectional areas, the following picture emerges interestingly. The average cross-sectional area of type 1 fibers was about 40% smaller in the world champion and that of type 2 fibers about 20% larger than in his training partner, with the result that type 1 fibers accounted for about 33% of the total area in the world champion and type 2 fibers for 67%, while type 1 fibers accounted for about 25% and type 2 fibers for 75% in his training partner. For a complete comparison, one would now have to take into account the absolute muscle mass, but this was unknown in this case. The results of this scientific case study thus also indicate that

- even "explosive" trainings slows a muscle down at the level of the muscle's molecular motors (MyHC isoform),
- in adult humans, the training methods used cannot explain most of the observed variability in the distribution of muscle fiber types, and
- for performance, the cross-sectional area of the fiber types is probably more relevant than their numerical distribution.

> **Box 5.3 Human Muscles Are Not Equal to Mouse Muscles!**
> 
> As I have pointed out to you, human skeletal muscles are composed mainly of type 1 and type 2A fibers and a minority of type 2X fibers. Mouse muscles, on the other hand, contain primarily type 2B and type 2X fibers and a minority of type 2A fibers. Type 1 fibers are rare in mice and primarily restricted to single muscles such as the soleus muscle. In contrast to humans, the spectrum of fiber types in

mouse, rat, rabbit, and guinea pig is broader and includes 1, 1/2A, 2A, 2A/2X, 2X, 2X/2B, and 2B. In human skeletal muscle, mitochondrial and oxidative enzyme content is typically highest in type 1 fibers and lowest in type 2X fibers. Mitochondria are small cellular organs (organelles) in which electrons generated during the chemical breakdown (dehydrogenation) of substrates such as glucose and fatty acids are transferred to oxygen ($O_2$). In the process, ATP is produced from ADP and $P_i$. This is why mitochondria are also referred to as the energy power plants of the cell.

In mouse and rat, this oxidative potential is highest in type 2A fibers and lowest in type 2B fibers, whereas type 2X fibers, which are glycolytic in humans, are highly oxidative in mouse and rat. By glycolytic here is meant that the fibers are well equipped to produce ATP relatively independently of mitochondria and $O_2$. Mouse skeletal muscle is therefore not the most appropriate experimental model for human muscle, and it is very important to be aware of these interspecies differences before attempting to extrapolate conclusions from studies using genetically modified (transgenic) animals or knock-out models to humans.

## 5.5 Changes in the Distribution of Muscle Fiber Types Due to Training or Inactivity

The majority of all studies on classical forms of training (i.e. endurance and resistance training) showed for adults that training only changes the distribution of hybrid fibers and type 2 fibers in terms of numbers. Regardless of the form of training (endurance or ressitance oriented, fast or slow movements), a shift from type 2X to type 2A fibers is observed, but not to type 1 fibers. In fact, many studies also show that the muscle fibers of highly trained individuals (whether endurance or resistance trained) are virtually devoid of MyHC type 2X. All of this suggests that classical training (i.e., usual in terms of training form and volume, etc.) can cause shifts in the distribution of fiber types, from type 2X to type 2A fibers, but not to type 1 fibers. It is likely that the majority of these shifts occur in or through the hybrid fibers, for example, by one fiber becoming more homogeneous in expression pattern. Unfortunately, the majority of human studies have quantified only the unique muscle fiber types, so that interesting information about the variability of the fiber type distribution may remain undiscovered.

Of course, it cannot be ruled out that extreme forms of muscle stress, for example cycling, where the thigh muscles are stressed for several hours a day (and this for several weeks, months and years), can also lead to shifts towards type 1 fibers. Either way, your muscle fibers will intrinsically (i.e., at the molecular motor class composition level) slow down with any increase in activity, whether endurance or resistance training, whether you train slow or fast. This is also true of athletes' "explosive" sprint training – it makes muscles intrinsically slower, meaning there is a shift in fiber type from 2X to 2A. This is ironic because many people train "explosively" in hopes that their muscle fibers will get faster in the process. However, the opposite is true. I know this sounds contradictory, but it's true!

Conversely, immobilization (bedriddenness, paraplegia, etc.) results in a shift from type 1 and type 2A to type 2X fibers. Muscle fibers in the vastus lateralis muscle of paraplegic individuals have virtually only MyHC type 2X one year after spinal cord injury (Biering-Sørensen et al. 2009). Similarly, so-called detraining (stopping training or training with relatively reduced volume/intensity) makes your muscle fibers intrinsically faster. In a study of young untrained men who completed a three-month resistance training program followed by three months of detraining, this was demonstrated (Andersen and Aagaard 2000). For the study, the protein content of the different MyHC types in the vastus lateralis muscle were examined before the start of the resistance training phase, after the resistance training phase and after the detraining phase. During the resistance training phase, the content of MyHC type 2X protein decreased significantly from approximately 9% to approximately 2%. At the same time, MyHC type 2A protein content significantly increased from approximately 42% to 49%. After detraining, the protein content of MyHC type 2X was significantly higher (almost twice as high!) at approx. 17% than before the resistance training phase, mainly at the expense of MyHC type 2A.

To put it bluntly, the average rate of ATP cleavage in your muscle fibers becomes faster when you mutate from a fit individual to a couch potato! This example shows that the proportion of type 2X motors can be increased through targeted modulation of muscular activity and inactivity. To what extent this affects athletic performance and health remains to be investigated. Nevertheless, these results suggest that trainers and coaches of competitive athletes should focus not only on training, but also on the phases (duration and extent) of relative inactivity (i.e. relative to baseline levels).

## 5.6 Why You Can Produce More Force Pliometrically than Miometrically

The maximum shortening velocity and the maximum isometric tension and – as a product of force amount and speed – also the maximum power of a muscle fiber type reflect the mixture of different MyHC isoforms in one and

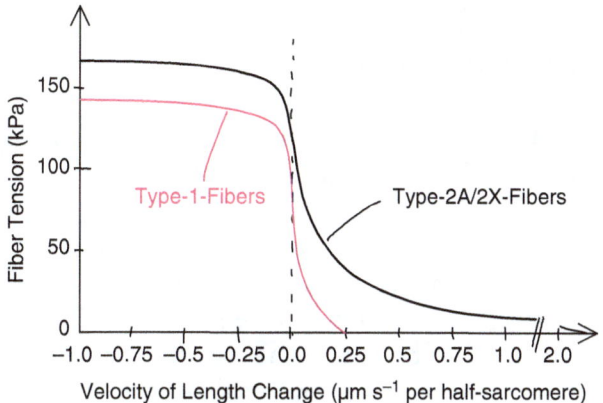

**Fig. 5.2** Force-velocity relationship in MyHC type 1 and MyHC type 2A/2X muscle fibers. The isometric (velocity = 0) force produced per muscle fiber cross-sectional area (fiber tension) is lower for type 1 fibers (red) than for type 2A/2X fibers (black). The tension under pliometric force production conditions (velocity < 0, active stretch) is highest for all fiber types, and the increase in tension relative to the isometric tension value is greater for type 1 fibers than for type 2A/2X fibers. In addition, the maximum velocity during miometric force production (velocity > 0, shortening) is much greater for type-2A/2X fibers than for type-1 fibers

the same fiber. In humans, type 1 vastus lateralis fibers can shorten approximately six times slower (in unloaded conditions) than type 2A/2X fibers. This difference coincides quite well with the six-fold difference in maximal isoform-specific MyHC ATPase activity (see above). Moreover, under isometric conditions, human MyHC type 1 fibers produce a tension of about 68 kPa (1 Pa = 1 N m$^{-2}$; force per cross-sectional area is a measure to consider fiber force independent of its cross-sectional area), whereas type 2A/2X fibers reach about 120 kPa (Fig. 5.2). The force-velocity relationship (Fig. 1.2) of a muscle presented in Sect. 1.6 therefore represents the combination of the velocity-force relationships of all activated muscle fiber types.

It is interesting to note, however, that Type 1 and Type 2A/2X fibers behave quite similarly under pliometric conditions with respect to maximum tension. Type-1 fibers then produce a tension of about 148 kPa and Type-2A/2X fibers about 166 kPa (Fig. 5.2). Thus, under pliometric conditions, type-1 and type-2A/2X fibers produce 1.4- to 2.1-fold higher tension than under isometric conditions. Why there is a general increase in tension under pliometric conditions and why this is greater in type 1 fibers than in type 2A/2X fibers is not yet scientifically clear. In any case, the physiological purpose of hybrid fibers could be that a hybrid MyHC composition within the same fiber, in addition to the mix of different muscle fiber types within the same muscle, allows a finer gradation of maximal shortening velocity and tension.

## 5.7 Summary: Does "Fast" Training Make Your Muscle Motors Faster?

Muscle fibers can be divided into groups based on their "motor type", among other things. In humans, three main types of muscle fibers are distinguished in this respect: Muscle fibers with type 1, type 2A and type 2X motors. Muscle fibers with 2X motors can produce force the fastest, those with 2A motors the second fastest and those with type 1 motors the slowest. If you start training as an untrained person, your fastest muscle fibers (type-2X fibers) will slow down by converting to 2A fibers. It doesn't really matter what type of training it is or how fast the movements are performed during training (explosive, fast or slow). Conversely, if you stop training as a trained person and become inactive, the opposite happens: the numerical proportion of the fastest muscle fibers (2X) increases at the expense of the type 2A proportion – the muscles become faster at the level of your molecular motors. I know this may sound confusing, but it's true. Consequently, if you train at "explosive" speeds and your movement speed does indeed improve as a result, the reason is hardly an increase in the number of 2X motors in your muscle fibers.

# 6

# Muscular Energy Bundles

## 6.1 The Dynamics of Muscular Energy Consumption

In human skeletal muscle, ATP consumption at rest is relatively low (approx. 0.007–0.008 mM ATP $s^{-1}$). The sum of all ATP-cleaving enzymes, so-called ATPases, is responsible for ATP consumption. At rest, ATP consumption is determined on the one hand by the sodium-potassium ATPase, which is responsible for maintaining the membrane potential, and on the other hand by ATP-consuming protein synthesis. Therefore, the individual MyHC fiber types hardly differ with respect to their ATP consumption at rest. However, the differences between the fiber types manifest themselves as soon as the muscle is put to work. Then, as part of the cross-bridge cycle, the MyHC ATPase accounts for approximately 70% of a fiber's energy consumption. The remaining 30% is accounted for by the ATPases that are needed for ion transport, for example for the return transport of calcium ions into the sarcoplasmic reticulum (see Sect. 2.4). It follows that the ATP or energy consumption of an active muscle fiber depends on the MyHC isoform: It is estimated that the maximum energy consumption for human muscle fibers under dynamic conditions (based on dry mass) is approximately 6.5 (type 1), 17.6 (type 2A) and 26.6 (type 2X) mmol $kg^{-1}$ $s^{-1}$. If the ATP consumption for ion transport is also taken into account, these figures must be corrected upwards by 30–40%. Based on the individual fibers, this then results in values around 1.7 (type 1), 4.7 (type 2A) and 7.2 (type 2X) mM ATP $s^{-1}$.

## 6.2 Matching Supply and Demand

However, skeletal muscle fibers only have about 4.7–5.1 mM of ATP stored (with type 2X fibers tending to be at the high end of the range and type 1 fibers at the low end), which means that chemical energy in the form of ATP would be exhausted after only a few seconds if it could not be renewed. However, you know from your own experience that under steady-state conditions (i.e., physiological equilibrium) you can easily use your muscles for several minutes to hours. In fact, [ATP] (the square brackets symbolize concentration) remains virtually unchanged during exercise. So how are supply and demand matched? The cleavage or consumption of ATP (i.e. demand) is mechanistically linked to the regulation of metabolic processes that can regenerate ATP (supply). This regulation, in turn, influences cross-bridge function via changes in [ATP], [ADP], [$P_i$], and [$H^+$]. With respect to energy, ATP thus represents the link between demand (ATP consumption by training and basic cellular processes) and supply (ATP synthesis) (Fig. 6.1). The difference between ATP consumption and synthesis corresponds to the muscular energy balance.

## 6.3 Muscle Fibers Have Several Resources for Regenerating Energy

On the ATP synthesis or regeneration side, three systems are available (Fig. 6.1). They differ in terms of maximum metabolic power (i.e. the amount of substance ATP and thus energy that can be produced per second) and metabolic capacity (i.e. the total amount of substance ATP that can be generated via the individual system):

- phosphagenic system: highest metabolic power but lowest capacity
- glycolytic system: lower metabolic power but higher capacity than the phosphagenic system
- mitochondrial respiration: lowest metabolic power, but by far the largest capacity

Clearly, the expression of these systems within a fiber must be matched to demand, that is, to the predominant myofibrillar ATPase activity (MyHC isoform). I will now discuss the different systems of ATP regeneration in the following and discuss fiber type-specific differences.

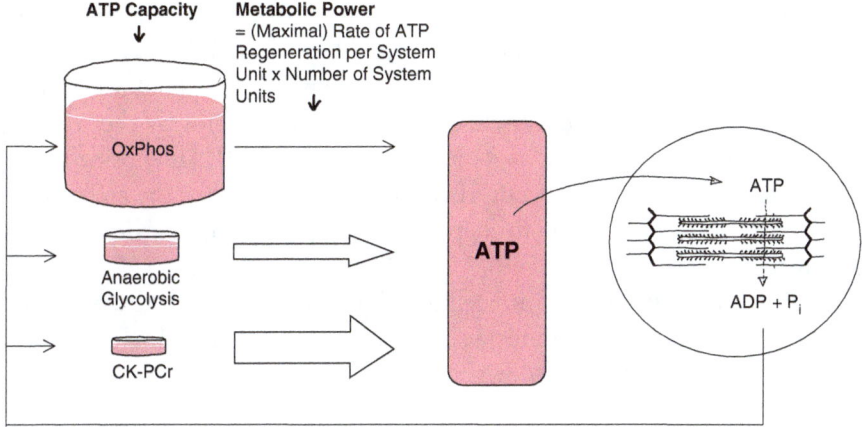

**Fig. 6.1** Muscular energetics. Muscle fibers require energy in the form of ATP to produce force. This energy is released during the cross-bridge cycle between actin and myosin when ATP is split. One molecule of ATP is converted into one molecule of ADP and one molecule of $P_i$. The reaction is mediated by the myofibrillar ATPase. The sum of all cross-bridge cycles or ATPase reactions thus represents the determining variable for the energy consumption (ATP demand) of a muscle fiber (right). Since the ATP storage in the muscle fibers would be exhausted very quickly during force production, i.e. the ATP supply would dry up quickly, ATP must be regenerated immediately and continuously. The three systems shown on the left are available for the regeneration of ATP. These systems differ in the amount of maximum ATP production capacity (moles of ATP that can be generated by the system, represented by the different size and filling of the ATP containers) and metabolic power, i.e. how much ATP can be produced per unit time. On the one hand, metabolic power depends on the number of ATP-producing units (system units). In the case of the oxidative phosphorylation system (OxPhos), this concerns the number of mitochondria. On the other hand, metabolic power depends on the maximum rate of ATP regeneration per system unit, i.e. in the case of OxPhos, on the maximum rate of ATP production per mitochondrion. The thickness of the arrows is symbolic of the maximum rate of ATP production per system unit. ATP, adenosine triphosphate; ADP, adenosine diphosphate; CK-PCr, creatine kinase-phosphocreatine system of ATP regeneration; $P_i$, inorganic phosphate

## 6.4 The Phosphagen System: A Firework of Energy

The phosphagenic system essentially involves two chemical reactions by which the muscle fiber can resynthesize ATP relatively quickly: the creatine kinase (CK) and adenylate kinase (AK) reactions. Both reactions occur in the sarcoplasm. CK is an enzyme that catalyzes the reaction of ADP and phosphocreatine (PCr) to ATP and creatine (Cr). Accordingly, the CK regenerates ATP from ADP and PCr, hence the system is also called the CK-PCr system of

ATP regeneration. However, the absolute amount of energy that can be produced (capacity) for this system is modest and limited mainly (to about 85%) by the size of the intracellular PCr store. The remaining 15% of ATP energy turnover during short-term muscle exercise is accounted for by the AK reaction, which produces 1 mole of ATP and 1 mole of AMP (adenosine monophosphate) from 2 moles of ADP. The mole is the SI unit for the amount of a substance and corresponds to approx. 602 quadrillion particles of the substance.

AMP is a very important intracellular signal molecule. On the one hand, AMP can be deaminated to inosine monophosphate (IMP). IMP stimulates glycogenolysis, i.e. the breakdown of glycogen (see below) into substances that are fed into glycolysis. In type 2 fibers, relative to type 1 fibers, the conversion of AMP to IMP occurs more rapidly, so [IMP] increases more in the same amount of time, leading to a stronger glycogenolytic signal. On the other hand, AMP activates AMP kinase (AMPK), which in turn facilitates both the transport of glucose (via glucose transporter 4, GLUT4) and fatty acids (via fatty acid transporters, FAT/CD36) into the muscle fiber and their metabolism in the mitochondria (see third system: mitochondrial regeneration of ATP). Via the alteration of AMPK activity, which is higher in type-1 fibers than in type-2 fibers, PGC-1α (*peroxisome proliferator-activated receptor γ coactivator 1-α*) signaling pathways are also affected, resulting in, among other things, new mitochondrial formation (mitochondrial biogenesis). The metabolites produced in the context of ATP cleavage and phosphagenic ATP regeneration therefore directly stimulate the other two systems (glycolysis and mitochondrial respiration).

If the phosphagenic system were the only system available, all PCr in the muscle would be degraded after 10 s and the store exhausted. However, since the other two systems (see below) also partially contribute to energy production from the beginning, PCr can contribute to ATP production for up to more than 20 s. Analogous to an electrical capacitor, which stores electrical charge (electrons) and consequently energy, PCr represents a biochemical capacitor, which stores a phosphate charge (energy). With the help of the phosphagenic system, we buffer rapid and short-term changes in ATP demand in everyday life (e.g. during the transition from sitting to walking, from walking to a short spurt, etc.). In resting muscle, [PCr] is slightly higher in type 2 fibers than in type 1 fibers. The total CK activity is slightly increased in type-2 relative to type-1 fibers. However, the level of activity of the different CK isoforms, which are named according to their localisation within the cell (Table 6.1), varies according to fiber type.

**Table 6.1** Comparison of the isoforms of creatine kinase

|  | Myofibrillar isoform | Mitochondrial isoform |
|---|---|---|
| Localization | Close to the myofibrils and the sarcoplasmic reticulum | Close to the mitochondria |
| Catalyzed reaction | Forward Response: PCr + ADP → ATP + Cr | Reverse Reaction: ATP + Cr → ADP + PCr |
| Highest activity | In type 2 fibers | In type 1 fibers |

Therefore, together with the slightly higher [PCr] in type 2 fibers, the regeneration of ATP via the phosphagenic system is probably more effective in type 2 than in type 1 fibers.

## 6.5 The Glycolytic System: Sugar-Sweet ATP Regeneration

The second system by which a muscle fiber can produce ATP involves the biological process of glycolysis (hence the name "glycolytic" system) (Fig. 6.1). Like the processes of the phosphagenic system, glycolysis occurs in the sarcoplasm. The starting molecule for glycolysis is glucose-6-phosphate, which can come from two sources.

The first source is the free glucose (simple sugar) in the muscle fiber. Free glucose enters the cell interior of the muscle fiber from the capillary blood via GLUT4 (glucose transporter 4), which are located in the sarcolemma. The glucose molecules in the blood originate on the one hand from the carbohydrates in ingested food. Based on study results with young healthy men, it is estimated that 85% of the total glucose transported from the blood into body cells is taken up by muscle cells (DeFronzo et al. 1981). On the other hand, glucose is produced in the body by new synthesis in the liver (hepatic gluconeogenesis from amino acids of muscular origin) and/or glycogen breakdown in the liver.

The second source is glucose-1-phosphate, which is the primary product of the breakdown of glycogen in muscle (glycogenolysis). Glycogen is the intracellular storage form of glucose and consists of many glucose units linked together in a branched chain form. Glucose-1-phosphate is converted to glucose-6-phosphate and then fed to glycolysis. All the enzymes of glycolysis in type-2 fibers have higher activity compared to those in type-1 fibers (on average twice, in individual cases up to ten times higher). Type-2 fibers can therefore produce ATP via glycolysis faster than type-1 fibers, thus have a higher glycolytic output (in human muscle, 2.5 mM ATP $s^{-1}$ for type-2 fibers and 1.2 mM ATP $s^{-1}$ for type-1 fibers). Also, relative to type 1 fibers, type 2 fibers have 16–31% greater glycogen stores at rest and higher glycogenolytic enzyme activity.

The latter has to do with the fact that the content of glycogenolytic enzymes (especially phosphorylase) is greater and the stimulation of glycogenolysis by degradation products (especially IMP, see above) is more effective in type-2 fibers relative to type-1 fibers. But beware: during conventional endurance training (prolonged activity at low to moderate power or speed), glycogen concentration typically decreases first in type 1 fibers. The reason for this is that primarily smaller motor units are recruited during this type of muscular activity (see Chap. 9). The situation is different for training sessions with high mechanical power and/or speed or very long-lasting muscular activity. With regard to resistance training, it is known that a single training session can reduce the glycogen content in the muscles used by 24–40% and that this reduction is primarily due to glycogen reduction in type 2 fibers (see Sect. 14.4). For a 65 kg male with 12% body fat, the mass of carbohydrate stores in the body is estimated to be 110 g of liver glycogen, 500 g of muscle glycogen, and 15 g of glucose in body fluids. This corresponds to a glycolytic energy potential of about 10.7 MJ (i.e. about 2500 kcal).

**Lactate: Hero or Villain?**
A major product of glycolysis is pyruvate. It has two possible fates: conversion to lactate (an anion; negatively charged ion) and/or feeding into the citrate cycle in the mitochondria. Therefore, until pyruvate or lactate is formed, the process of glycolysis also occurs in the sarcoplasm (as do the reactions of the phosphagenic system). The conversion of pyruvate to lactate is catalyzed by the enzyme lactate dehydrogenase (LDH). LDH consists of four subunits (polypeptide chains). If the single polypeptide chain is encoded by the gene *LDH-A*, it is called the M polypeptide chain isoform (M for muscle). If the polypeptide chain originates from the *LDH-B* gene, it is called the H isoform (H for heart). In total, there are five LDH isozymes (i.e. protein isoforms), LDH-1 to LDH-5, which differ in the composition of their polypeptide chains: LDH-1 consists of four H subunits ($H_4$), LDH-2 of three H and one M subunit ($H_3 M_1$), the composition of LDH-3 is $H_2 M_2$, of LDH-4 it is $H_1 M_3$ and finally of LDH-5 it is $M_4$.

If the LDH isoform contains more M than H subunits, the conversion of pyruvate to lactate predominates (i.e. the chemical equilibrium is on the side of lactate). In the opposite case, the conversion of lactate to pyruvate predominates. Type 1 fibers primarily express (produce) the isoenzymes LDH-1 to LDH-3, whereas in 80% of type 2 fibers, only LDH-5 is present. LDH-3 and LDH-4 account for the remaining 20%, but no clear differences between type 2A and type 2X fibers can be identified in this regard. Nevertheless, the different LDH expression pattern between fiber types coincides with the tendency for pyruvate to be converted to lactate in type-2 fibers and lactate to be converted to pyruvate in type-1 fibers. When the pyruvate resulting from glycolysis is converted to lactate, it is called anaerobic glycolysis because no oxygen ($O_2$) is used in the process (which does not mean that no oxygen is present). Anaerobic glycolysis can regenerate 2–3 moles of ATP per mole of glucose-6-phosphate.

Lactate is therefore – contrary to what one unfortunately often reads or hears – by no means a waste product of the anaerobic metabolism! Both at rest and during training or competition, the muscle is the primary site of lactate production as well as lactate oxidation. According to current scientific understanding, the faster, more glycolytic fibers produce and export lactate, which is taken up and oxidized by the slower, more oxidative fibers. This process is called the cell-to-cell lactate shuttle. The lactate exported by the glycolytic muscle fibers can be taken up by the oxidative fibers located in the same muscle or transported via the bloodstream to other muscles or to the liver. In the liver, the lactate is converted to pyruvate, which is then used to produce glucose via gluconeogenesis. Other vital organs also use lactate as a substrate for energy production, including the heart, brain and kidneys. In addition to the cell-to-cell lactate shuttle, there is also the more controversial hypothesis of the intracellular lactate shuttle (i.e. there is no scientific consensus on this), according to which lactate is translocated directly from the sarcoplasm into the mitochondria, converted into pyruvate and oxidized.

> **Box 6.1: Does Lactate Cause Muscle Soreness?**
> 
> No. Muscle soreness is the result of (micro)injury to muscle tissue (see Sects. 7.3 and 7.4). The moderate decrease in intracellular pH associated with the accumulation of lactate may lead to a slight decrease in generated fiber force, but is not responsible for the phenomenon of "muscle soreness".

It is important that the lactate, as a negatively charged ion, is always transported through the sarcolemma together with a proton (hydrogen cation, $H^+$). This occurs via specific transport proteins, so-called monocarboxylate transporters (MCT), of which there are also different isoforms. In human muscle, expression of MCT1 is highest in type 1 fibers, lower in type 2A fibers, and virtually absent in type 2X fibers. Conversely, the expression of MCT4 is low in type-1 fibers and higher in type-2 fibers. According to the cell-to-cell lactate shuttle hypothesis, one molecule of lactate produced in each glycolytic muscle fiber is cotransported with one proton of MCT4 into the blood and taken up via MCT1 into the oxidative fibers of the same muscle or other muscles.

## The Correct Interpretation of the Term "(an)aerobic"

Instead of being converted to lactate, the pyruvate produced in glycolysis can also be introduced into the mitochondria. This is done by the pyruvate dehydrogenase (PDH) complex, which is located in the outer mitochondrial membrane. The PDH complex decarboxylates pyruvate to acetyl-coenzyme A (acetyl-CoA, activated acetic acid). Acetyl-CoA is the starting material used in the mitochondrion to produce or regenerate energy in the form of ATP with the help of oxygen (i.e. aerobically). Therefore, when pyruvate is metabolized from glycolysis in the mitochondria, it is referred to as aerobic glycolysis. Via aerobic glycolysis, theoretically 32 mol ATP can be regenerated per mol pyruvate. In addition to the conversion of pyruvate by the PDH complex, acetyl-CoA can also be produced in the mitochondria via the process of β-oxidation from fatty acids.

The terms "aerobic" and "anaerobic" should therefore simply be understood to mean that the production of energy or ATP occurs with or without the use of oxygen, regardless of how much oxygen is present in the cells. This means, for example, that anaerobic glycolysis can occur even at normal oxygen partial pressure in the muscle fiber. Therefore, the terms "aerobic glycolysis" and "anaerobic glycolysis" should not be interpreted to mean that these metabolic pathways are engaged *because* oxygen is present or absent. Rather, the relative contribution of each system to the regeneration of ATP depends on the rate at which ATP must be regenerated to produce and maintain external mechanical power or speed.

## The Mitochondrial Porter for Aerobic Glycolysis

The PDH complex therefore represents, so to speak, the entry portal through which carbohydrates can be metabolized aerobically at all. The opening of this portal is controlled by pyruvate dehydrogenase kinases (PDKs). PDKs therefore perform a switch function: the stronger the activity of the PDKs, the more closed the PDH portal. It is therefore not surprising that PDKs are more active in type 1 fibers than in type 2 fibers. This means that in type-1 fibers the PDH portal is more closed, which is equivalent to a switch in substrate use from carbohydrate to fat. This in turn means that there is increased formation of acetyl-CoA from fatty acids (instead of pyruvate).

As mentioned above, the fatty acids enter the muscle fibers from the blood (e.g. mobilized from the fat cells) via fatty acid transporters called FAT/CD36. There are significantly more FAT/CD36 in human type 1 fibers than in type 2 fibers. Inside the muscle fibers, the fatty acids are activated, i.e. converted into acyl-CoA, and then transported into the mitochondria. To do this, they must be briefly bound to carnitine (acyl-CoA) for passage through the mitochondrial membrane. Carnitine therefore takes on the mandatory role of a shuttle in fat metabolism. Without a mitochondrial carnitine shuttle, no fat could be metabolized in the mitochondria. However, carnitine also has another important function. If more acetyl-CoA molecules are produced per unit of time during high metabolic demand (during high-intensity muscular activity) than can be shuttled into the citrate cycle, there is an accumulation of acetyl-CoA. This accumulation then shifts glycolysis from aerobic to anaerobic, i.e. towards increased formation of lactate (instead of acetyl-CoA) from pyruvate, and at the same time inhibits fatty acid oxidation, i.e. the formation of acetyl-CoA from acyl-CoA via β-oxidation. Carnitine now buffers the excess accumulation of acetyl-CoA at the onset of high-intensity exercise by creating the acetyl residue as acetylcarnitine from the mitochondrion. The size of the intracellular carnitine store can therefore influence or limit performance in training and competition.

> **Box 6.2: Does L-Carnitine Increase Fatty Acid Oxidation During Endurance Training?**
>
> As more than 25 years of research in this field suggest, the sole (oral or intravenous) intake of L-carnitine does not increase muscle carnitine content. Recently, however, it was demonstrated for the first time in young men that, first, the content increased after 24 weeks of supplementation of L-carnitine in simultaneous combination with high sugar intake and, second, the increased carnitine content in muscle led to increased fat and reduced carbohydrate oxidation at low-intensity exercise performance. At high-intensity exercise performance, the different metabolic pathways were found to be better matched, which reduced anaerobic energy provision. Overall, these effects led to an increase in endurance performance. However, it is to be hoped that stimuli other than sugar or insulin will be discovered that have the same activating effect on the transport of L-carnitine, because it is highly questionable whether the long-term high daily sugar intake will not lead to health problems that far outweigh the potential positive effects on fatty acid oxidation during exercise. Until all health effects have been studied, these results should therefore be taken with extreme caution and considered only for elite endurance athletes, if at all.

## 6.6 Mitochondrial Respiration: Why We Need Oxygen

Inside the mitochondria, acetyl-CoA is formed from acyl-CoA via the process of β-oxidation. As already described, acetyl-CoA is the starting material for aerobic ATP production in the mitochondria. Acetyl-CoA and $O_2$ can be used to regenerate ATP from ADP and $P_i$. In the citrate cycle, acetyl-CoA gives rise to both carbon dioxide ($CO_2$; diffuses into the blood and is exhaled through the lungs) and reduction equivalents (hydrogen/electron carriers). The latter move along the respiratory chain from protein complex to protein complex and are finally transferred to oxygen ($O_2$), and water ($H_2O$) as well as heat are released. This produces energy in the form of an electrochemical potential. The energy is used to synthesize ATP from ADP and $P_i$. Since $O_2$ serves as an electron acceptor in this process and ADP is phosphorylated to ATP, it is referred to as oxidative phosphorylation or mitochondrial respiration (third system for ATP regeneration, Fig. 6.1).

How much $O_2$ is needed therefore depends on the mitochondrial respiration rate. The $O_2$ comes from the blood, more precisely from haemoglobin ($O_2$-binding molecule) in the red blood cells (erythrocytes). From there it diffuses into the muscle fibers, where it is either used directly or transferred to myoglobin ($O_2$-binding molecule or $O_2$-storage in the muscle fibers). In human muscles, the myoglobin content in the oxidative fibers is, as expected, about 50% higher than in the glycolytic ones. The better the capillarisation (i.e. the supply of fine blood vessels to the muscle fibers), the better the supply of substrates (e.g. fatty acids, glucose, amino acids), the exchange of gases ($O_2$ and $CO_2$) and metabolic products (e.g. lactate and protons) and the removal of heat. Depending on the type, a single muscle fiber is surrounded or supplied by more or fewer capillaries. The values vary depending on the method of measurement and calculation. In untrained muscle, a single type 1 and type 2A fiber is surrounded by approximately 4.8 capillaries, while a type 2X fiber has 2.9 capillaries. In endurance athletes, however, these values (number of capillaries surrounding a fiber of a given type) can be much higher (type 1: 7.8, type 2A: 6.6, and type 2X: 4.5). If one relates the determined number of capillaries to the number of muscle fibers, one arrives at a ratio of approx. 1.3–2.5 capillaries per fiber, depending on the training condition and type of training.

The $O_2$ in the blood comes from the ambient air. You know this from your own experience: If you sit on your bike or go jogging and slowly increase your cycling power or running speed a little every 3–4 minutes, starting from a low level of exertion, your heart rate (number of heartbeats per minute), stroke volume (blood volume ejected by the left ventricle per heartbeat), breathing volume and breathing rate will also increase. Increased breathing causes more $O_2$ to be inhaled and more $CO_2$ to be exhaled per unit time – the oxygen uptake measured at the mouth increases. It therefore stands to reason that this oxygen uptake corresponds to the product of cardiac output and oxygen extraction (the arteriovenous $O_2$ difference). Oxygen extraction, in turn, depends on the mitochondrial respiration rate and the mitochondrial volume (number and size of mitochondria) in the cells. The larger this volume and the rate of mitochondrial respiration in your muscles and the larger your cardiac output (mainly due to the dimension of your left ventricle), the more oxygen can be used.

## 6.7  Mitochondria: Small but Mighty!

Mitochondrial volume can vary depending on muscle fiber type, especially when considering muscle fibers from untrained individuals. For example, the volume of mitochondria in type 1, type 2A, and type 2X fibers is 6, 4.5, and 2.3% of the muscle fiber volume, respectively. Also, the activity of mitochondrial enzymes (of the citrate cycle, electron transport chain, etc.) in the untrained state is higher in type-1 fibers than in type-2 fibers. Note, however, that this ratio can change significantly with training. Indeed, in highly trained endurance athletes, it can be observed that the oxidative potential (e.g. expressed by the activity of oxidative enzymes) of type 2A fibers in thigh muscles is at least as great as that of type 1 fibers. Mitochondria are not all the same, by the way. In both type-1 and type-2 fibers, there are two distinctly different types of mitochondria that differ in terms of localization, morphology, and biochemical properties. You must think of these two mitochondrial populations as a continuous reticular structure rather than sharply demarcated organelles. The subsarcolemmal mitochondria (located just below the cell membrane of the muscle fiber) look narrow and lamellar and appear to exhibit greater plasticity (changeability) in response to stimuli such as training or inactivity than the smaller and more compact mitochondria located between the myofibrils near the sarcoplasmic reticulum.

The capacity for mitochondrial ATP regeneration from fatty acids is practically unlimited. Even the above-mentioned man with the relatively low body fat percentage of 12% still has approx. 7.8 kg of subcutaneous fat and 161 g of intramuscular fat with a body mass of 65 kg. This corresponds to an energy potential of approx. 311.9 MJ (i.e. approx. 74,500 kcal)! You read that right – even in healthy individuals, fat is stored in the muscle fiber (analogous to glycogen), in the form of tiny lipid droplets (fat droplets near the mitochondria). This allows fatty acids to be taken up more quickly for mitochondrial respiration during repetitive muscle use. In type 1 fibers, these lipid droplets account for approximately 0.5% of the fiber volume, and in type 2 fibers, less than 0.1%. Endurance athletes have larger volumes of lipid droplets than untrained or resistance-trained individuals. Glycogen and lipid droplets are dynamic stores designed to be cyclically depleted and replenished (in the course of hunger → exercise → food intake → recovery, etc.). Lipid droplets as a dynamic storage form of fat inside muscle fibers are clearly distinguishable from the pathological condition of fat infiltration. Chronic excessive energy intake and/or insufficient energy expenditure results in the accumulation of fat in the body, mainly in the form of subcutaneous and visceral fat. The latter is also known as intra-abdominal fat – fat that accumulates in the abdominal cavity and is a risk factor for chronic metabolic (e.g. type 2 diabetes) and cardiovascular disease. If the triglycerides are not stored in their intended location (in the white fat cells) or if the uptake capacity of the white fat cells is exhausted, the triglycerides are stored ectopically inside other organs (i.e. not in their physiological location), including muscle, liver or pancreas. Depending on their quantity and type, these ectopic lipids have a toxic effect on the functioning of the corresponding organs and thus on our organism.

## 6.8 Integration of the Three Systems for the Regeneration of ATP

As discussed, ATP is cleaved at different rates in individual muscle fibers during force production depending on the predominant MyHC isoform. Immediately, ATP is regenerated in all fiber types by the phosphagenic system. Because type 2 fibers consume ATP faster (producing ADP and $P_i$) than they can regenerate, and the two chemical reactions of the phosphagenic system (CK and AK reactions) are virtually in chemical equilibrium, stereotypical changes occur in the chemical concentrations of ATP, ADP, $P_i$, PCr, Cr, AMP, and $H^+$. [PCr] decreases, whereas [Cr] and [$P_i$] increase. Once [PCr] decreases to a low level, [ATP] also begins to decrease in single fibers, while [ADP] increases substantially. In the process, [AMP] increases via the AK reaction and [IMP] also increases via its deamination. As discussed, the increase in [IMP] stimulates glycogenolysis and glycolysis (more so in type-2 fibers than in type-1 fibers), while the increase in [AMP] leads to increased substrate import into the muscle fiber and triggers intracellular signaling cascades.

The increase in [ADP] and [Cr] stimulates mitochondrial respiration in all fiber types (Fig. 6.1), except that the mitochondria of type 1 fibers are much more sensitive to [ADP] and [Cr] compared to type 2 fibers. Therefore, it takes longer in type-2 fibers, that is, higher [ADP] and [Cr] must be reached, until mitochondrial respiration can be initiated. This is also referred to as the metabolic inertia of type 2 fibers. This temporal delay in the activation of mitochondrial ATP regeneration can also be demonstrated during resistance exercise. During high-intensity resistance exercise, for example on the knee extension machine, the breakdown of PCr and anaerobic glycolysis generate approximately 80% of the total amount of ATP required during the first 30 s. The contribution of these systems decreases with increasing intensity. The contribution of these systems decreases with increasing exercise duration – between 30 and 120 s it is approx. 45% and from 120 s onwards it is still approx. 30% and this until the exercise is stopped (what this means for practice, see Sect. 13.7).

The decrease in anaerobic ATP regeneration is accompanied by an increase in aerobic ATP resynthesis (aerobic glycolysis). As previously mentioned, in humans, energy expenditure even during high-intensity exercise in type 1 fibers is about 1.5 mM ATP $s^{-1}$ (for comparison, in type 2X fibers it is up to about 7 mM ATP $s^{-1}$). For a muscle composed of different fibers (vastus lateralis muscle), the average (i.e., across all fiber types) mitochondrial ATP regeneration rate at maximal muscle stimulation is estimated to be about 1.4 mM ATP $s^{-1}$. It follows that even at peak exertion, type 1 fibers (as opposed to fast fibers) can maintain a balanced energy balance (approximately 1.5 mM ATP $s^{-1}$ consumption and production each). In relation to the knee extension exercise described above, this means that the type 1 fibers cover their ATP requirement during high-intensity resistance exercise shortly after the start of the exercise purely via mitochondrial respiration.

## 6.9 Summary: ATP Molecules Resemble Rechargeable Batteries

In order for your muscle fibers to do work in everyday tasks, training and sports, they need to be continuously supplied with energy. This is energy that is converted from energy-rich chemical compounds (ATP molecules) inside the muscle fibers during chemical reactions. Muscle activity in this sense is therefore always the result of the conversion of chemical energy into internal mechanical work (cf. Sect. 1.10) and heat.

The ATP molecules function similarly to rechargeable batteries. So that your muscles do not run out of juice during muscular activity, these batteries must be continuously recharged. For recharging, there are different types of battery chargers within the muscle fibers, which differ in terms of the speed and capacity of recharging (Fig. 6.1). One type of battery charger is the mitochondria, which are responsible for recharging by oxidative phosphorylation. A peculiarity of this type of battery charger is that it functions only with oxygen, and this oxygen must consequently be delivered to the muscle fibers from the inhaled air via the blood. The mitochondrial battery charger can only recharge ATP relatively slowly, but its substrate capacity is almost inexhaustible. During low-intensity activity, the ATP molecules can thus be recharged exclusively via the mitochondrial charging stations.

If the internal mechanical work per unit time, i.e. the internal mechanical power, and thus the speed of the energy conversion processes in the muscle fiber are persistently high, then two other types of battery chargers must also provide support: The CK-PCr response and anaerobic glycolysis (Fig. 6.1). These two types of battery chargers are relatively fast, but their substrate capacity is limited. Thus, during sustained high-intensity activity, all three battery charging systems are active simultaneously, but their relative contribution to ATP regeneration differs both at the onset and during the course of exercise performance. Finally, if the rate of discharge of the ATP batteries is greater than the rate of recharge across all available battery charging stations, metabolic intermediates accumulate in the muscle fiber, inhibiting force generation. Muscle fiber fatigue and exercise termination occur. This temporary relative fatigue is thus the price you have to pay if you want to maintain a very high muscle power for a maximum length of time.

# 7

# Why You Fatigue During Exercise

## 7.1 The Different Components of Neuromuscular Fatigue

Neuromuscular fatigue is a complex phenomenon caused by both central (brain and spinal cord) and peripheral factors (muscles). In the context of muscles and training, the term "fatigue" is usually defined as a reversible decrease in performance. Here, the term "performance" means force, torque, power, speed, etc. By "reversible" is meant that the measured decrease in performance recovers over time. At the muscle fiber level, fatigue has several components that affect the excitation-contraction coupling already mentioned (see Sect. 4.1). These include disturbances in the ion concentration outside (potassium) and inside (sodium) the muscle fibers, the accumulation of *reactive oxygen species* (ROS) and the decrease (ATP, PCr) or increase (ADP, $P_i$, $H^+$) of metabolites.

## 7.2 Metabolites as Fatigue Mediators

While disturbances in ion concentration mainly interfere with the initiation and propagation of action potentials at the sarcolemma and its invaginations (termed T-tubules), changes in ROS and/or metabolite concentration impair myofibrillar force production. Thus, the increase in $[P_i]$ and decrease in [ATP] inhibit the release of $Ca^{2+}$ from the sarcoplasmic reticulum. In turn, the reuptake of $Ca^{2+}$ into the sarcoplasmic reticulum is disrupted by the increase in $[P_i$

], [ADP] and [ROS] and the decrease in [ATP]. The $Ca^{2+}$ sensitivity of troponin C decreases with the increase of $[P_i]$, [ROS] and $[H^+]$. Incidentally, the negative logarithm of proton concentration ($[H^+]$) corresponds to pH. The pH in muscle is about 7 at rest, but can drop to about 6.5 at very high metabolic power, thus moving toward "more acidic". Finally, $[P_i]$ and [ADP] directly inhibit the cross-bridge cycle in terms of force and velocity, respectively.

## 7.3 Microtraumata as Fatigue Mediators

Another possible cause of muscle fatigue or decline in performance is microscopic muscle injury (microtrauma). The occurrence of microtrauma is specifically associated with force production in long muscle fibers (which does not necessarily equate to a long muscle-tendon unit, see Sect. 1.4). "Long" in this context means that the muscle fibers must generate force at a greater length than usual. In principle, this is possible with mio-, iso- and/or pliometric use. In particular (but not exclusively), pliometric muscle fiber use at long fiber lengths, i.e. use when the fibers are stretched during force production, is indisputably associated with the occurrence of microtrauma and muscle soreness.

A morphological feature that occurs consistently with microtrauma is that the normal periodic myofibrillar structural pattern (the sequence of A and I bands and sarcomeres separated by Z-disks, etc., see Sect. 2.5) is lost. Under the electron microscope, the structural pattern appears "smeared". This is accompanied by damage to the myofibrillar cytoskeleton, i.e. the proteins that stabilise the structure of the sarcomeres. The microtraumata described occur in localized regions of the affected muscle and often spread over only a few sarcomeres.

Interestingly, the mechanical and/or metabolic (i.e. chemical) fatigue factors discussed above can also result in altered signaling to the motor neurons in the spinal cord. Specifically, there may be a reduced *motor drive* through the central nervous system. This effect is mediated by so-called muscle afferents, i.e. thinly myelinated (group III) and non-myelinated (group IV) nerve fibers inside the muscle. These increase their firing frequency (firing rate) when metabolites accumulate in the muscles, which stimulate the receptors of the nerve fibers (ergoreceptors), and feed sensory feedback back to the central nervous system. As a result, there is a reduction in the activation of muscle fibers by the central nervous system, which in turn contributes to the decrease in performance. This is true for both maximal and submaximal performance, with a slower increase in firing rate during submaximal performance.

## 7.4 From Muscle Mice to Sore Muscles

First of all, the classical theory of how cross-bridges work (see Sect. 5.2) cannot explain many of the mechanical phenomena observed during pliometric force production. In fact, relatively little is known about the physiology of pliometric force production or "eccentric muscle contraction". However, it is undisputed that pliometric force production is associated with the occurrence of microtrauma or muscle soreness. There are several theories regarding the actual cause of microtrauma due to pliometric force production, the most exciting of which I would like to present to you in more detail from both a theoretical and experimental perspective. The theory is known as the *popping sarcomere theory* and was put forth in 1990 by Australian electrical engineer David Morgan (Morgan 1990). Morgan postulated that microtraumata resulted from an uneven distribution (an inhomogeneity) of sarcomere forces along myofibrils. In principle, such an inhomogeneity of sarcomere forces may be due to an inhomogeneous length distribution and/or minute differences in the cross-sectional areas of the sarcomeres.

Can you still remember the length-force relationship we looked at in Chaps. 2 and 3 (Figs. 2.1b and 3.1)? In this context, the inhomogeneous length or force distribution means that the sarcomeres inside a muscle fiber are located at different points of the length-force relationship at the beginning of fiber activation. As a reminder, short sarcomeres are on the ascending branch and long ones are on the descending branch, while those of intermediate length are on the plateau of the length-force relationship (Fig. 2.1b). "Ascending" here means that the force of a short sarcomere increases with active elongation due to progressively larger filament overlap (more active cross-bridges). The reverse is true for "descending" sarcomeres. They become weaker with stretching. For sarcomeres on the plateau, the degree of overlap is optimal and thus the force is maximum.

Now, if a sarcomere on the ascending branch is serially connected to a sarcomere on the descending branch (i.e. they follow each other) and if both sarcomeres are stretched with the same force production, the force of the short sarcomere increases and that of the long sarcomere decreases. Therefore, the shorter sarcomere can resist stretching better than the longer one because of the increasing force. In other words, in this case, most of the strain is absorbed by the long sarcomere. Similarly, in the case where a sarcomere on the plateau is connected to a sarcomere on the descending branch. In this case, too, the longer (i.e., weaker) sarcomere is stretched more than the shorter (i.e., stronger) one. According to Morgan's hypothesis, the inhomogeneity in sarcomere force or length during pliometric force production thus results in a disproportionately large elongation of long sarcomeres (Morgan 1990). In this process, the long sarcomeres would be stretched such that filament overlap would be lost. The longer and weaker sarcomeres attempt to compensate for the loss of force by increasing the rate of elongation (see the force-velocity relationship, Fig. 1.2). The rate of elongation of the lengthening sarcomeres therefore increases abruptly, causing the sarcomeres to suddenly *pop*, hence the term "*popping sarcomeres*". Important: As various other independent study results also show, it is not primarily the amount of external force, but the extent of sarcomere stretching during pliometric force production that is responsible for the microtraumata. Thus, contrary to popular belief, muscle soreness is not so much the result of exceptionally forceful muscle use, but of muscle use at unusually large muscle lengths. Overall, the predictions of the theory are confirmed by both theoretical calculations and experiments, but there are also study results that speak against this theory. It remains to be seen whether the controversy can be resolved by the research community in the coming years.

## 7.5 Summary: The Lore of Being Sore

Who isn't familiar with it – the notorious delayed-onset muscle soreness (DOMS)? The term "DOMS" is generally understood to mean the feeling of muscle pain, swelling and stiffness that becomes noticeable after unaccustomed muscle strain. DOMS does not set in immediately after exercise or training, but typically reaches its maximum after about 24–48 h and is usually gone after 4 days. However, muscle recovery is then far from complete and can take several weeks. The time course depends on the type and number of causative events. These are the smallest muscle fiber injuries, so-called micro traumas. These occur when the muscle fibers generate force when stretched abnormally, for example when you press against an object in a stretched position or when you walk down a steep hill. So contrary to popular belief, muscle soreness is not causally related to any temporary buildup of lactate in the muscle fibers. Many people perform stretching exercises before and after resistance exercise to prevent DOMS from developing. You can save yourself this time and effort with a clear conscience. In fact, the best available scientific data clearly shows that stretching does not reduce, much less prevent, muscle soreness. Why should it? Micro-injuries are not fundamentally "bad". On the contrary, they are at the origin of the muscle adaptation that protects you from precisely such micro-injuries, namely the increase in muscle fiber length due to the addition of sarcomeres in series (see Sect. 10.2). In this sense, a mild occurrence of DOMS is certainly not a bad exercise effect.

# 8

# The Molecular and Cellular Muscle Universe

## 8.1 Muscle Regeneration: A Balancing Act

It is currently thought that microtrauma affects the sarcolemma and/or sarcoplasmic reticulum, increasing permeability to $Ca^{2+}$ (calcium) ions (and signaling molecules). The large increase in intracellular $Ca^{2+}$ concentration may subsequently trigger proteolysis (the enzymatic dissolution) of structural proteins and lead to loss of muscle force. The mechanically induced injuries are associated with inflammatory processes (i.e., an immigration of inflammatory cells such as macrophages and neutrophils), which may further exacerbate the tissue injuries. In addition, the inflammatory cells release chemical mediators such as bradykinins and prostaglandins, which bind to the extracellular pain receptors and are thus causally involved in the perception of pain. Thus, the inflammatory process that may be used to repair the tissue damage may simultaneously increase the injury. Overall, successful muscle repair is a balancing act between degeneration and regeneration (see next section).

> **Box 8.1: Does It Make Sense to Exercise When the Muscles Are Sore?**
> Not in the same way that led to muscle soreness. In the case of resistance training, muscle soreness stops being noticeable after 2–7 days, depending on the extent of microtrauma. However, keep in mind that the repair process can take several weeks depending on the extent of the injury. Now, if you exercise a "sore" muscle the same way again (i.e., same exercise and same exercise execution), you are shifting the balancing act between degeneration and regenera-

tion towards degeneration and the repair process may be disrupted. This can lead to muscle tissue being replaced by *fibrofatty tissue*, resulting in a decrease in muscle function. It is still unclear today whether the formation of replacement tissue is the result of impaired regeneration or represents an alternative form of scarring. However, there is nothing to be said against light exercising of the affected muscles with predominantly miometric force production, for example light endurance training on a bicycle, cross trainer or arm ergometer.

**Box 8.2: Does Stretching Prevent or Reduce Muscle Soreness?**

One reason people perform stretching exercises immediately before and after resistance training is to prevent muscle soreness or its severity. However, the best available scientific evidence (Herbert et al. 2011) clearly shows that stretching does not reduce, much less prevent, muscle soreness in adults. This is true across all cases studied (lab *vs.* field studies, stretching type and extent, athletes or untrained, men and women, study quality) and it is therefore highly unlikely that this body of data will be altered by future studies. So, for the purpose of muscle soreness prevention, if you do stretching exercises immediately before and after resistance training, you can save that time for other things with a clear conscience. In order to temporarily alleviate muscle soreness (a sensation, *mind you*), passive stretching of the affected muscles to reduce passive tension may be helpful, as has been shown with the biceps brachii muscle (Reisman et al. 2005).

## 8.2 DNA: The Mother Molecule of All (Muscle) Proteins

As mentioned, muscle fibers can be "traumatized" over long fiber lengths during pliometric force production. The microtraumatic extent depends on the degree of stretching and the number of active stretch cycles. Training-induced adaptive signals may therefore well add up. It is likely that in our daily lives, natural wear and tear often results in minor microtraumatic events in the muscle (e.g., descending a staircase with unusually high steps, or sprinting to catch a train, etc.) that we do not usually experience as muscle soreness. Such minor injuries can be repaired without causing cell death, inflammatory reactions, or histological (affecting the tissue) changes. For example, minute injuries to the sarcolemma, such as may occur during spontaneous pliometric force production, can be efficiently mended by intracellular vesicles. In contrast, more extensive injuries, such as those caused by myotoxins (peptides in snake venom) or genetic defects (muscular dystrophies), involve the death (necrosis) of muscle fibers and inflammatory processes. Similarly, in negative training, depending on the extent of injury, there is in principle the possibility of (partial) necrosis of individual muscle fibers, although in humans substantial fiber necrosis after training has only been demonstrated in a few studies.

However. New cell material is needed to repair the damaged muscle fibers, because we have seen that degeneration leads to the breakdown of cell components. The template for the production of this cell material comes from DNA (deoxyribonucleic *acid*), which is found in the nuclei (nucleic DNA) and mitochondria (mitochondrial DNA) of muscle fibers. Muscle fibers, unlike most other cells in our body, are multinucleated, meaning they contain multiple DNA-containing nuclei. The nuclei of non-regenerating muscle fibers are located just below the sarcolemma and are distributed along the entire length and circumference of the fiber. Within a muscle fiber, the number of its nuclei or their DNA content principally determines the transcriptional capacity of that fiber. Injury or necrosis of muscle fibers can result in the loss of nuclei and thus DNA, which in principle leads to a decrease in transcriptional capacity. None of this would necessarily be a problem for muscle regeneration if the muscle fibers were able to divide and renew themselves.

---

**Box 8.3: What Is DNA and How Are Muscle Proteins Made?**

DNA (*deoxyribonucleic acid*) is an immensely long molecule which is found in condensed form (chromosomes) in the cell nuclei of humans (and eukaryotes in general) and in which the genetic instructions needed for the structure and functioning of all cells of the living organism are encoded. The totality of the genetic information of a cell or an organism is called the genome. However, the actual production of proteins takes place outside the nucleus. Since DNA cannot leave the nucleus under normal circumstances, it must be transcribed into a chemical form that can be exported from the nucleus. This form is called RNA (ribonucleic *acid*). The process of transcribing or copying DNA into RNA is called transcription (Fig. Information flow from DNA via RNA to protein). A segment of DNA that is transcribed as a single unit and that encodes a discrete heritable property in the form of a protein or RNA is called a gene (see, for example, *MYH genes* in Sect. 5.3 or *LDH genes* in Sect. 6.5).

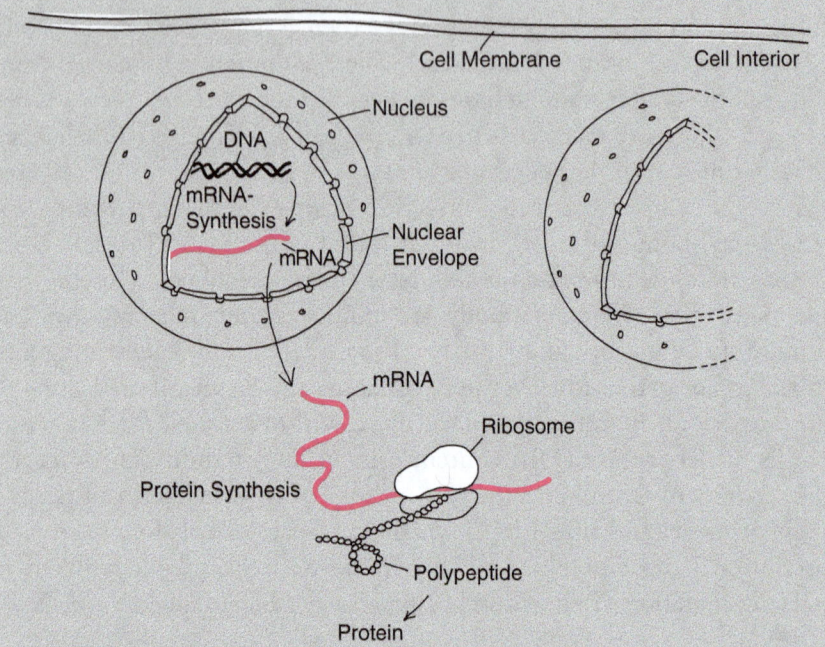

### Flow of information from DNA via RNA to protein

In eukaryotic cells, mRNA is produced from DNA in the nucleus. The mRNA molecules are transported through the nuclear membrane into the cytoplasm, where they bind to ribosomes (shown here greatly enlarged and isolated). The ribosomes "scan" the mRNA molecules, translating the information into the specific amino acid sequence of polypeptides or proteins. Note that unlike most other cell types in our body, a single muscle fiber (muscle cell) contains many nuclei. DNA, deoxyribonucleic acid; RNA, ribonucleic acid; mRNA, messenger RNA ("messenger ribonucleic acid").

The human genome contains approximately 25,000 genes. The majority of genes in the DNA of a cell encode proteins, which in turn make up the main component of cells. The RNA molecules that are copied from these genes are called mRNA (*messenger RNA*). However, for a minority of genes, the RNA molecules themselves are the end product. These RNAs, which do not encode proteins, serve as enzymatic and structural components of many cellular processes, much as proteins do.

Transcription from DNA to mRNA can therefore be understood as a simple information transfer: Since DNA and mRNA are chemically and structurally very similar, DNA can serve as a direct template for the base-paired synthesis of mRNA. In principle, the process of transcription is analogous to the transcription of a handwritten note into an electronic text. Both the language and the form of the text do not change and the symbols used are very similar.

In contrast, the conversion of mRNA information into a protein represents a translation (Fig. Flow of information from DNA via RNA to protein), i.e. a translation into another language with different symbols. The sequence of nucleotides in the mRNA is translated into a sequence of amino acids (protein building blocks). The four mRNA nucleotides are matched by 20 different amino acids – i.e. one nucleotide does not encode exactly one amino acid. It has been shown that the translation of mRNA into protein follows the rules of the genetic code: The nucleotide sequence of mRNA is read and translated in groups of three (triplets). Each triplet forms a codon and each codon determines an amino acid or even a stop signal. In addition, the genetic code is redundant, which means that a particular amino acid can be encoded by several different nucleotide triplets.

On the one hand, the amino acids for the production of a particular type of muscle protein come from the recycling of amino acids that are released when other proteins are broken down. On the other hand, the amino acids come from the proteins that we take in with food and digest, or the body manufactures them itself (these amino acids are called non-essential amino acids, in contrast to the essential amino acids that must be supplied). The building, breaking down, and remodeling of muscle protein must therefore be understood first as a dynamic process and second as a locally resolved process. Dynamic means that at any given moment, including right now as you read this text, protein is being built up and broken down in your muscle fibers. "Locally resolved" means that protein synthesis and degradation rates are different for different protein fractions or functional protein groups (mitochondrial, sarcoplasmic, myofibrillar, ion/fatty acid/glucose transport-specific proteins, etc.). For example, mitochondrial protein synthesis may increase or decrease at the expense or in favor of myofibrillar protein synthesis. If one does not differentiate between the various protein fractions, one simply speaks of mixed muscle protein.

A cell, such as a muscle fiber, can regulate and thus change the expression of its genes depending on the current need or on the (patho-)physiological situation (e.g. training and nutritional stimuli), on the one hand by controlling mRNA production (transcription). The composition of the mRNA population in a muscle fiber can therefore vary depending on the situation. On the other hand, the muscle fiber can also vary the rate at which mRNA is translated into protein (translation), i.e. it can increase or reduce the rate of protein synthesis.

Both mechanisms, individually or in combination, can lead to altered protein composition and quantity in the muscle fiber, which in turn can alter its functional properties. It should not be forgotten, however, that protein composition and quantity are also dependent on the mRNA and protein degradation that also takes place (which can also be influenced by various stimuli).

## 8.3 All Muscle Fibers Are Muscle Cells, But Not All Muscle Cells Are Muscle Fibers

The problem is that the muscle fibers of an adult human (and mammals in general) are in a post-mitotic stage, which means that they can neither synthesize DNA nor undergo cell division (mitosis). Thus, they cannot reproduce or renew themselves. Consequently, muscle fiber regeneration would not be possible and we would lose muscle fibers and therefore muscle mass and force with each severe microtrauma. Fortunately, there are muscle stem cells that have the ability to proliferate when stimulated and thus provide the nuclei or DNA necessary for muscle repair.

This pool of muscle stem cells consists largely of satellite cells. This type of muscle cell was first observed by Alexander Mauro in electron microscopic studies about half a century ago (Mauro 1961). Satellite cells are embedded in the extracellular matrix between the sarcolemma and the basement membrane and are arranged in a satellite-like fashion around the muscle fibers (hence their name). Unlike multinucleated muscle fibers, they are mononuclear, meaning they have only one nucleus. When viewed in muscle cross-section, under resting conditions, meaning not after training and/or injury, you can typically count about five to fifteen satellite cells per 100 muscle fibers. However, this value can vary greatly and depends on age, training condition, muscle (group) and fiber type, but not gender. Older people have on average fewer satellite cells than younger people (see Sect. 19.6), trained people have more than untrained people, and the trapezius and tibialis anterior muscles have more satellite cells than the vastus lateralis, biceps brachii or masseter muscles. There tend to be more satellite cells around type 1 muscle fibers than around type 2 fibers. The exact significance of these differences is still not clear. The distribution of satellite cells along muscle fibers is also not random. On the one hand, there is a higher density of satellite cells at the ends or at the muscle-tendon junction (see Sect. 10.2.1). On the other hand, in adult humans about 90% of the satellite cells are located at a distance of only about 20 µm from a blood capillary.

## 8.4 When Satellite Cells Are Awakened

If microinjuries occur, the dormant satellite cells are activated, i.e. they begin to proliferate by cell division. The activation of satellite cells is not limited to the specific site of microtrauma. Indeed, localized damage at one end of muscle fibers leads to activation of satellite cells along the entire fiber and migration of these satellite cells to the site of regeneration. The activation of satellite cells is therefore also accompanied by emphasized cell mobility (along the muscle fiber, between muscle fibers, or even tissues) and it is thought that cell adhesion must be reduced for this to occur.

Proliferating satellite cells and their progeny are called *myogenic precursor cells* (MPCs) or adult myoblasts. The majority of these mononuclear MPCs undergo the irreversible myogenic differentiation process, at the end of which there is either fusion with injured muscle fibers (as single MPCs or as myotubes, i.e. several united MPCs) or mutual fusion and formation of new muscle fibers.

## 8.5 The Gift of Self-Renewal

A characteristic of stem cells and thus also of satellite cells is the ability to self-renew. Thus, depending on the type of division (symmetric or asymmetric), proliferating MPCs give rise to new satellite cells that are needed to replenish the pool of satellite cells. Self-renewal of satellite cells is fundamental for long-term, i.e. lifelong, muscle integrity (see Sect. 19.6). Muscle regeneration involves the following overlapping steps:

1. Inflammatory reaction as a result of microtrauma and the associated muscle degeneration
2. Activation, proliferation, differentiation and fusion of satellite cells
3. Maturation and remodeling of newly formed or repaired muscle fibers

Skeletal muscles thus respond to microtrauma with highly orchestrated degeneration and regeneration processes. These processes take place at the level of molecules, cells and tissues.

If the degeneration and regeneration processes run ideally, the result is the reconstruction of innervated and vascularised (i.e. supplied with capillaries) muscle that can produce force. Under normal conditions, regenerated muscle fibers or muscles are both morphologically and functionally indistinguishable from uninjured muscle material. Incidentally, the process of muscle regeneration in adult humans is similar to the prenatal (before birth) formation process of our muscle fibers. These are formed during intrauterine (i.e. in utero) development by fusion of mononuclear mesodermal myogenic precursor cells.

---

**Box 8.4: What Is Muscle (Fiber) Hypertrophy?**

Muscle fiber hypertrophy is defined as the increase in muscle fiber volume, with or without a concomitant increase in the number of nuclei within the same fiber. If the number of nuclei in the fiber remains the same during the increase in volume, then the so-called myonuclear domain increases. The myonuclear domain is thus defined as fiber volume per fiber nucleus:

$$\text{Myonuclear Domain} = \frac{\text{Volume of the muscle fiber}}{\text{number of nuclei in the fibre volume}}$$

Experimentally, however, the myonuclear domain is usually defined as muscle fiber cross-sectional area divided by the number of nuclei detected in this cross-sectional area. If the number of nuclei increases proportionally with volume increase, muscle fiber hypertrophy can occur with a constant myonuclear domain. Therefore, several mechanisms, acting individually or in combination, can in principle be considered for muscle fiber hypertrophy: In the case of muscle fiber hypertrophy without an increase in the number of nuclei, it is sufficient if training increases the muscle protein synthesis rate at a constant degradation rate and/or the intracellular water content. The latter may be the case, for example, in the initial phase of creatine supplementation.

In these examples, the myonuclear domain increases. It is assumed that there is an upper limit to the size of the myonuclear domain, i.e. that a single nucleus can only cover a limited "protein territory" (Fig. Radial muscle fiber hypertrophy and Fig. Longitudinal muscle fiber hypertrophy). This upper limit is estimated to be around 2000–2500 $\mu m^2$ per nucleus (determined experimentally). Once this limit is reached for each nucleus, it is speculated that further hypertrophy is only possible if additional DNA is introduced into the muscle fiber. Since muscle fibers are in the post-mitotic phase (see text), this can only be done by fusion with satellite cells. This fusion decreases the size of the myonuclear domains inside the muscle fiber (or, in other words, increases the transcriptional capacity), since the same cell volume is now distributed among a larger number of nuclei. This in turn allows further hypertrophy until the myonuclear domains are again at their limit (Fig. Radial muscle fiber hypertrophy and Fig. Longitudinal muscle fiber hypertrophy).

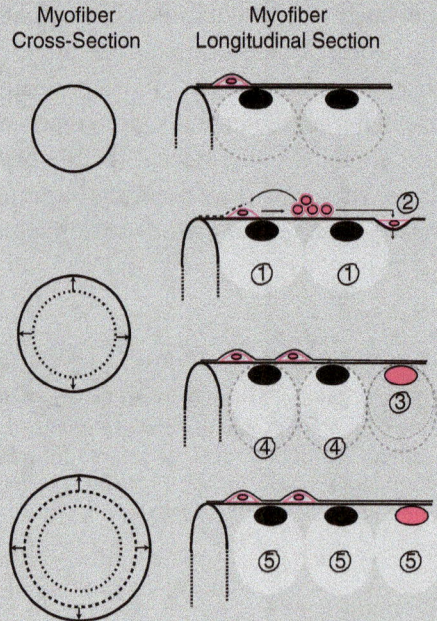

**Radial muscle fiber hypertrophy**

In the right panel, the black ellipses represent the cell nuclei of the muscle fiber, while the red circles or ellipses represent satellite cell nuclei or cell nuclei derived from satellite cells. The gray areas symbolize the size of the current effective myonuclear domain. The dashed lines symbolize the theoretical maximum possible size of the myonuclear domain. When resistance training is initiated, the myonuclear domain of all cell nuclei ① expands in an initial phase by increasing protein synthesis. At the same time, the satellite cells are activated, whereupon they divide (multiply) and fuse with the existing muscle fiber ②. This increases the number of cell nuclei in the muscle fiber, which means that the DNA content and thus the transcriptional capacity of the muscle fiber increase ③. The myonuclear domain decreases in the meantime due to the increase in the number of cell nuclei ④, which lays the foundation for further hypertrophy by expansion of the myonuclear domain ⑤. If the newly synthesized proteins or sarcomeres are incorporated radially (i.e. parallel to each other) while the fiber length remains constant, this is referred to as radial muscle fiber hypertrophy (According to Toigo and Boutellier 2006).

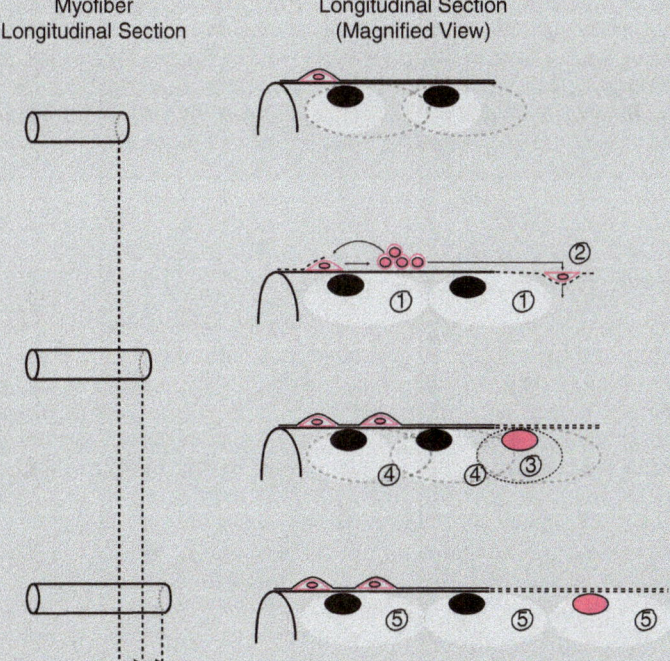

**Longitudinal muscle fiber hypertrophy**

Steps ① to ⑤ correspond to those in Fig. Radial muscle fiber hypertrophy. If the newly synthesized proteins or sarcomeres are incorporated longitudinally (lengthwise) while the cross-sectional area remains the same, this is called longitudinal muscle fiber hypertrophy. Explanation of the symbols see also Fig. Radial muscle fiber hypertrophy (According to Toigo and Boutellier 2006).

Thus, muscle fiber hypertrophy with an increase in the number of fiber cell nuclei requires the involvement of satellite cells, which, as described earlier, are the source of the new fiber cell nuclei. In a narrower sense, of course, we are interested in muscle fiber hypertrophy due to the increase in intracellular protein content. The myofibrillar proteins constitute by far the largest fraction of the protein mass of a muscle fiber. This means that the muscle mass gain from training comes from the increase in myofibrillar protein mass and not, for example, from the increase in the number of mitochondria or similar.

It is very important that you understand the definition given above because it is also relevant to the possible ways in which a muscle fiber can hypertrophy geometrically. The muscle fiber can be seen in a very simplified way as a cylinder and the volume of a cylinder is defined by its length multiplied by its cross-sectional area. Thus, the volume of a muscle fiber may increase as its length and/or cross-sectional area increases. Consequently, muscle fiber hypertrophy can be radial (in width, Fig. Radial muscle fiber hypertrophy) and/or longitudinal (in length, Longitudinal muscle fiber hypertrophy). In longitudinal fiber hypertrophy, the sarcomeres are incorporated longitudinally, that is, in series. In this case, the myofibrils or muscle fibers become longer. The increased number of sarcomeres in series causes the unloaded maximum shortening velocity of the fiber to increase (see Sect. 3.1). In radial fiber hypertrophy, the sarcomeres are incorporated in parallel, causing the myofibrils or muscle fibers to become thicker. Maximum fiber force increases (see Sect. 3.2). Depending on the stimulus, longitudinal and radial fiber hypertrophy can occur simultaneously.

### Box 8.5: What Is Muscle Fiber Hyperplasia?

Fiber hyperplasia is when existing muscle fibers divide, resulting in an increase in the number of muscle fibers. As discussed, postnatal muscle fibers are postmitotic and therefore do not divide. Thus, muscle fiber hyperplasia is not a primary mechanism of muscle enlargement by exercise in adult humans. However, as explained, satellite cells can divide and proliferate (and thus hyperplasize), with the possible result of, among other things, new muscle fibers being generated (myogenesis) to replace necrotic fibers. This normally occurs in a highly orchestrated manner (degeneration and regeneration) and is unlikely to end in an overall increase in the total number of muscle fibers.

With current experimental techniques, it is impossible to definitively answer the question of whether the total number of fibers in a muscle changes as a result of training. If this should be the case, however, it is hardly due to hyperplasia of muscle fibers, but rather to satellite cell-mediated myogenesis. It is true that there are several animal studies, particularly in avian species and cats, in which putative muscle fiber hyperplasia has been observed during certain forms of mechanical loading (Kelley 1996). However, more recent studies strongly challenge this interpretation and postulate that the increased number of fibers counted was not due to hyperplasia but to longitudinal fiber hypertrophy of intrafascicular-terminating muscle fibers (i.e. muscle fibers that extend over only a fraction of the total muscle length, see Sect. 4.5) (Paul and Rosenthal 2002). Muscle hypertrophy, i.e. the increase in volume of a muscle, therefore involves both the hypertrophy of muscle fibers and the hyperplasia of satellite cells in the long term – the latter possibly in connection with the formation of new muscle fibers.

### Box 8.6: What Is Muscle Fiber Splitting?

Interestingly, so-called split fibers, i.e. fibers that split or branch, can be observed in muscles of patients with neuromuscular diseases (for example, Duchenne muscular dystrophy) and elderly people. The same applies to "powerlifters" who consume anabolic steroids (Eriksson et al. 2005). It is thought that split fibers occur when myotubes do not fuse completely with the muscle fiber, for example only at one end, and that they indicate an abnormal regenerative capacity of the muscle.

### Box 8.7: What Is Muscle (Fiber) Atrophy?

In the absence of training stimuli and/or adequate dietary protein intake, muscle atrophy (radial and/or longitudinal) occurs, i.e. loss of muscle mass. In humans, the primary mechanism of muscle mass loss is a reduction in the rate at which muscle protein is synthesized. If the rate of muscle protein degradation remains the same, which is the case in healthy individuals into old age and regardless of sex, the result is a negative net balance (see Figs. 11.1 and 19.1) for muscle protein. As a result, protein mass decreases over time until eventually muscle function is impaired. In addition, muscle denervation can occur if the muscles are not used for a long time, for example during immobilisation or similar. In this case, the motoneurons in the spinal cord perish. In a first phase, the muscle fibers belonging to this motoneuron can be reinnervated collaterally by axons of other motoneurons. This leads to an increase in the number of innervated motor units (see Sect. 4.6) and a tendency for fine motor skills to decrease. However, if the process of denervation continues, in the long term not only motor neurones but also the associated muscle fibers perish. The number of muscle fibers in the muscle decreases.

### Box 8.8: Do Muscles Have a "memory"?

A commonly observed phenomenon is that when individuals resume resistance training after a prolonged period of inactivity (i.e., detraining), they regain their previous peak strength faster than was required to initially build strength. This effect is called *muscle memory*. The reason for this was long thought to be mechanisms related to motor learning in the central nervous system. However, it is known that hypertrophied muscles can maintain their condition over several months of detraining. For example, in a resistance training study with elderly subjects, it was shown that peak force 2 years after stopping training was still 9–14% higher than at the beginning of the study. Further, in a group of women, it was shown that a 30–32 week period of detraining resulted in a marked loss of peak force previously gained during 20 weeks of resistance training, and that the lost peak force was restored as early as 6 weeks after resuming resistance training (retraining). These facts suggest the possibility of a local memory mechanism in the muscle.

> As discussed, during muscle fiber hypertrophy there is a long-term satellite cell-induced increase in the number of nuclei and thus an increase in transcriptional and translational capacity (Box 8.3). Animal experiments show that such newly incorporated nuclei are retained by the muscle fibers even during several months of atrophy. If the atrophied muscle fiber is now trained again, i.e. when training is resumed, it starts with a greater capacity for protein synthesis, so to speak. More protein can therefore be synthesized per unit of time from the start, which could explain the faster onset of training effects during retraining. Muscle memory is therefore located in the number of nuclei of muscle fibers.
>
> Muscle memory carries with it important implications. Older individuals who have had a lifetime of structured resistance training should have a higher anabolic potential due to a higher number of nuclei. Given that muscle mass and function may decline in older individuals (see Sect. 19.6), an intact or higher anabolic potential is certainly advantageous. In other words, the (re)initiation of resistance training in these individuals is likely to result in a stronger anabolic response, i.e. be more effective, than in other individuals. It is therefore clearly recommended to "fill up" the muscle fibers with nuclei through resistance training before senescence sets in.

## 8.6 Muscle Spindles Also Contain Muscle Fibers

Muscle spindles are proprioceptive sensory organs that act as stretch-sensitive mechanoreceptors to monitor changes in muscle length. When the muscle is stretched, the proprioceptive signal generated in the muscle spindles increases as a function of stretch amplitude and duration and is transmitted via afferent neurons to the spinal cord where, among other things, stretch reflexes are triggered. Muscle spindles consist of a few thin muscle fibers called intrafusal (i.e., located within the spindle) fibers. The intrafusal fibers are innervated by both sensory neurons (group Ia afferent neurons) and γ-motoneurons, and their MyHC composition is complex. The spindles are surrounded by a capsule. Muscle spindles, as mentioned, play an important role in monitoring muscle length. It is therefore hardly surprising that, in addition to muscle (fiber) length (number of sarcomeres in series), adjustments in muscle spindles or their sensitivity can also contribute significantly to extensibility or mobility.

## 8.7 Characterisation of Human Muscle Tissue

I have now told you quite a bit about human skeletal muscle cells and their properties. But how do you get the material in the first place? Understandably, we cannot simply cut out whole muscles from living humans for research purposes. However, there are several methods to obtain small(er) muscle samples, that is, to biopsy a muscle. In the clinic, open biopsy is often used, in which a piece of muscle (about 0.5–1 cm long and high) is usually cut out intraoperatively (i.e., during surgery). However, this method is not suitable for minimally invasive, routine, location-independent, and repeated sampling as needed for scientific studies for several reasons. In addition, the amount of material obtained significantly exceeds the amount of material typically required in research, which must be avoided from an ethical point of view.

In research, therefore, the preferred technique is needle biopsy, which was invented by Jonas Bergström (1962) and has always been a suitable alternative to open biopsy. The muscle most commonly biopsied in human exercise studies is the vastus lateralis (outer thigh muscle). This is because this muscle is easily accessible (it is on the surface) and the biopsy site is well away from major blood vessels and nerves. Typically, Bergström needles with a diameter of 5 mm are used. The entire procedure is performed under sterile conditions. First, the biopsy site is selected (typically above the junction line between the knee and hip joint or above the fascia lata, between approximately 25–50% of the length of this junction line as viewed from the knee).

The affected skin area is then sterilized in a circular fashion over a large area. The skin and the subcutaneous tissue (dermis and subcutis) outside or above the muscle fascia are then made temporarily insensitive to pain by infiltration with lidocaine. A scalpel is then used to make an approximately 4–5 mm long stab incision through the skin, subcutaneous tissue and muscle fascia. The sterile biopsy needle is then carefully inserted through the incision into the muscle and pushed approximately 1 cm deep towards the head (cranial). Study participants feel deep pressure at this time and sometimes there are single muscle twitches. The needle is then advanced further and once at the target site, three small pieces of muscle are usually "snipped" with the needle device so that approximately 50–150 mg of muscle tissue (varying depending on the method) can be easily removed with a biopsy.

After removal, the wound is treated medically and the tissue obtained is treated for its subsequent processing (molecular and cellular examinations). This step is extremely important because all analyses depend on the quality of the starting material. The study participants are then given precise instructions on how to treat the site in the following days (no water contact, etc.). After the local anaesthetic has worn off, the patient feels a pain for a few days, comparable to a sore muscle. By the way, I know this from my own experience, because my muscles have been biopsied several times. During this time you should take it easy on the muscle. In the long term, only a small skin scar may remain. Muscle function is not affected by the biopsy. In 0.15% of cases, however, minor complications (haematoma, local skin infection or similar) can occur.

In scientific studies, tissue is now taken from the same study participants and from the same muscle at specific time intervals, for example before and after a training phase lasting several weeks or before and after (up to 3–4 time points) an acute training intervention. This involves moving the puncture site a few centimeters at a time. Muscle biopsy allows us to assess adaptations at the cellular level as well as decipher the molecular mechanisms of adaptations. Obtaining human muscle tissue (and more importantly, processing it properly) is therefore a very important research tool. Only by understanding the relationship between training stimulus, adaptations and mechanisms of adaptation will we be able to develop individualized, targeted, effective and time-efficient training methods for rehabilitation and therapy of patients as well as for enhancing the performance of athletes. Please note that all scientific questions concerning research into diseases or the structure and functioning of the human body must be submitted to the relevant ethics committee for approval. In addition, all studies must be conducted in accordance with GCP (Good Clinical Practice), i.e. they must meet international ethical and scientific standards for the planning, conduct, documentation and reporting of clinical trials. In Switzerland, there is the HFG (Humanforschungsgesetz, Human Research Act), a federal law on research involving humans, which aims to protect the dignity, personality and health of humans in research. It is intended to create favourable conditions for research involving human subjects and to help ensure the quality of such research and guarantee transparency. Research must also comply with the requirements of the Declaration of Helsinki, the declaration of the World Medical Association on ethical principles for medical research involving human subjects.

## 8.8 Summary

Training-induced growth of skeletal muscle in adulthood is primarily the result of muscle fiber hypertrophy, i.e. the increase in volume or mass of muscle fibers. In turn, resistance training-induced muscle fiber mass gain is primarily due to the increase in myofibrillar muscle protein over time. The primary basis for the mass gain is the boosting of muscle protein synthesis by increasing the translation of mRNA to protein. Increased translation rates can be achieved by at least two mechanisms (Fig. 8.1a):

(a) An increase in ribosomal efficiency, i.e. more translation per ribosome

 and/or

(b) An increased ribosomal capacity through ribosomal biogenesis (i.e. the de novo synthesis of ribosomes).

The most recent scientific data show that both translation enhancement mechanisms are involved in resistance training-induced muscle hypertrophy. According to the myonuclear domain theory, hypertrophy of muscle fibers occurs with or without the addition of muscle cell nuclei: In muscle fibers with a small myonuclear domain, volume increase up to the theoretical upper limit of the myonuclear domain occurs without the addition of cell nuclei (i.e. DNA) (Fig. 8.1b). Thereafter, any further hypertrophy is possible only with the simultaneous addition of new nuclei. The size of the myonuclear domain remains unchanged (Fig. 8.1b).

Postnatally, however, muscle fibers cannot undergo nuclear division (mitosis) and thus cannot replicate DNA. Muscle fibers can therefore not renew and/or multiply on their own. For this, they depend on satellite cells, the mononuclear muscle stem cells. Following the myonuclear domain theory, it is they that act as "DNA donors", thereby allowing the addition of nuclei and fiber hypertrophy while maintaining a constant myonuclear domain (Fig. 8.1b). It is undisputed that satellite cells play an indispensable role in the lifelong maintenance of muscle tissue, as the regenerative capacity of a muscle is largely determined by them. The precise role of satellite cells in adaptation to training stimuli, particularly in exercising humans, is less well studied and the general validity of myonuclear domain theory in this context is not entirely undisputed.

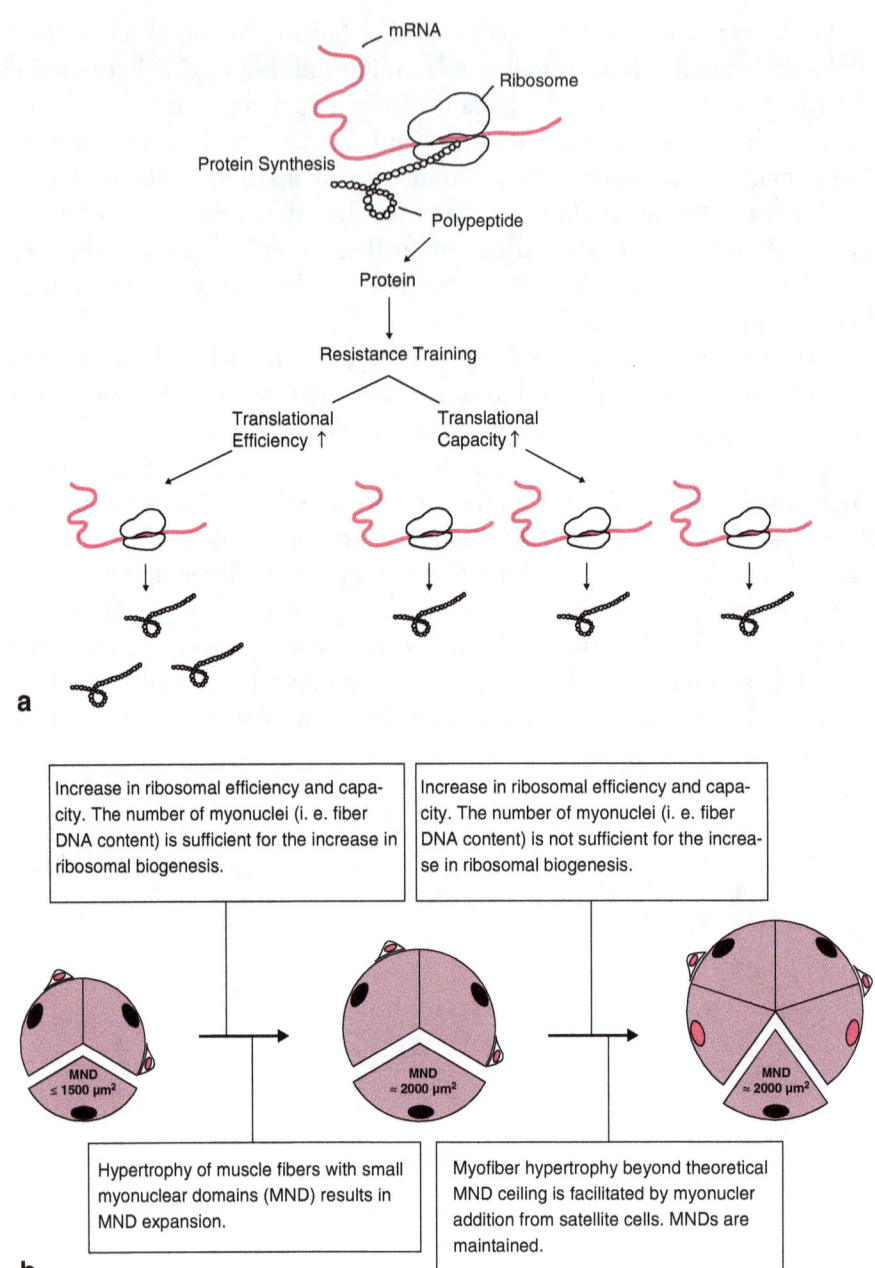

**Fig. 8.1** Enhancement of mRNA-to-protein translation speed through the strength-training-induced increase in ribosomal efficiency and/or ribosomal biogenesis

# 9

# How You Can Influence Which Muscle Fibers Are Used in Training

## 9.1 Back to the Motor Units

As explained in Sect. 4.7, three types of motor units can be roughly distinguished (see Fig. 4.2): FF (fast fatigable), FR (fastfatigue resistant) and S (slow). The physiological properties of a motor unit result directly from the properties of the motoneuron and the innervated muscle fibers. For example, Burke et al. (1973) showed in the same experiments that the FF-type motor unit consists of rapidly shortening muscle fibers and has a high content of glycolytic enzymes. They named these muscle fibers FG (*fast glycolytic*). They called FR-type motor units made of fast fibers that have both oxidative and glycolytic enzymes FOG (*fast oxidative glycolytic*). Finally, S-type motor units included slow oxidative muscle fibers, so they were called SO. In the context of the MyHC classification scheme, this corresponds to the following assignment, according to which FF consist of type-2X, FR of type-2A, and S of type-1 muscle fibers. However, please always be aware that the properties of human motor units and muscle fibers are not discrete categories, but rather a continuum of properties. Consider the hybrid fibers mentioned in Sect. 5.3, which express several MyHC isoforms simultaneously. Also, in humans, unlike in cats (with discrete groups of motor units), the properties of motor units are more continuously distributed.

## 9.2 How Is the Force of a Muscle Modulated During Voluntary Force Production?

If you are interested in building muscle mass and force, then you need to ask yourself how you get the central nervous system to activate as many muscle fibers as possible during training, and what exactly the individual fiber needs to "experience" in order to adapt. In other words, what are the mechanisms that dictate the recruitment of motor units during voluntary muscle use, and what parameters can you control during your training to achieve the desired effects? If you have exceptional genetics for building muscle mass and force, these questions need not concern you much. But if you are one of the remaining 98% of people, then addressing the question of how it all works is certainly more worthwhile than blindly following any training programs or emulating idols.

Considered in isolation, the force of an activated muscle depends on the number of activated (i.e. recruited) motor units (i.e. the number, MyHC type and size of the force-producing muscle fibers) on the one hand, and on the frequency (firing rate, see Sect. 4.2) with which action potentials are triggered in the cell bodies of the α-motoneurones (and consequently on the cell membrane of the muscle fibers) on the other. The greater the recruitment and the higher the firing frequency, the higher the resulting muscle force. Conversely, as recruitment and firing frequency increase, so does the amount of muscle force. What does this mean for training?

## 9.3 Muscle War Zone: Recruit and Fire!

As a first example, consider the case where you are pushing against an immovable object (i.e., performing isometric force production). You start by applying very little pressure to the object and then slowly but steadily increase the pressure to the voluntary maximum possible. What happens inside the muscle? As the motor drive or effort increases, there is an increased recruitment of motor units. As the pressure increases, more and more motor units, and therefore muscle fibers, are used, cumulatively. Now take the following case as a second example: In front of you are three dumbbells of different mass (small, medium and large). At intervals of a few minutes, you now perform a biceps curl (i.e. an arm flexion at the elbow joint) with the light, medium and very heavy dumbbells (in this order). The number of motor units recruited, and therefore muscle fibers used, increases the heavier the dumbbell (for the same curl execution). It follows from the two examples that the recruitment of motor units increases with increasing muscle force. As explained, this is true both within an isometric muscle action with slowly increasing muscle force and when comparing a constant low muscle force with a constant high muscle force.

## 9.4 How Do Recruitment and Increase in Firing Frequency Encode the Level of Force?

In any case, recruitment is completed before the peak voluntary force for the corresponding motor task is reached. This upper limit of recruitment can vary depending on the muscle. For most larger muscles (e.g. biceps brachii, tibialis anterior and vastus lateralis), motor units are recruited until approximately 85–95% of peak voluntary force is reached. This means that for large muscles that produce a force of about 85–95% of peak voluntary force, all motor units that can be used for the specific motor task have been recruited. Accordingly, if you are holding or slowly moving a load somewhere that is ≥85–95% of the specific peak force, you now know that all muscle fibers that can be used for that motor task are active. For smaller muscles (e.g., hand muscles), the recruitment of motor units is complete at approximately 30–50% of the voluntary peak force.

Once all motor units are activated (at approximately 85–95% or 30–50% of peak voluntary force), any further increase in force (up to 100%) occurs exclusively via increases in the firing frequency of the motor units or α-motoneurons. Thus, in larger muscles, force is encoded over a larger range via recruitment than in smaller ones (up to 85–95% *vs.* 30–50%), while conversely, the range of pure frequency encoding is larger in smaller muscles (approximately 30–100%) compared to that in larger ones (approximately 85–100%). Until the recruitment limit is reached (85–95% or 30–50% of the voluntary peak force), frequency coding of the force always takes place at the same time, although it contributes less to the increase in force compared to recruitment coding (see Sect. 4.2) (Box 9.1).

> **Box 9.1: The Nebulous Intramuscular Coordination**
> The misconception of intramuscular coordination metaphorically states that resistance training leads to the activation of "dormant" muscle fibers and that this is one of the reasons why muscle force increases. The increase in intramuscular coordination is an action of the central nervous system to better organize the existing muscle fibers, or something like that.

> Well, unless you believe in Snow White and the Seven Dwarfs, you can forget that romantic notion. For maximal voluntary effort (peak voluntary force), motor unit recruitment is complete (within the specificity of the motor task) for most muscles and states. This is because the tonic recruitment threshold is 85–95% of peak voluntary force, even for large muscles. So once a value of 85–95% of peak voluntary force is reached, all task-specific motor units are recruited. Therefore, if you measure more peak voluntary force after a training period of several weeks, this means that, firstly, the cross-section of the muscle fibers used has increased and/or, secondly, the rate at which action potentials are triggered in the axon hills of the motoneurons has increased (increase in firing frequency) and/or, thirdly, you have learned motorically to activate the antagonist muscles less strongly when using the agonists.

## 9.5 What Do Autonomous Reserves Have to Do with Hibernation?

In textbooks on training theory, one stumbles over the term "autonomically protected reserves" again and again. This refers to a reserve of strength that can only be tapped under extreme conditions (e.g. danger of death or under the influence of pharmaceuticals) and is normally protected by the autonomic nervous system. That additional force can be mobilized under certain extreme conditions is known from anecdotal examples. However, the attempts to explain this are often very fanciful. According to the general idea, this additional force comes from dormant or protected motor units that can only be recruited in extreme cases. The muscle fibers belonging to these motor units would, according to this theory, be used very rarely if at all (unless you use your muscles often to extricate yourself from life-threatening circumstances).

The question therefore arises why, of all things, the muscle fibers of such motor reserve units should not atrophy over the long period of disuse, because this is exactly what normally happens in humans. However, there are several animal species, for example bats, squirrels, bears, for which hibernation is an important survival strategy. During hibernation, these animals experience long periods of physical or muscular inactivity and food abstinence. Surprisingly, the loss of muscle mass during hibernation is minimal in these animals. The reasons for this are still unknown. So unless you carry hibernator genes, it seems unlikely that reserve strength comes from otherwise "dormant" motor units. A more plausible explanation for the reserve force can be derived from our earlier considerations. As we have seen, the instantaneous (i.e., existing at the time of recruitment) firing rate decreases as recruitment proceeds (Fig. 9.1). This means that the larger high-threshold motor units are switched

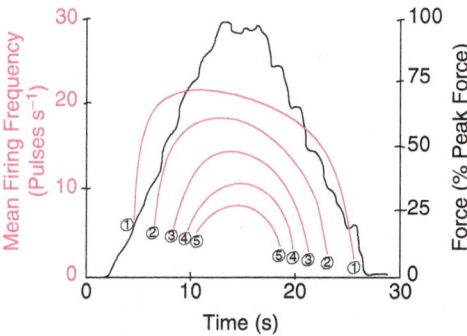

**Fig. 9.1** Force coding by recruitment and increase of firing frequency of motor units. The black line is associated with the y-axis on the right and shows the increase in force during isometric force production for a defined movement task from 0 to 100% of the peak voluntary force (approximately for the first 15 s) and the subsequent decrease in force during slow relaxation (approximately for the second 15 s) over time. The red lines are associated with the left y-axis and symbolize the firing frequency for five motor units that differ in size, with ① being the smallest motor unit and ⑤ being the largest. That is, as the force increases, more and larger motor units are recruited. At 100% of peak voluntary force, all five motor units and their associated muscle fibers are active. As the force decreases, the motor units are derecruited in reverse order, i.e., the larger ones first, then the smaller ones. The firing frequency of all activated motor units increases with increasing force and decreases with decreasing force. The larger motor units are recruited at a low firing frequency and under normal conditions the relative increase in frequency is greater for the smaller motor units than for the larger motor units. (According to De Luca and Contessa 2012)

on at a lower firing rate, even though they could theoretically fire at a much higher frequency (as evidenced by electrostimulation). Accordingly, these motor units have a greater reserve in the sense of increasing the firing rate. Extremely stressful situations could cause hyperactivation of the firing frequency of the high threshold motor units. This mechanism of hyperactivation could explain the additional muscular force that can be developed under extreme conditions.

## 9.6 The Tonic Recruitment Threshold

Now imagine that you are standing in front of a railing and holding its bar with an underhand grip. Initially, you press against the railing with very little force and then very slowly (in slow motion) increase the muscle force up to the voluntary peak force, as if you wanted to tear the railing out of the ground. As explained above, motor units are continuously recruited during this process, and at about 85% of peak voluntary force, all motor units that can be recruited for this motor task are active. Very importantly, however, is the following: For this example (slow increase in force), a recruited motor unit remains active (i.e., its α-motoneuron fires action potentials) until the end. The force (or threshold of force) at which a single motor unit is recruited during a slow increase in force is called the *tonic recruitment threshold*. "Tonic" refers to the fact that when this threshold is crossed, the same motor unit remains continuously active as long as the force is greater than or equal to the force threshold. Quite obviously, therefore, each motor unit has a characteristic tonic recruitment threshold in terms of muscle force. Motor units that remain tonically active only at a relatively high force value are called *high threshold motor units*. Conversely, motor units that exhibit tonic activity at a relatively low force level are *low threshold motor units*. I will consistently refer only to these two types of motor units in the following discussion of "switching on and off" motor units during exercise.

## 9.7 The Regular Recruitment of Motor Units

Milner-Brown et al. (1973) were able to show that motor units with a high threshold develop a higher twitch force than those with a low threshold and that the motor units are recruited in the order from the weakest to the strongest. Thus, the order in which motor units are switched on (i.e., recruited) and switched off again (i.e., derecruited) is strongly correlated with their "size" (see Sect. 9.8). Each newly activated motoneuron in order of increasing size has a slightly lower firing frequency at the time of recruitment than the preceding motoneuron. For all recruited motoneurons, however, the firing frequency increases until 100% of the peak voluntary force is reached. The scheme of force coding during slow isometric force increase from 0 to 100% of peak voluntary force by recruitment and increase of firing frequency thus follows the principle of an onion skin (Fig. 9.1) and the force level at which all motor units are activated differs for small and large muscles (Fig. 9.2).

## 9.8 Mechanism of Recruitment of Motor Units

The size characteristics of motor units are the surface area of the cell body of the α-motoneuron (or the radius of the cell body), the diameter and conduction velocity of the axon, and the number, type, and cross-sectional area of the innervated muscle fibers. Thus, a high-threshold motor unit has an α-motoneuron with a large cell body and a large-caliber axon, whereas the cell

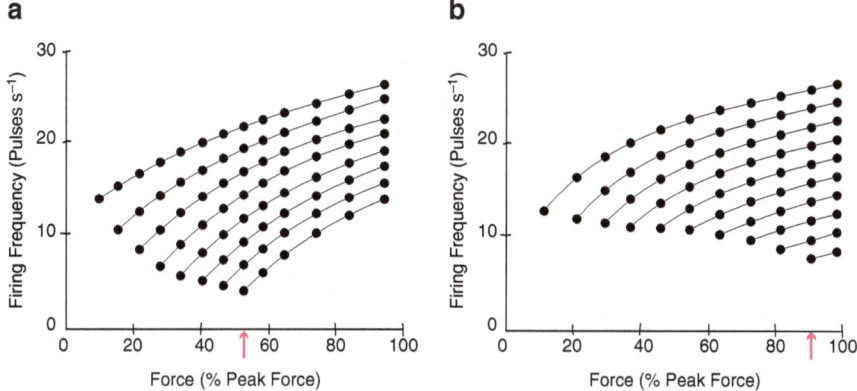

**Fig. 9.2** Recruitment limit for small and large muscles. (a) Force coding for a small skeletal muscle (e.g. the hand muscle) with isometric force production between 0 and 100% of the peak force. (b) Force coding for a large skeletal muscle (e.g. the vastus lateralis, outer thigh muscle) with isometric force production between 0 and 100% of the peak force. In both cases, force encoding occurs via recruitment and increase in firing frequency the principle of an onion skin (see also legend of Fig. 9.1). Note that for the small muscle, recruitment is already completed at a lower force value than is the case for the large muscle (indicated by the red arrows). The increase in force after recruitment is completed is exclusively due to the increase in the firing frequency. (According to De Luca and Contessa 2012)

body or axon of an α-motoneuron belonging to a low-threshold motor unit are smaller or smaller-caliber (Fig. 9.3). The innervation number of high-threshold motor units is large, and that of low-threshold units is smaller. High threshold motor units tend to innervate type 2 muscle fibers, low threshold motor units tend to innervate type 1 fibers. But why is greater motor drive, or muscle force, required to recruit high-threshold motor units than low-threshold units? Quite simply, in order for an action potential to be triggered at all in the trigger zone of the α-motoneuron (at the transition from cell body to axon), the membrane of the cell body must be depolarized sufficiently strongly, that is, suprathreshold. In this context, the threshold value for the triggering of the action potential is to be understood as a modulable quantity.

In other words, the membrane potential of the cell body must be shifted in the direction of positive values to such an extent that the threshold value for triggering the action potential is reached. This occurs by influx of singly positively charged sodium ions ($Na^+$) through $Na^+$-ion channels in the cell membrane of the α-motoneuron cell body. The $Na^+$ influx, and thus the influx of positive charge, makes the membrane potential, which is negative at rest, more positive. The trigger zone is where all changes in membrane potential

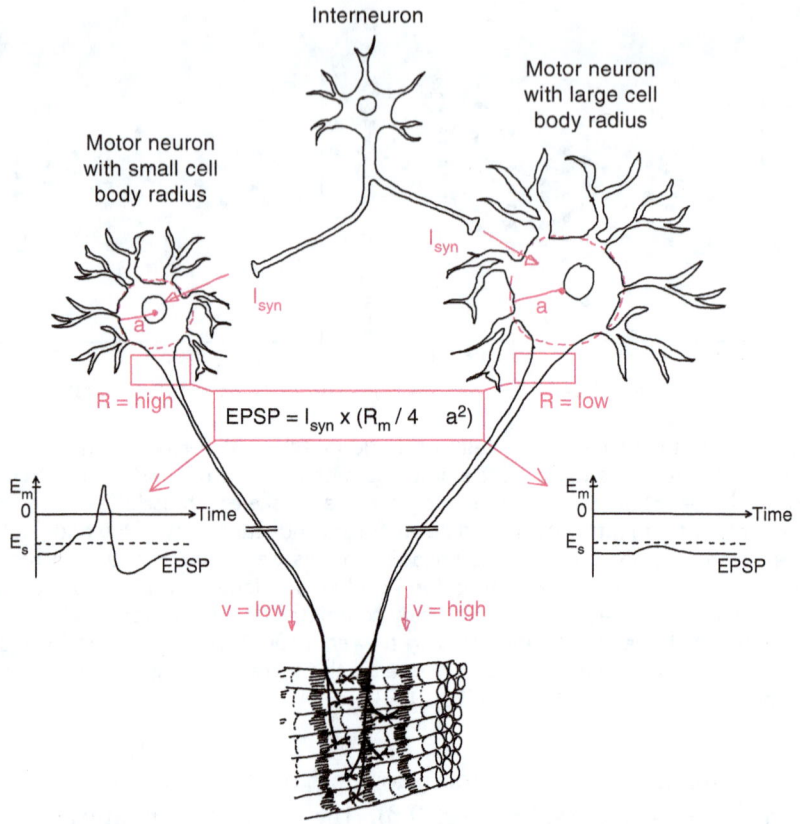

Fig. 9.3 Physical basis of motor unit recruitment. The schematic representation shows a small (left) and large (right) motoneuron in the spinal cord. In this example, both motoneurons receive the same synaptic input current ($I_{syn}$) from an interneuron. In the example shown, the synaptic input current, which is proportional to the force effort, is relatively small. This results in an action potential being triggered only in the axon hillock of the small motoneuron, which propagates to the associated muscle fibers and leads to fiber force production. For action potentials to be triggered at the axon hillock, the excitatory postsynaptic potential (EPSP) must rise above a critical threshold ($E_s$). If this is the case, the sign of the membrane potential ($E_m$) briefly reverses from negative ($E_m < 0$) to positive ($E_m > 0$). The EPSP is thus dependent on $I_{syn}$ and the electrical resistance (R) of the motor neuron cell body. The latter is proportional to the membrane resistance ($R_m$), but inversely proportional to the idealized spherical area ($4\pi a^2$) of the motoneuron cell body. The smaller the radius (a), that is, the smaller the motoneuron, the greater the resistance (R). Conversely, the larger the radius, the smaller the resistance. Small motor units are therefore recruited at relatively low input current. This is also the reason for their designation as low threshold motor units (analogously, large threshold motor units). Note that the conduction velocity (v) along the thin axon of the smaller motor neuron (left) is lower than that of the thick axon (right). (According to Enoka and Pearson 2013)

are accounted for (there are also stimuli that hyperpolarize the membrane, i.e., make it more negative). If the membrane potential in the trigger zone exceeds a certain positive value, an action potential is triggered and the signal is transmitted to the muscle fibers.

## 9.9 Where Brain Meets Muscle

Motor drive from the central nervous system reaches the α-motoneurons in the form of action potentials via the release of neurotransmitter molecules. These neurotransmitters bind to receptor proteins in the cell membrane of the α-motoneuron, which leads directly or indirectly to the opening of the $Na^+$ ion channels and thus to $Na^+$ influx. The change in membrane potential this causes is called the excitatory postsynaptic potential (EPSP; Fig. 9.3). If you produce a strong motor drive and/or a lot of muscle force, the amount of neurotransmitter released increases and so does the EPSP (note: in certain cases the force output is minimal despite a very large motor drive; see Sect. 9.12). Because of the larger cell body surface area of high threshold motor neurons, membrane resistance to potential change is greater than for those with lower surface area. This means that for a given synaptic input current (amount of neurotransmitter), the EPSP is smaller in high threshold motoneurons than in low threshold motoneurons (Fig. 9.3). For the same synaptic input current, the probability of triggering an action potential in the trigger zone and thus activating innervated fibers is smaller for high-threshold motor units relative to those with low thresholds. In other words, EPSP is directly proportional to synaptic input current (the amount of neurotransmitter) and membrane resistance, but inversely proportional to the radius of the cell body (i.e., size) of the α-motoneuron (Fig. 9.3). Whether or not an action potential is triggered in the trigger zone, and consequently whether or not the muscle fibers belonging to this motor unit are activated, therefore depends primarily (i.e. if the membrane resistances are similar) on the amount of synaptic input current (the strength of the motor drive or the amount of neurotransmitters), the surface size of the motoneuron cell body and the relative position of the threshold potential, *a priori* independently of how much force the muscle actually produces.

All cell bodies of the α-motoneurons are known to be located in the spinal cord. If you now press against an immobile object with the least amount of force, the motor drive generated by the central nervous system is small. This small motor drive hits both the low threshold and high threshold cell bodies simultaneously in the form of a small release of neurotransmitters. You now

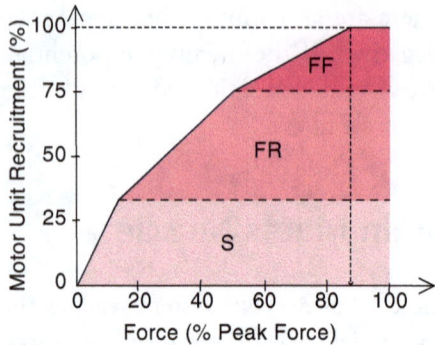

**Fig. 9.4** Influence of muscle force on the recruitment of motor units: the size principle. The number and size of the motor units recruited increase with increasing force exertion. Recruitment is "summative", that is, the larger motor units are added in *addition to* the smaller motor units already recruited in order of increasing size. Note that recruitment is completed at a varying percentage of peak voluntary force depending on the size of the muscle. Thereafter, any further increase in force occurs solely by increasing the firing frequency of the motor units. For larger muscles (as in the example shown), recruitment is exhausted at approximately 85–95% of peak voluntary force, meaning that all motor units that can be recruited for the specific movement task are activated. For smaller muscles, this force threshold is about 30–50%. Note that the labeling of the motor units (S, FR, and FF) in this diagram is emblematic of their threshold level of excitation-from low (S), meaning low threshold, to high (FF), meaning high threshold. S, *slow;* FR, *fast fatigue resistant;* FF, *fast fatigable*

know what result this leads to: Only for the low-threshold motor neurons is the relatively weak synaptic input current sufficient to raise EPSP above the threshold necessary to trigger an action potential. Consequently, only low threshold motor units are recruited. Only with increasing motor drive are high threshold motor units recruited in addition to low threshold motor units. Or, in short, the smallest motor neuron is activated first, the largest last. This effect is known as the "size principle of motor neuron recruitment" and was first described by Derek Denny-Brown and Joe Pennybacker in 1938 (Denny-Brown and Pennybacker 1938) and later by Elwood Henneman (1957) (Fig. 9.4). Incorrectly, the initial description is often attributed to Henneman in the literature, which is why the size principle has also become known over the years as the "Henneman's Size Principle".

## 9.10 How Is the Rate of Force Development Encoded by Recruitment and Frequency?

As you have just learned, during slow isometric force development, you need to use 30–50% (smaller muscles) or 85–95% (larger muscles) of the peak voluntary force, depending on the muscle, to recruit all the motor units available for the motor task. As discussed, following the size principle, the high threshold motor units are recruited after the low threshold motor units. Consequently, the type 2 fibers are activated only at higher force, after most type 1 fibers have already been activated. However, you now know from Sect. 1.6 that muscle force decreases with increasing shortening speed because of the force-velocity relationship. This would mean that, due to the (too) low force during explosive or ballistic force development, you could only activate a few to no type 2 fibers or recruit motor units with a high threshold value, which would not make sense from a movement functional point of view.

With an increase in the rate of force development, the motor units must therefore be recruited earlier. The reason for this is that there is a constant (i.e. invariable) time delay of several milliseconds between the triggering of the action potential in the trigger zone of the motoneuron and the force generated by the motor unit taking effect in the muscle. In other words, mechanical recruitment, that is, force development, occurs with a delay relative to the time of electrical recruitment (action potential in the axon hillock of the α-motoneuron). Now, in order for the same motor unit to be mechanically recruited at different rates of force development (i.e., as at low rates), it must be electrically activated at an earlier time. How is this possible, or by what mechanism are high threshold motor units and type 2 fibers recruited or activated by the central nervous system during rapid force development? This occurs by temporarily lowering the recruitment threshold to a value below the tonic threshold.

Desmedt and Godaux (1977) showed that during ballistic force production against a resistance corresponding to only 30% of the peak voluntary force, most motor units were recruited in the tibialis anterior muscle. The reduction in recruitment threshold necessary for this occurred in all motoneurons, that is, both high and low threshold motoneurons, in such a way that the size principle retained its validity (Desmedt and Godaux 1977). Motor units of both thresholds are also recruited during ballistic, i.e. explosive, force development, but practically simultaneously (Fig. 9.5). Because of the larger diameter of high-threshold axons, their conduction velocity is greater than that of low-threshold ones, so that when an action potential is

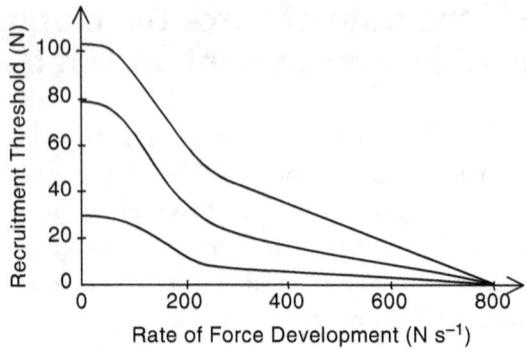

**Fig. 9.5** Effect of rate of force development on recruitment threshold and recruitment order. This schematic shows for three motor units the force (called the recruitment threshold) at which they are recruited as a function of the rate of force development. During force development from 0 to 100 N at low speed, the motor units are recruited following the size principle in the order of their tonic recruitment threshold. As the speed increases, the recruitment threshold decreases for all three motor units. The greatest reduction in threshold occurs for the largest motor unit (the unit with the highest tonic recruitment threshold). Note that even with very rapid, explosive force development (slightly below 800 N s$^{-1}$), the recruitment order is preserved, except that the motor units are recruited virtually simultaneously regardless of their size

elicited in the trigger zone at approximately the same time, the electrical signal from the high-threshold motoneurons arrives in the muscle before the signal from the low-threshold motoneurons (Desmedt and Godaux 1977). Unfortunately, this has been or is often incorrectly interpreted to mean that only explosive movement execution can selectively train type 2 fibers and that you must train fast or explosively in resistance training to activate the fast type 2 fibers and make them faster through training. Neither of these claims is true: even if you train explosively, you will slow down at the level of the MyHC isoforms (see Sect. 5.5). However, it is true that fast movements are a strategy to recruit high-threshold motor units and thus activate type 2 fibers (Fig. 9.6).

However, you must be aware of an important, practical point. If the force you have produced and are holding with a high rate of force development is below the tonic recruitment threshold of the motor units used in the force increase, these units will not remain active, i.e. they will be derecruited (switched off). Thus, of the motor units that were used for the rapid increase in force, only those remain active (i.e., continue to fire action potentials) for which the target force held is greater than their tonic recruitment threshold.

Motor units can therefore in principle exhibit two types of activity: If the force produced is above the tonic recruitment threshold for a motor unit,

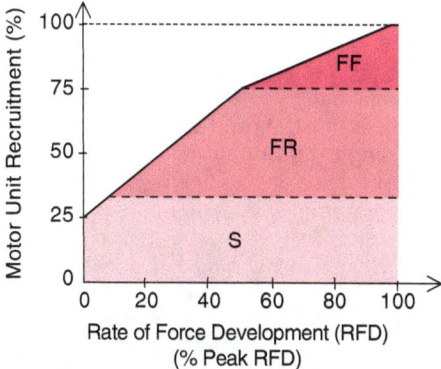

**Fig. 9.6** Influence of the rate of force development on the recruitment of motor units. As the rate of force development increases (for a given external force, e.g., 30% of peak voluntary force), the number and size of motor units recruited increase. Recruitment is summative, that is, even at the highest rapidity, the larger motor units are recruited in *addition* to the smaller motor units already recruited in order of size. The size principle of recruitment therefore holds even during the fastest voluntary force development. Note that the labeling of the motor units (S, FR, and FF) in this schematic is emblematic of their threshold of excitation-from low (S), meaning low threshold, to high (FF), meaning high threshold. S, *slow;* FR, *fast fatigue resistant;* FF, *fast fatigable*

then that motor unit exhibits tonic activity, that is, it fires action potentials continuously. If the force produced is below the tonic recruitment threshold for that motor unit, then it may be phasically active, and this occurs whenever the rate of force development increases or is high. Recent research results suggest that to increase muscle protein synthesis (and thereby increase muscle mass in the long term), it is not sufficient to switch high threshold motor units on and off a few times (as occurs during fast or explosive movements in resistance training), but that these motor units (and thus also the previously recruited low threshold motor units) must be tonically active for a certain period of time (cf. Sects. 9.6 and 13.7) or that their muscle fibers are fatigued by the tonic activity of the motor unit (Box 9.2).

**Box 9.2: How Can You Develop Muscle Force Rapidly?**

An important reason why appropriate training increases the rate of force development is that the instantaneous firing rate of the motor units in the corresponding muscle increases. This means that the motoneurons of the involved motor units fire at a higher frequency when they are recruited after the training phase (→ more action potentials per unit time in the muscle cell membrane → steeper increase in the intracellular calcium ion concentration per unit time →

more force per unit time; see Sect. 4.2). For example, 12 weeks of ballistic training (10 sets of 5 repetitions each on 5 days per week against 30–40% of peak voluntary torque with maximal voluntary movement speed) of the anterior tibialis muscle (anterior tibialis muscle) results in an increase in the intramuscularly measured firing rate of single motor units (from approximately 69 to 96 Hz) and an increase in the rate of torque development of 82% (Van Cutsem et al. 1998). In addition, the electromyographic signal (i.e., the sum of all muscle fiber action potentials measured on the skin surface over the muscle) is advanced by a few milliseconds (Van Cutsem et al. 1998). Similarly, for the same motor task (lifting the foot), lower values (48% compared to 100% in younger people) for the rate of torque development are measurable in older people than in younger people. This reduction is associated with a peak firing rate of the motor units in the tibialis anterior muscle that is reduced by approximately 30% (Klass et al. 2008).

## 9.11 Practical Relevance: Force Magnitude and Rate of Force Development

I have now already presented two strategies or mechanisms that you can use to control which muscle fiber spectrum (either type 1 fibers only or type 1 plus type 2A fibers or type 1 plus type 2 fibers) you target in training:

- The more force you produce, the more motor units of both thresholds are recruited according to the size principle, i.e. the more type 2 fibers are activated in addition to the type 1 fibers. If the force is greater than 30–50% or 85–95% of the peak voluntary force, all motor units are recruited and thus all type-1 and type-2 fibers are activated.
- The higher the rate of force development for a given target force (e.g. as fast as possible from 0 to 100 N), the more motor units of both thresholds are also recruited according to the size principle, i.e. the more type 2 fibers are activated in addition to type 1 fibers.

In both cases, however, a recruited motor unit remains active only if the force produced is higher than the tonic recruitment threshold for that motor unit (Fig. 9.7).

The first case has the following meaning for practice: If you perform a single biceps curl standing upright (upper arm parallel to the side of the torso), from full extension to full flexion, you know from Sect. 2.8 that the muscle force, the moment arm and therefore the muscular torque are a function of the joint angle position and the external torque. The latter is given by the weight of the dumbbell and its perpendicular distance to the elbow joint. This

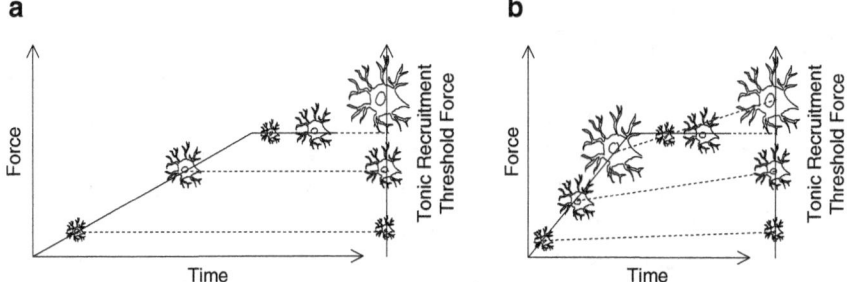

**Fig. 9.7** Recruitment of motor units with different tonic recruitment thresholds as a function of the rate of force development. (**a**) In the case of very slow force development, motor units (represented schematically by the different size of the cell body of their motor neurons) are recruited at the force corresponding to the tonic recruitment threshold (right). Note that the largest motor unit whose tonic recruitment threshold is above the achieved target force is not recruited in this case (slow force development). Thus, on the plateau of force, only those motor units whose tonic recruitment threshold is less than or equal to the force on the plateau are active. (**b**) In the case of very fast force development, the recruitment threshold is reduced for all motor units. Note that in this case the largest motor unit is also recruited, but only phasically. At the plateau of force, only those motor units whose tonic recruitment threshold is less than or equal to the force at the plateau remain active. Accordingly, the largest motor unit is derecruited again if the final force reached and maintained during the rapid increase in force is not greater than or equal to the tonic recruitment threshold for that specific motor unit. Thus, motor units exhibit tonic activity if the force produced is greater than or equal to the tonic recruitment threshold. Phasic activity of motor units is said to occur when the same motor units are temporarily recruited (i.e. derecruited after the increase in force) by a very rapid development of force

means that these quantities vary depending on the angular position in the elbow joint. This is an important point for understanding training: internal muscle force varies depending on joint position, despite a constant external load (as is usually the case in training). As you progress through the *range of motion* (ROM) during miometric force production in a non-fatigued state (e.g. first repetition), internal muscle force will increase or decrease depending on joint angle. Somewhere in the ROM (exactly where is not known and also varies with the type of curl execution) the internal muscle force reaches its relative maximum value. At all other joint angles, the force is either less or equal.

Let us now assume that this relative peak is ≥85% of the peak voluntary force. In this case, all motor units that can be recruited for this motor task or biceps function are recruited. If internal muscle force in the nonfatigued state falls below 85% of peak voluntary force anywhere in ROM, partial derecruitment of motor units occurs. Thus, with miometric force production in the non-fatigued state, the extent of recruitment varies as a function of the internal force curve. This means that recruitment, and thus the number of muscle fibers used, can vary within a single repetition of an exercise. Full recruitment and thus activation of all fibers only occurs in the non-fatigued state if the muscle force generated in the corresponding angular position is greater than the aforementioned 30–50% or 85–95% of the voluntary peak force.

The second case has the following significance for practice: If you now perform the biceps curl described above ballistically and thus treat the dumbbell as a projectile, the internal muscle force varies not only depending on the angular position, but also depending on the momentum that you give the dumbbell through the impulse. The greater this momentum, the more the dumbbell will continue to move uniformly in a straight line by itself. This in turn means that you will have to use less force to maintain the movement, with the consequence that motor units will be derecruited due to the decrease in force. If all motor units are recruited at the beginning of the ballistic movement with a resistance of 30% of the voluntary peak force, the recruitment decreases as the momentum of the dumbbell increases. Therefore, during a ballistic muscle activity or an explosive movement, especially the high threshold motor units show a phasic activity as long as the produced force is not higher than the tonic recruitment threshold for the motor units concerned (Fig. 9.7).

## 9.12 Do You Want Big and Strong Muscles? Weaken Them!

Finally, I would like to discuss the third strategy for recruiting motor units, which is perhaps the most important for muscle building training: local muscle fatigue. Let me illustrate this with an example. Suppose the motor task were to push isometrically with both shins against the lever arm of a dynamometer (torque meter) in a seated position at a fixed knee joint angle of 90° (i.e., attempt a knee extension), first within 5 s to 50% of the previously acquired peak voluntary torque, then hold for 1 s, in 5 s back to 20%, then hold this for 50 s, and then pause for 6 s. This cycle would be repeated as many times as necessary. This whole cycle would then be repeated until you couldn't get back to the initial 50% despite maximum effort. Let's also assume that I would determine the voluntary peak torque anew each time during the 6 s pause intervals.

## 9  How You Can Influence Which Muscle Fibers Are Used in Training

What would happen in the course of the repetitions? Externally, nothing, except perhaps that your facial expression would not have become happier with increasing fatigue. The measured external torques are always the same, by the way, analogous to your workout in the gym: the external resistance held or moved normally remains the same (except for specialized equipment) from the first to the last repetition. What is measurable in our example, however, is the decrease in peak voluntary torque measured externally in the pauses between repetitions from repetition to repetition. In other words, the thigh muscles fatigue more with each repetition, which manifests itself in a decrease in peak voluntary torque from repetition to repetition.

What happens inside the vastus lateralis muscle (external thigh muscle) in terms of recruitment and increase in firing frequency of motor units? In this regard, let us first consider the slow increase in peak voluntary torque from 0 to 50% and the subsequent slow decrease to 20%. First, the number of motor units recruited increases with each repetition, that is, with increasing fatigue. Moreover, with each successive repetition, the same motor unit is recruited at a smaller torque, which means that fatigue, similarly to rapid force development, leads to a decrease in the recruitment threshold. In addition, as fatigue increases, the firing rate tends to increase. Once torque is reduced from 50% to 20%, the motor units are derecruited in reverse order. However, this occurs more slowly in the fatigued muscle in that the motor units, once recruited, are derecruited later due to the decrease in the recruitment threshold. If we now consider the 50-second hold at 20% of peak torque, we notice something similar. With each repetition, the number of motor units recruited at the beginning of the 50-second hold increases. Further, the number of motor units recruited also increases with increasing time under tension (from 0 to 50 s). Finally, the firing rate of all motor units recruited increases with increasing time under tension.

This all makes sense: at a force of less than 85% of the voluntary peak force, not all motor units are recruited. If these motor units now become fatigued, there would inevitably be an external drop in force if additional motor units were not recruited to compensate for this drop in force. With increasing fatigue of the motor unit and thus increasing fatigue of the muscle fibers, on the one hand the motor drive increases, whereby, in accordance with the size principle, more and more motor units with a high threshold value are recruited (Fig. 9.8). On the other hand, in the course of fatigue, there is also a decrease in the recruitment threshold, so that motor units with a high threshold can be brought into operation at a lower torque during repeated loading. This is all necessary to maintain external torque as internal fatigue increases. You can also think of this situation as follows. Peak voluntary muscular torque decreases

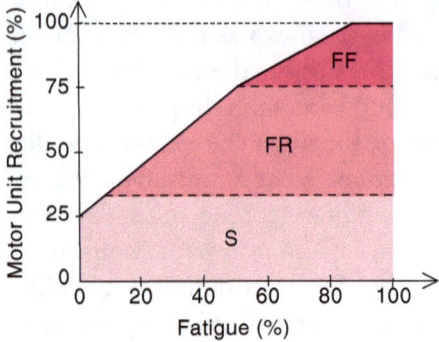

**Fig. 9.8** Influence of muscle fatigue on the recruitment of motor units. During muscle fatigue, that is, as the muscle weakens (decrease in peak voluntary force), progressively more and larger motor units must be recruited to maintain mechanical output (external force). Note that even in this case, recruitment follows the size principle and at a certain level of fatigue or decrease in peak voluntary force, all motor units that can be recruited for the specific movement task are recruited. The labeling of the motor units (S, FR, and FF) in this scheme is emblematic of their threshold level of excitation-from low (S), meaning low threshold, to high (FF), meaning high threshold. S, *slow*; FR, *fast fatigue resistant*; FF, *fast fatigable*

from repetition to repetition, while external torque remains more or less constant. This means that the external torque increases from repetition to repetition relative to the peak internal torque. So there is a relative increase in force or torque, so to speak, with increasing fatigue, and we have seen that recruitment increases with an increase in force up to a muscle-specific threshold of complete recruitment. Once all motor units have been recruited, external torque can only be maintained as long as the muscular torque produced by all fibers is not less than the external torque. This example shows that an increase in motor drive does not necessarily lead to greater muscular force or external torque.

Therefore, for high threshold motor unit recruitment, the increase in motor drive is more important than the actual external mechanical result. Accordingly, if you exercise at a low force (i.e., with a lower training resistance) relative to the force value of complete recruitment (30–60% or 85–95% of peak voluntary force), you can still activate all the muscle fibers that can be used for the motor task, provided that you hold or move the resistance until you can't anymore, that is, until exhaustion (Fig. 9.8). I will show you later that the effective time under tension of the FF-type motor units until exhaustion is a central variable for increasing muscle protein synthesis and thus for stimulating the processes required for muscle growth (Box 9.3).

> **Box 9.3: "Lift weights like grandma, you'll have muscles like grandma!" Is that Really so?**
>
> This popular saying is often quoted by coaches and trainers. However, its content is wrong. To get strong and large muscles, contrary to popular belief, you do not necessarily need particularly big loads or muscle forces. What is primarily required is a large motor drive, that is, a large effort of force, regardless of the mechanical result of that effort. This leads, if it lasts long enough (i.e. in the course of fatigue or exhaustion), to the orderly recruitment of more and larger motor units (according to the size principle) and thus to the activation of type 2 fibers. You can therefore choose a moderately heavy load in resistance training, relative to the peak voluntary force. You simply have to move or hold this resistance until it is no longer possible despite maximum effort, i.e. until *motor task failure*. However, the effective time under tension should be neither too short nor too long. You will find out why this is the case in Chap. 13.

## 9.13 Can Type 2 Fibers Be Selectively Activated?

The general consensus is that the order in which motor units are recruited during voluntary muscle efforts follows the size principle (Heckman and Enoka 2012). However, there are also the hypotheses that the recruitment scheme is more flexible under certain conditions.

The first hypothesis is that fast muscle efforts in the style of explosive or ballistic movements preferentially lead to the recruitment of high threshold motor units (i.e. fast motor units). As I explained to you above using the results of Desmedt and Godaux (1977), contrary to this view, the size principle of recruitment also holds for the fastest (i.e., ballistic) muscle efforts, even though this decreases the recruitment threshold for all motor units. Thus, the rate of force development does not affect the order of recruitment of motor units.

The second hypothesis is that as the length of the muscle-tendon unit changes during force production (i.e., depending on whether force production is mio-, iso-, or pliometric), the recruitment order also changes. This assumption is more plausible because the synaptic input acting on a cell body of a motoneuron may be different during isometric compared to anisometric (i.e., mio- or pliometric) force production (e.g., Tax et al. 1989). However, contrary to this assumption, it has been demonstrated that the recruitment order is not different for isometric and miometric force production (Desmedt and Godaux 1979). For pliometric force production, the situation seems to be less clear.

Nardone and Schieppati (1988) and Nardone et al. (1989) showed that the same motor units are not used in the calf muscles during pliometric force production as during miometric force production. Firstly, the authors reported that 15 and 50% of the motor units in the soleus (clod muscle) and M. gastrocnemius (twin calf muscle) were recruited only during pliometric muscle use, second, that these motor units had a high threshold, third, that the recruitment of these motor units was accompanied by the derecruitment of motor units recruited during the miometric phase, and fourth, that the putative selective recruitment occurred mostly during high movement speed. In contrast to the results of Nardone and Schieppati (1988) and Nardone et al. (1989), most subsequent studies failed to find a difference in recruitment order when comparing miometric and pliometric muscle actions. This is true for both lifting and lowering loads (e.g., Stotz and Bawa 2001), decelerating a negative torque produced by a dynamometer (e.g., Altenburg et al. 2009), or force production against elastic resistance (e.g., Christova and Kossev 2000). In summary, the order with which motor units are recruited is relatively constant for the different types of muscle use (iso-, mio- and pliometric) and follows the size principle. For specific motor tasks involving pliometric force production, the recruitment order may differ in some circumstances.

## 9.14 Neuroanatomical Muscle Cartography

Unlike the two ideas above, there is definitely more scientific evidence that recruitment order, or recruitment in general, is a function of motor task. Take for example the case of the first dorsal interosseous muscle (belonging to the finger joint musculature as part of the Mm. interossei dorsales). This muscle counts about 150 motor units in humans (i.e., the innervation number is about 150) and performs two functions: abduction and flexion of the index finger relative to the corresponding metacarpophalangeal joint. Desmedt and Godaux (1981) were now able to show that 8% of the approximately 150 motor units in the first dorsal intercalary muscle changed their rank within the recruitment order depending on the function, and this was true under both static and dynamic conditions. This can be explained by the fact that the cell bodies of the motoneurons may receive altered synaptic input from the central nervous system depending on function (abduction or flexion). "Altered" here may mean that depending on the motor task or function, the (poly-)synaptic excitation and/or inhibition signals may be different, which may facilitate or impede the triggering of an excitatory postsynaptic potential (EPSP) (hyperpolarization *vs.* hypopolarization).

The extensor digitorum communis muscle (simple finger extensor), which extends the index, middle and ring fingers, is more complex than the first dorsal intercostal muscle in that it has multiple muscle heads, tendons and attachment sites. The innervation number for the simple finger extensor is about 270. It appears that the motor units of complex muscles are organized into subgroups that may have a different composition depending on the perceived function. You can also think of it as the totality of all motor units forming and deploying different teams of motor units depending on their function. The recruitment of motor units in the finger extensor has been studied for different isometric muscle functions: extension of the index finger, middle finger, ring finger or two fingers together (index plus middle finger or middle plus ring finger), or extension of the wrist with the fingers relaxed.

It was possible to measure that a separate subgroup of motor units was recruited in the finger extensor muscle during the extension of each individual finger. For the simultaneous extension of two fingers, the two subgroups were again recruited together. Finally, all motor units together formed the pool of motor units used for wrist extension. Within the corresponding subgroups (single finger, two fingers, etc.), the motor units were recruited according to the size principle. Now, if a motor unit is recruited as the twentieth unit when the index finger is extended because of its size, for example, the order in which the motor units are recruited may be different when the index and middle fingers are extended simultaneously. The reason for this is that when the functional subsets of motor units are combined, the cards are reshuffled with respect to the size of the motor units. If all of the additional motor units used in simultaneous index and middle finger extension are larger than the one mentioned, their position in the recruitment order remains unchanged. However, if a few of the additional motor units used are smaller, then the named motor unit is recruited later, that is, it occupies a different, higher position in the recruitment order (Bawa 2002).

These observations raise the suspicion that muscles may have anatomical neuromuscular compartments corresponding to subgroups of motor units. The biceps brachii muscle (two-headed arm muscle) clearly exhibits such anatomical-neuromuscular compartments. Both the long (laterally located) and short (medially located) heads are innervated separately by corresponding branches from an arm nerve (musculocutaneous nerve). Both heads are in turn subdivided into smaller compartments, which are innervated by further nerve branches. Roughly speaking, each biceps head is subdivided into three anatomical neuromuscular compartments from medial (towards the middle of the body) to central and lateral (towards the outside) (Fig. 9.9).

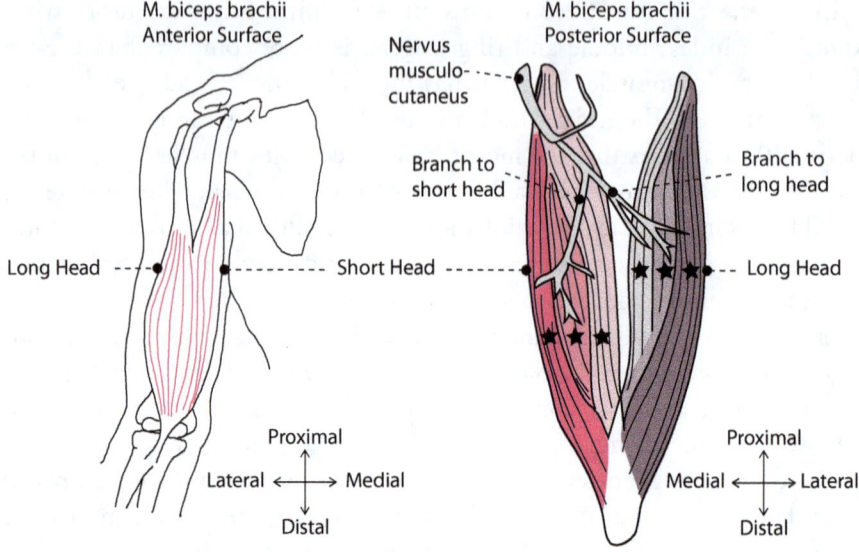

**Fig. 9.9** Anatomical neuromuscular compartments of the two-headed humerus muscle (M. biceps brachii)

The biceps brachii muscle is therefore divided into six anatomical-neuromuscular compartments. The two biceps heads have different points of attachment to the scapula and merge differently with the insertion tendon at the elbow joint. Interestingly, the motor units located laterally within the long head of the biceps were shown to be recruited during elbow flexion and the motor units located medially were recruited during supination (i.e., outward rotation of the hand by rotation of the forearm) or linear combinations of flexion and supination. In contrast, the centrally located motor units were recruited for nonlinear combinations of flexion and supination (ter Haar Romeny et al. 1984). How is this possible?

A simple explanatory model (summarized in Fig. 9.10) would be that the pool of α-motoneurons in the spinal cord belonging to the long biceps head consists of three subsets:

- Cell bodies receiving synaptic input from supraspinal centers exclusively during flexion
- Cell bodies receiving synaptic input during both flexion and supination
- Cell bodies that receive synaptic input exclusively during supination

The lateral motor units (or muscle fibers) therefore only receive flexion input and cannot be recruited by supination. The central motor units (or muscle

# 9 How You Can Influence Which Muscle Fibers Are Used in Training

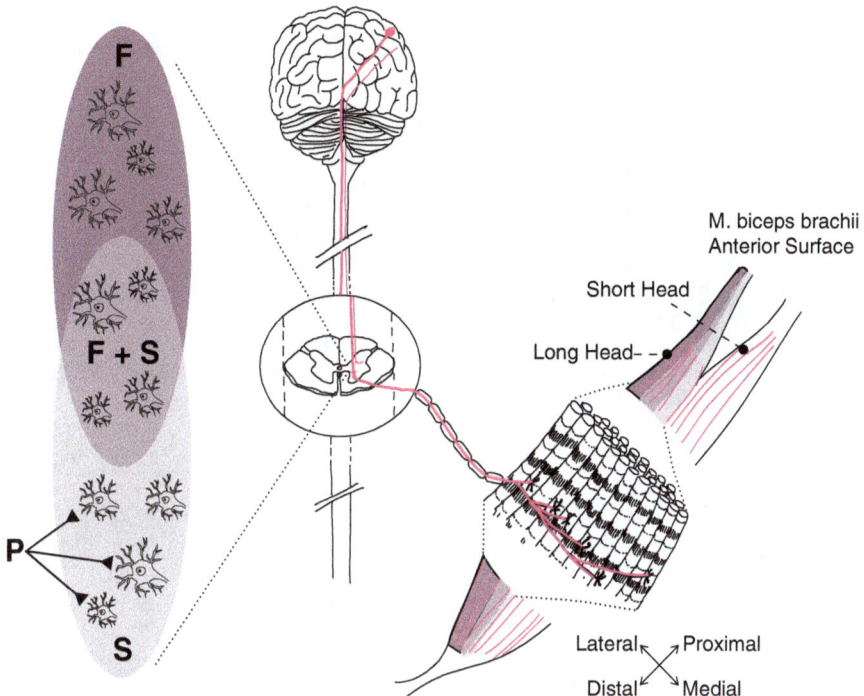

**Fig. 9.10** Somatotopic representation of the anatomical neuromuscular compartments of the long head of the biceps as pooled cell bodies of motoneurons in the spinal cord

fibers) can receive both flexion and supination input. If a cell body receives both inputs simultaneously, linear stimulus summation occurs, that is, the probability of triggering an action potential in the trigger zone increases. The medial motor units (and thus the medially located muscle fibers) receive only supination input and cannot be recruited during flexion alone (ter Haar Romeny et al. 1984). If arm flexion is performed with the wrist pronated, on the one hand there is selective inhibition of flexion input and inhibition of the supination cell bodies (hypopolarization), with the result that the flexion force of the biceps muscle decreases. Despite this inhibitory effect of pronation on biceps function, peak voluntary force during flexion with pronated wrist is still approximately 85% compared to flexion with supinated wrist. This points to the well-known fact that the brachialis muscle is the main elbow flexor and not the biceps brachii muscle as is generally assumed (Boxes 9.4 and 9.5).

### Box 9.4: Why You Should Train the Same Muscle with Different Exercises

If you train a muscle with a specific motor task to the point of voluntary exhaustion (e.g. the extensor digitorum communis muscle by extending the index finger against resistance), all motor units that can be recruited for this motor task are used, but not those for extending the middle and ring fingers. This means that in the extensor digitorum communis muscle, by extending the index finger to exhaustion, you activate only the muscle fibers that can be activated for this purpose. Performing exactly the same exercise several times therefore hardly leads to the recruitment of additional motor units and therefore also not to the activation of more muscle fibers (always provided that you train to exhaustion and the effective time under tension is within a reasonable range; see Sect. 13.7). However, in order to recruit or train as many motor units of a muscle as possible, you must exhaust as many anatomical functions of the extensor digitorum communis muscle as possible, i.e. also the extension of the middle and ring fingers and the wrist.

Therefore, if you want to train as many muscle fibers of a muscle as possible (and this is certainly a goal in terms of building muscle mass and strength), then it is recommended to train several anatomical functions or motor tasks (exercises) for the same muscle instead of repeating the exact same exercise countless times. Repeating the same exercise several times only makes sense in terms of muscle hypertrophy if you either did not recruit all the motor units when you first performed it and/or the motor units that were recruited were not active for long enough (i.e. the effective time under tension was too short; cf. Sect. 13.7). The former can occur if you do not perform the motor task or exercise to voluntary exhaustion. The second may occur if the movements are performed in a fast/explosive/ballistic manner and/or the selected training resistance (expressed as a percentage of peak voluntary force, peak voluntary torque or similar) is too high (see Sects. 9.12 and 13.7).

### Box 9.5: Sport-Specific Resistance Training? What Is That?

Sport-specific strength training represents the well-intentioned attempt to achieve specific training effects for the sporting movement or the muscles used in it. For this purpose, an attempt is made to simulate the athletic movement against a resistance on machines, cable pulleys, with dumbbells, etc. Not only the trajectory of the movement is tried to be imitated, but also the speed of the movement. However, the concept of sport-specific strength training is also an example of how good faith coupled with ignorance can lead to nonsense.

We have seen from the example of the long head of the biceps that it has three anatomical-neuromuscular compartments, which are somatotopically mapped in the spinal cord (and in the brain) in the form of at least three pools of motor units, which are specifically used depending on the function or motor task (e.g. flexion, supination, flexion plus supination, with or without anteversion and internal rotation, etc.). There are therefore no motor units in the long biceps head for rowers, nor those for artistic gymnasts or climbers. Now, in order to achieve the greatest possible transfer of training effects from the gym to your sport, those muscle fibers that have adapted as a result of resistance training must be used in movements specific to the sport. In addition, the muscle adaptations must be such that they have a positive effect on the sport-specific movement task. This is not necessarily the case. If the length-force relationship of your muscles has adapted to the typical sport-specific stress pattern (see Sect. 2.8) and you now use resistance training to effect a length adaptation over larger or smaller joint amplitudes, this can have a detrimental effect on the length-force relationship within the muscle and on the length-force coordination between the muscles involved.

In principle, you increase the chance of transferring adaptation effects to the sport if you train as many muscle fibers as possible in resistance training. However, this means that you train as unspecifically as possible. By "non-specific" I mean that in strength training you use the same muscle with several different movement tasks (anatomical functions). In this sense, provocatively speaking, the most non-specific is exactly the most sport-specific resistance training. What is important to pay attention to, however, is that the typical joint amplitudes in resistance training, especially (but not exclusively) in training phases close to competition, correspond to those in the sport. Otherwise, there is the possibility of a loss of coordination, i.e. the development of force depending on the joint angle within a muscle and between several muscles is no longer optimal, for example to accelerate an object to the maximum (see Box 3.1).

## 9.15 Force Transmission Between Neighbours

The inhomogeneous activation of a muscle via anatomical-functional or motor units related to the motor task implies that all motor units available for this task are recruited following the size principle when the exercise is performed correctly. However, this does not necessarily mean that all motor units of the muscle are recruited. Within the same muscle head or muscle fascia, not all fibers are usually active during force production, and the question therefore arises as to how force can be effectively transmitted to the tendons despite inhomogeneous activation. With a revealing experiment, Sybil Street was able to show that muscle force is also transmitted laterally between the muscle fibers (Street 1983).

From a frog muscle, Street removed a muscle fiber bundle together with the tendons at both ends. At the left end of the tendon, she attached the muscle fiber bundle to a force sensor. From the middle to the right end of the bundle, she removed all fibers except for one, which also inserted into the tendon attached to the force sensor at the left end. Now she attached the free end of this one fiber to the right end with an appropriate apparatus, stimulated the fiber there electrically and recorded the force measured by the sensor at the left end. She then detached the fiber at the right end again and instead attached the ends of the muscle fibers, which had been clipped in the middle, to the pad. Street then stimulated the same muscle fiber at the right end again (*but without attaching it*). The result was astonishing: even without the attachment of the stimulated muscle fiber, the measured force was still 75% of the value measured in the attached state.

These results were interpreted to mean that the fiber activated in the unattached state (unable to transmit force longitudinally) transmitted the force produced laterally to the adjacent attached muscle fibers, which in turn transmitted the force to the force sensor. The experiment demonstrates that muscle fiber force can be transmitted to adjacent fibers to a significant degree.

Lateral (or transverse) force transmission therefore plays a no less important role alongside longitudinal force transmission. These lateral connections also ensure that the neighbouring muscle fibers remain aligned with each other despite inhomogeneous activation. The lateral connections are made up of protein complexes called costameres. The costameres are located at the level of the Z-disks (see Sect. 2.5) and are anchored to them. They are therefore arranged at regular intervals along the muscle cell membrane, analogous to the Z-discs. Costameres form a connection between various intramyocellular structural proteins and the extracellular basement membrane, which is a specialized connective tissue. This is rich in laminin, proteoglycan and collagen IV and is anchored to the extracellular matrix by a collagen VI-rich network.

## 9.16 Tensional Integrity and Mechanotransduction: To What Extent Do Muscle Fibers Have Integrity?

According to the cellular model of *tensional integrity* (*tensegrity*), muscle cells or cells in general are pre-stressed structures. In general terms, however, the model, which was first described by the architect R. Buckminster Fuller (1961), describes a building principle according to which a structure stabilises its form through sustained tension. In terms of a living cell, this model means that tensile forces are resisted by micro- and intermediate filaments of the cytoskeleton and counterbalanced by structural, compression-resistant cellular elements (internal microtubular struts and anchors in the extracellular matrix). In this context, the individual filaments may also perform a dual function depending on the structural context (Ingber 2003a, b). The mechanical forces for pretension or compression, by which the shape of a muscle fiber is stabilized, derive in part from the actin-myosin force (active). On the other hand, passive forces also contribute, for example the osmotic force, which also determines the water content and thus the internal pressure (see Sect. 23.4).

The intermediate filaments (fine "traction cables") connect the many subcellular structures (cell nuclei, mitochondria, sarcomeres, sarcoplasmic reticulum) with each other or form a structural lattice for them. Through their material properties, they confer rigidity to the entire cytoskeleton. The concept of tensional integrity can also be applied to our bodies. Here, the bones represent the compression-resistant elements, while the muscles, tendons and ligaments are the tension-resistant structures. In this example, the shape or posture of our body is the result of the muscular tensile forces that push or stabilize the compression-resistant skeletal components against each other in the face of gravity.

If a single muscle fiber now produces force or is passively stretched, this leads to a change in the tension conditions inside the cell, with the result that the shape of the cell changes, i.e. a deformation (e.g. shortening) occurs. This change in tension inside the cell is carried by the muscle fiber at the appropriate points along its length via the lateral connections into the surrounding muscle fibers, i.e. the deformation propagates into the surrounding muscle fibers. However, the magnitude of the mechanical deformation of the surrounding fibers decreases from the site of origin. If the tensional integrity of a muscle fiber is disturbed in a site-specific manner, the surrounding fibers will also experience this to a certain extent.

## 9.17 Can a Muscle Be Specifically "Sculpt"?

"Sculpting" can be understood as the voluntary formation of sub-areas within a muscle, for example, in the case of the pectoralis muscle, the lower, upper, inner or outer part. The presence of task-specific subsets of motor units (see Sect. 9.14), intrafascicularly terminating muscle fibers with myomyonal connections (see Sect. 4.5), and microtraumata occurring at different locations along the length of the muscle or fiber (see Sects. 7.3, 7.4 and 8.1) clearly indicates that the local (within a muscle or along/inside a muscle fiber) loading during exercise is fundamentally inhomogeneous. So even if you try to repeat the same exercise in exactly the same way, it is likely to be difficult to reproduce the microscopic events around lateral and longitudinal force transmission. This also becomes clear in light of the fact that your workouts are, after all, "making history" within the muscle, meaning that the workout leads to adaptations that in turn influence force production and transmission.

In addition, local forces can propagate to adjacent fibers in at least two ways, further reducing the local discriminatory power of the training effect. We have seen that the cytoskeletons of adjacent muscle fibers are laterally coupled via the extracellular matrix (see Sects. 9.15 and 9.16). Changes in tension integrity within a muscle fiber are therefore directly (i.e. mechanically) linked to those of surrounding fibers. For example, if a muscle fiber is activated and produces force, the resulting fiber deformation leads to passive forces in surrounding muscle fibers that may not be activated. These passive forces can also theoretically lead to adaptations, depending on the molecular context.

Therefore, from a theoretical point of view, a muscle fiber does not necessarily have to have been activated in principle in order to be able to adapt to an unknown degree. Propagation effects can also occur with microtrauma: As explained in Sect. 8.1, microtrauma increases the permeability of the cell membrane of muscle fibers. This allows signalling molecules (known as cytokines or growth factors) to pass from the inside of a fiber to the outside, where they can act on neighbouring cells (e.g. satellite cells or other muscle fibers) in the immediate vicinity. This type of signal transmission is also referred to as paracrine signal transmission. The satellite cells in particular are activated, among other things, by such cytokines released by the injured muscle fiber. But also in the neighbouring, not directly activated muscle fibers, the binding of these signal molecules to receptors on the cell membrane can lead to the triggering of signal transduction cascades, which result in structural and/or metabolic adaptations.

In summary, this means that the experienced training stimulus can vary locally depending on the type and degree of stress or is not fully homogeneous. As a consequence, the adaptations to this training stimulus acting on the intramuscular site can also be heterogeneous to a certain degree. For example, it is known from experiments with cats that the cross-section of a muscle fiber can vary along its length.

So it stands to reason that if, in the example of the biceps muscle, you only train exactly one anatomical function with more or less always the same force vectors in the muscle, the externally visible adaptations (locally different size/length and therefore shape) will also tend to be specific. The problem starts where experts and gurus would have you believe that there is a magic exercise for every conceivable muscle that will result in the desired sculpting for all of them. Forget it. Each of us has learned throughout our development to use his/her muscles in a certain way. So if doing exercise X correlates with effects X in one person, that doesn't mean there is a causal relationship between exercise and effect that applies to everyone. You have to find out for yourself which exercises or exercise executions literally "set your muscles on fire" during training and where the muscle soreness is felt depending on the exercise.

## 9.18 Summary

In a narrow sense, the size principle of motor unit recruitment states that motor neurons are recruited in the order of their recruitment threshold. The recruitment of each motor unit requires that the excitatory postsynaptic potential evoked by excitation of the respective motoneuron exceeds its individual threshold potential for recruitment. Accordingly, all influences that lead to an increase in the excitatory postsynaptic potential and/or to a decrease in the threshold potential favor the recruitment of the corresponding motor unit. In this context, the excitatory postsynaptic potential is directly proportional to the synaptic input current, i.e., the voluntary effort, and inversely proportional to the size of the cell body of the corresponding motor neuron. In other words, the excitatory postsynaptic potential increases with increasing input current and/or decreasing cell body surface area (see Fig. 9.3). Large motor units, or motoneurons with a large cell body, are thus recruited only when either the neuronal excitatory strength (i.e., motor drive) increases and/or the threshold potential is reduced (Fig. 9.11).

From the analogy between the gradual adjustment of the brightness of a theatre stage and the gradual adjustment of muscle force (see Sect. 4.2), it follows that switching on lamps to increase brightness corresponds to the process of increasing force via the recruitment of additional motor units. If we now refine this analogy, the following applies: The dimmable light switches of the large stage lamps (≈ cell body of the large motor units) are harder to operate, or they have a larger switch pressure (≈ recruitment threshold potential), than those of the small stage lamps. Turning on the dimmable light switches in the control room is done as a function of the severity of their operability, i.e., the easy-to-operate light switches are turned on first, followed by the hard-to-operate ones. Finally, you have two options in the control room to turn on more and larger lights: You increase the effort with which you generally press all dimmable light switches (≈ increase in neural excitability) and/or you use a technical trick to decrease the switch pressure (≈ recruitment threshold potential) required to turn on the lamps.

In training practice, you can influence these two factors, and therefore the recruitment and number of muscle fibers used, by using at least three recruitment strategies: The amount of force, the degree of fatigue, and the rate of force development. You will learn how to use these recruitment strategies

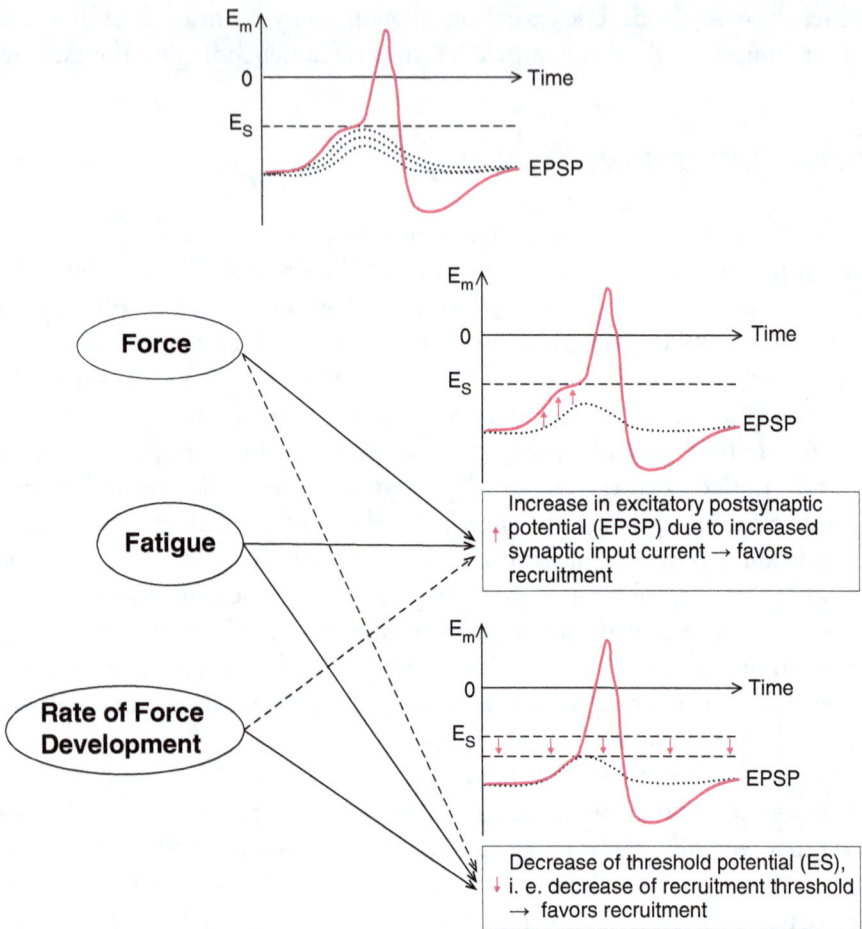

**Fig. 9.11** Mechanisms (EPSP and $E_s$) and strategies for motor unit recruitment during exercise (level of force, fatigue, and rate of force development)

individually or in combination in Chap. 13, but always be aware that the recruitment of motor units within a skeletal muscle must be understood at the neuromuscular compartment level: If only one of several neuromuscular compartments is activated during an exercise, the recruitment principle ("from small to large") applies to all motor units within that neuromuscular compartment. Once multiple neuromuscular compartments are engaged simultaneously, the recruitment principle applies to the totality of motor units in the activated neuromuscular compartments. Conceptually, this can be thought of as forming a single compartment from the motor units in the different neuromuscular compartments in this case, and listing the motor units in order of size "from small to large." The order of recruitment then corresponds to the order of this listing.

The existence of neuromuscular compartments is relevant in practice because the specific use of these neuromuscular compartments depends on the required movement function of the muscle. For example, the biceps muscle not only has the task or function of flexing the arm, but also of rotating the wrist outward or lifting the arm forward when the arm is flexed. If, for example, you perform the biceps curl with the wrist turned inwards (i.e. with the back of the hand facing the ceiling), the muscle fibers of the biceps muscle that are only used for the outward rotation of the hand will not be trained. The reason for this is that the neuromuscular compartment required for this function is virtually "switched off" during this exercise. As a consequence, the strain on the so-called brachialis muscle, which is located below the biceps muscle, increases. However, a muscle grows most strongly in its entirety if all its individual components, i.e. its muscle fibers, grow to the maximum possible extent and the upper arm circumference grows most strongly if each upper arm muscle (e.g. biceps, triceps, brachialis etc.) is trained in accordance with these guidelines. In conclusion, it is therefore recommended that you train those muscles that have different movement functions with different exercises accordingly, i.e. perform several, functionally different exercises per muscle.

# 10

# When Resistance Training Meets Muscle Plasticity

## 10.1 How Do Muscles Adapt To Resistance Training?

Resistance training generally leads to adaptations along the entire neuromuscular axis, that is, from the central nervous system to the muscle fiber. I will discuss here primarily those adaptations in the muscles or muscle fibers and the motor neurons that are related to increasing muscle mass and strength. At the individual muscle fiber level, most studies have shown that resistance training (understood as a general classification of training activity) results in muscle fiber hypertrophy and a change in muscle fiber type. Box 8.4 explains that muscle fiber hypertrophy is defined by an increase in muscle fiber volume (i.e. it is independent of whether there is an increase in the number of nuclei and therefore DNA content within the same fiber).

However, we are primarily interested in muscle fiber hypertrophy in the narrower sense, which results from an increase in intracellular protein content. Resistance training results in an increase in myofibrillar protein mass, which leads to an increase in muscle mass. In principle, there are two possible mechanisms for increasing myofibrillar protein mass, which act individually or in combination:

- Increase in protein synthesis rate (i.e. increase in translation or translation efficiency; see Boxes 8.3 and 8.4) in muscle at the same degradation rate.
- Increase in the number of cell nuclei through fusion with satellite cells and thus increased transcription rate (see Box 8.4).

In the long term, therefore, the extent of muscle fiber hypertrophy depends on the abilities to respond to resistance training stimuli with strong activation of translation and strong activation, proliferation, replenishment, and fusion of satellite cells. The actual muscle hypertrophy is then the summed adaptation of all muscle fibers.

Since a muscle fiber can be roughly approximated as a cylinder (volume equals length times cross-sectional area), there are three ways for a muscle fiber to hypertrophy (see Box 8.4):

- Increase in length with constant cross-sectional area (longitudinal hypertrophy)
- Increase in cross-sectional area with constant length (radial hypertrophy)
- simultaneous increase in length and cross-section (longitudinal and radial hypertrophy)

## 10.2 Length Adaptation (Longitudinal Hypertrophy or Atrophy) in Animals and Humans

In longitudinal fiber hypertrophy, the sarcomeres are incorporated lengthwise, that is, in series, and the myofibrils gain length. The average sarcomere length remains the same or decreases slightly. In longitudinal fiber atrophy, the number of sarcomeres decreases in series, with the average sarcomere length remaining unchanged.

It is obvious that in addition to thickness growth, there is also length growth of muscles. It is obvious that your muscles (like your bones) are longer today than they were at the time of your birth, and it is usually obvious that the longer muscle-tendon unit is not simply the result of a greatly lengthened tendon, but also of a growth in the length of the muscle. But does length growth also occur in adult humans? If so, does it really happen by addition of sarcomeres in series, does this apply to all muscles and in response to which (training) stimuli?

**What Happens with Chronic Passive Stretching or Shortening of Animal Muscles?**
Let me first go back to the origin of the first experiments on the subject, which were conducted in the early 1970s by Pamela Williams and Geoffrey Goldspink (Williams and Goldspink 1971, 1973). The two muscle cell

biologists studied the effect of chronic, passive (i.e., the muscle does not produce any force in the process) stretching on the muscles of mice. The two researchers immobilized the ankle of the mice for 4 weeks in such a way that the soleus muscle (the muscle located under the gastrocnemius muscle) was fully stretched, and measured the resulting change in the number of sarcomeres in series along the entire muscle.

The change was impressive: the number of serial sarcomeres increased by about 20% in the relatively short period of time, so that the average "resting" sarcomere length in the stretched muscle was about the same as that in the normal, untreated muscle. Please note the sequence of events that must have occurred to achieve this result: The muscle-tendon unit of the soleus muscle was stretched as a result of immobilizing the ankle in dorsiflexion (the top of the foot was brought toward the tibia). This stretched all structures, including the individual sarcomeres. In the next step, the muscle registered this deviation (in this case, increase) in sarcomere length from the "resting" sarcomere length and produced new sarcomeres to shorten the length of the stretched sarcomeres back to normal.

In a similar experiment, the researchers immobilized the soleus muscle in a fully shortened position (ankle in plantar flexion). The result was that the number of sarcomeres in series decreased by 40% during the four-week immobilization period. The length-tension relationship (see Fig. 3.1a) for the immobilized muscles was also recorded, i.e. at which muscle length which tetanic tension could be generated. It was found that the maximum tetanic tension occurred at the muscle length corresponding to the muscle length during immobilization. The conclusion from these results, which is widely supported in basic research, is that muscles can change the number of serial sarcomeres as a result of chronic stretching and that this occurs in such a way that in the usual joint position (in the case of the soleus muscle: large joint angle = shortening, small joint angle = stretching) the sarcomeres have a length that is optimal for force production (Fig. 2.1b; see also Sect. 2.8).

Finally, it was observed that the muscle immobilized with shortened muscle length was significantly stiffer, that is, more resistant to passive stretching, than the untreated muscle and that this increase in stiffness was accompanied by an increase in collagen content. The described increase in stiffness could represent a protective mechanism to prevent injury in shortened muscles. Incidentally, the control centre for the described adaptation processes very probably lies in the muscle itself, because the outcome of the experiments was the same even with prior removal of the nerve.

Follow-up experiments revealed other important findings. For example, Tabary et al. (1972) showed that the age of the animals had an influence on the change in the number of serial sarcomeres. They immobilized the soleus muscle in young and old rabbits in a stretched position for 18 days and examined the changes in muscle fiber and tendon length. As expected, muscle-tendon unit length increased dramatically in both age groups. Whereas in young rabbits the increase in muscle-tendon unit was due to a decrease in muscle fiber length accompanied by an increase in tendon length, old rabbits increased muscle-tendon unit length solely due to an increase in muscle fiber length. From these experiments, it appeared that depending on the age of the animals, one or the other tissue type (muscle or tendon in this example) was more amenable to length adaptation during a chronic passive stretch. One can now speculate on the significance of these results for children exposed to extreme forms of passive stretching, for example ballet students.

In the experiments described above, where do you think the serial sarcomeres were incorporated into the muscle? Distributed throughout the muscle or in very specific locations? The answer is that most sarcomeres were added at the two ends of the muscle fibers, at the muscle-tendon junction (Williams and Goldspink 1971). That the adaptation occurred primarily at the muscle-tendon junction is interesting in that the mitochondrial content and protein synthesis rate are greater there than in the rest of the muscle. In addition, we saw in Sect. 8.3 that there are also more satellite cells at the ends of the muscle fibers.

It is clear from the animal experiments described that immobilisation leads to muscle atrophy when the muscle length is short. This can be problematic, because after accidents and/or operations it may be necessary to immobilize individual muscles with a cast in a shortened position. Could the atrophy be reduced or at least attenuated if the muscle were passively stretched per day? Pamela Williams investigated this very question when she repeated the immobilization experiments on mice described above. Again, she immobilized the muscles at short muscle length, only she removed the cast daily for 0.25, 0.5, 1, or 2 h, during which time she slowly moved the muscle passively through its entire *range of motion* (ROM). It was found that with only 0.5 h of passive movement or stretching per day, the decrease in ROM and the number of serial sarcomeres could be prevented (Williams 1988). Even 0.25 h per day was better than no passive exercise at all. It was also shown that there was a strong correlation between the potential ROM in the joint and the number of serial sarcomeres, suggesting that the changes in ROM were due to changes in the muscle and not just the connective tissue and tendons. Finally, it has been shown in other experiments that intermittent passive motion over all ROM and/or all muscle activity prevents an increase in muscle collagen content.

However, the adaptations described above do not necessarily occur according to rules that are valid for all muscle types and species. Spector et al. (1982) were able to reproduce the results in the rat qualitatively (for the direction of the changes) for the soleus and gastrocnemius muscles, but the tibialis anterior muscle showed virtually no response to immobilization in a lengthened or shorted position. This muscle-specific adaptation of leg muscles is often attempted to be explained by their functional role. Thus, it is speculated that the muscles belonging to the postural musculature, such as the soleus and gastrocnemius muscles, are more plastic, i.e. more amenable to adaptation, than muscles that are used less frequently. No experimental data are available on the muscles of the upper extremity.

**The Length Adaptation is in the Service of the Optimal Sarcomere Length**
Why don't muscles simply lengthen during chronic passive stretching by extending their sarcomeres in length rather than increasing their number in series? The answer is that, from a mechanical point of view, it makes sense for the sarcomeres to operate close to or at the plateau of their length-force relationship (Fig. 2.1b; see also Sect. 2.8.3), because at this length their force is maximal. From a control point of view, it makes sense for the sarcomeres to be active on the ascending branch of the length-force relationship because they are naturally more mechanically stable there. On the other hand, it seems to make less sense if the sarcomeres operate on the descending branch of the length-force relationship, because it has been postulated that sarcomeres on this part of the curve become mechanically more unstable with increasing length (see Sect. 7.4).

In summary, it is therefore conclusive that primarily the length of the individual sarcomeres is controlled, that is, the lengthening of a fascicle is achieved by the addition of sarcomeres of approximately equal length and not by stretching the existing sarcomeres. The latter would reduce the mechanical stability of the muscle. In fact, most muscles operate at a stereotypical sarcomere length, which is controlled. This is evidenced by the fact that the number of serial sarcomeres in a given muscle is very consistent for similarly sized individuals or animals of the same species and is a very plastic and tightly regulated quantity (Burkholer and Lieber 2001).

Thus, the scientific data strongly supports the simplifying assumption that muscle length adapts to strain such that sarcomeres operate at optimal length, that is, at or near the plateau of the length-force relationship. At the optimal length, the filament overlap is optimal and the resulting force is maximal. An analysis of 36 independent studies of 52 different muscles from eight different species (including humans) showed, as a first approximation to the subject, that a typical muscle operates at 94 ± 13% of the optimal sarcomere length (Burkholder and Lieber 2001). As expected, this range covers a substantial portion of the ascending branch, the plateau, and a small portion of the descending branch of the length-force relationship. Projected onto the curve, the span is therefore not centred, but shifted a little to the left towards the ascending branch.

It is important to understand that a muscle adapts its length by addition and subtraction of serial sarcomeres to the current demand (training or inactivity, etc.). If only muscle performance is required, then all adaptations will be aligned with this. However, if joint stability or fixation is the primary concern, the musculoskeletal system will adapt to this, even at the expense of producible muscle performance.

What are the functional consequences of adjusting fiber length in humans? If muscle fiber length increases by increasing the number of serial sarcomeres, then on the one hand the rate of length change (e.g., maximal unloaded shortening velocity) increases, potentially manifesting in an increase in movement speed. On the other hand, ROM increases, provided, of course, that it is not limited by the joint or reduced articulation. In addition, the ability of a muscle fiber to generate force increases with increasing fiber length for any given shortening speed (Fig. 3.1b; see Sect. 3.1).

Finally, a longer fiber may be protective against microtrauma. Why should more sarcomeres in series protect against microtrauma? If you activate two muscle fibers with the same average sarcomere length but different numbers of sarcomeres in series and stretch them the same distance (pliometric activity), the change in length in the fiber with more serial sarcomeres can be accommodated by more sarcomeres, meaning each individual sarcomere is stretched less. The fiber with fewer sarcomeres in series therefore has a greater chance of local microtraumata occurring due to the postulated force and length inhomogeneity according to the *popping sarcomere theory* (see Sect. 7.4).

## Can Human Muscle Be Lengthened by Chronic Passive Stretching?

Or, to put it another way, does chronic passive stretching also lead to adaptation of the number of serial sarcomeres in humans, analogous to the animal model? This question is justified, because we have seen that muscles from other species do not always represent a good model for human muscle (see Box 5.3). As you can imagine, it is extremely difficult and only possible under exceptional circumstances to collect such data experimentally in humans. In rare cases, however, the opportunity presents itself. One such case was described by Richard Lieber's group (Boakes et al. 2007). Specifically, it was the case of a then 16-year-old girl who underwent a procedure to lengthen her right femur by 4 cm. This procedure, called bone distraction, was performed to correct a severe imbalance in leg lengths that had developed due to a previous fracture in the growth plate of the right femur.

Generally, this surgical measure is used to lengthen bones by up to 20 cm. Among the reasons that make such a procedure necessary are, for example, developmental disorders or traumatic diseases that lead to a strong lateral difference in the length of bones in the lower and upper body. Bone lengthening is assisted by a device that is inserted into the bone marrow, lengthens itself at a certain rate by a certain distance during the distraction phase (in the case described, about 0.5 mm per day and by a total of 4 cm, which corresponded to a bone lengthening of 10%) and thus pushes the bone apart in the longitudinal direction.

In the case described, the researchers determined the sarcomere lengths in the vastus lateralis muscle intraoperatively (i.e. during surgery) when the distraction device was inserted and also when it was removed 12 months later, using a special technique (measuring the diffraction of laser beams). In addition, they used ultrasound to determine the fascicle length of the vastus lateralis muscle before, during, and after the 3-month distraction phase and 9 months after the subsequent consolidation phase. Keep in mind that fascicle or muscle fiber length is equivalent to muscle length only in spindle-formed muscles (Fig. 3.3). The results clearly showed that fascicle length had increased from 9.1 to 19 cm(!) during the distraction phase and then remained unchanged or stable during the consolidation phase (i.e., during bone healing or distraction osteogenesis) (it was 18 cm at the end of the consolidation phase). By now, it should be clear to you that this result is not yet evidence of specific adaptations such as an increase in the number of sarcomeres in series. Indeed, one possible explanation for the increase in fascicle length would simply be that the individual sarcomeres were stretched and remained in that stretched position. A second option would be that the fascicles became longer by adding new sarcomeres in series, as we know from animal experiments. However, thanks to intraoperative measurement of sarcomere lengths by laser diffraction, this point could be elucidated.

The average sarcomere length in the vastus lateralis muscle of the girl decreased from 3.64 to 3.11 µm over the 12 months. The number of serial sarcomeres can now be calculated from the fascicle length divided by the average sarcomere length. Consequently, the number of serial sarcomeres increased

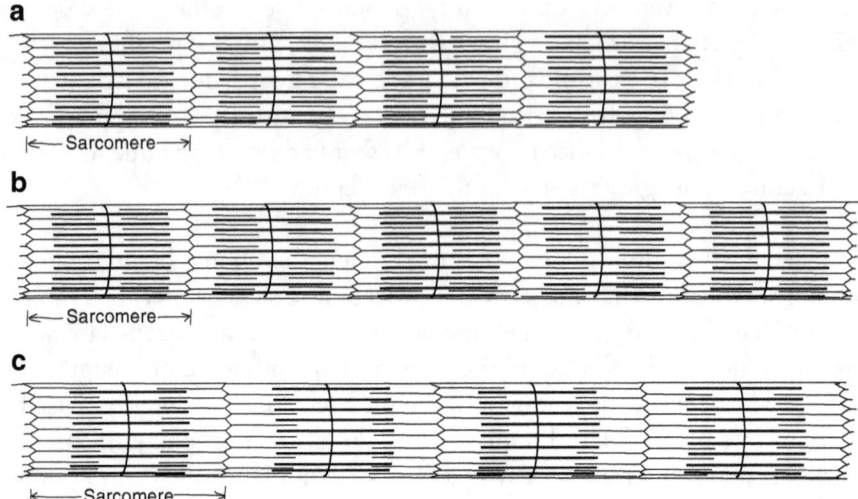

**Fig. 10.1** Fascicle length increase with chronic passive stretching. Fascicle length, given by the number and length of individual sarcomeres, can in principle increase from baseline (**a**) if either the number of sarcomeres in series (**b**) and/or the average sarcomere length increases (**c**). Under physiological conditions, (**b**) is the predominant mechanism because a muscle adjusts its length via the addition or subtraction of sarcomeres in series such that the individual sarcomeres can operate near the plateau of their length-force relationship. This optimizes the mechanical output for the typical length stress, which can be specific depending on the sport or activity pattern

from an initial 25,000 (9.1 cm/3.64 µm) to 58,650 (18 cm/3.11 µm). Broken down to a day, this corresponded to a daily synthesis or incorporation of approximately 350 serial sarcomeres. In this case, the number of serial sarcomeres increased more than enough to compensate for the change in bone length during the three-month distraction phase and the subsequent nine-month consolidation phase by chronic passive stretching. These data show unequivocally and definitively that in humans the number of serial sarcomeres *can* increase in response to chronic passive stretching (Fig. 10.1) (Box 10.1).

> **Box 10.1: Muscle Lengthening Through Passive Stretching?**
> The data from animal and human experiments are clear: The number of serial sarcomeres *can* increase in response to chronic passive stretching as a function of muscle type and age. But do these experimental results translate to real-world conditions in humans? Can they be extrapolated to measures such as stretching, flexibility training and massage? Probably not, or only with great caution. We have seen that the passive stretching stimuli applied in the animal and human experiments described above (passive stretching for practically 24 h per day for

several weeks) were extreme. It is therefore hard to imagine that a person who has to eat, sleep and do a few other things during the day in addition to training can achieve these changes. Perhaps such an adaptation is possible in professional ballet dancers or circus performers who do several hours of passive stretching a day from an early age, but hardly in the average person. In any case, this evidence would still have to be provided.

The situation is therefore similar to the discussed case of increasing the number of type 1 fibers with training (more precisely the controversial conversion of type 2 to type 1 fibers; see Sect. 5.5). There, too, it is possible in rabbits to achieve a change in muscle fiber type from type 2 to type 1 fibers with 24 hours of electrical stimulation per day. Even if a human muscle could be stimulated analogously, it would probably take even longer to effect such a transformation. Even in the case of fiber type transition, however, it is conceivable that the extreme training programs (many hours per day for several years) of professional cyclists, triathletes, etc. could lead to such adaptations. But again, scientific evidence is lacking. Nevertheless, this does not exclude the possibility that novel or combined training stimuli, which have not yet been investigated at all, could lead to such adaptations.

**From Electrically Stimulated Rabbit Muscles to Rats on a Treadmill**
It is well known that muscle force production can be mio-, iso- or pliometric (see Sect. 1.5). All three forms of force production can take place at different muscle lengths. For example, you can use your muscles isometrically for several seconds in a fully stretched or shortened position. Or you may start a miometric action from a long/short muscle length. Or you pliometrically lower a load to full muscle stretch or stop before. Of course, there are several combination variations.

The impressive effectiveness of the combination of stretching and force production was demonstrated in an experiment in which the tibialis anterior muscle of rabbits was stretched and electrically stimulated continuously for 4 days (Williams et al. 1986). It was shown that the muscle fibers or muscles became about 11% longer during these 4 days (from about 52 to about 60 mm) and that this was due to the addition of more than 2000 serial sarcomeres (from a total of about 18,000 to 20,600). They also had rats run on a treadmill either uphill (miometric force production) or downhill (pliometric force production) and then measured the adaptations in the number of serial sarcomeres as well as the shift in the maximum of the length-tension relationship (= indirect indicator of length adaptation). In one study, rats were trained either miometrically or pliometrically for 15–30 min daily on a treadmill for one week. Based on an average number of serial sarcomeres of 3259 in the vastus intermedius muscle, running downhill resulted in an increase to 3526 serial sarcomeres in just one week, whereas running uphill resulted in a decrease to 3140 serial sarcomeres (Lynn and Morgan 1994). If the group running uphill continued training for a further 2 weeks, the number of serial sarcomeres no longer changed, i.e. it had already adjusted to the new functional requirements after one week and conserved this state as long as the stimulus was applied.

Parallel to the increase (downhill race) or decrease (uphill race) in the number of serial sarcomeres, the maximum of the angle-torque relationship also shifted towards a longer (downhill race) or shorter (uphill race) muscle-tendon unit. In other words, the highest torque was measured after the one-week training period (15–30 min per day) in the case of downhill racing at an angular position corresponding to a longer muscle-tendon unit (and vice versa for uphill racing; Lynn et al. 1998). Through these results, the idea emerged that the mode of force production was crucial for the adaptation of the number of serial sarcomeres. More specifically, the hypothesis stated that (only) pliometric muscle actions would lead to length adaptation. However, the results of Pamela Williams presented above, according to which serial sarcomere addition followed isometric force production at large muscle length, impressively demonstrate that it does not necessarily have to be pliometric force production. Other animal studies (e.g., by Koh and Herzog 1998) also argue that the absolute muscle length or length excursion at which force is produced is a primary stimulus for length adaptation.

**Resistance Training and Fascicle Length Adaptation in Humans: Do You Pay Enough Attention to Force Production with Great Muscle Lengths?**
In summary, the relationship between mechanical forces (passive and/or active) and muscle length can be understood as a control loop with negative feedback. In this control loop, sensors (the controllers) inside the muscle fibers record the sarcomere deformation and analyze it in terms of a comparison between the actual value (controlled variable) and the setpoint value (command variable). The setpoint corresponds to the optimal sarcomere length. The controller responds to deviations of the actual value from the setpoint via actuators (molecular and cellular mechanisms of protein synthesis and degradation; see Box 8.3 and Chap. 11) by adjusting the manipulated variable (number of sarcomeres in series), which returns the actual value to the setpoint. The deformation of the sarcomeres thus represents the controlled variable in this system, which is kept constant (Box 10.2).

### Box 10.2: A Muscle Protein as the Backbone of the Sarcomere

The muscle protein titin is the largest known protein in the human body with a molecular mass between 3000 and 3800 kDa. Titin filaments are extremely long, up to 1.5 μm in length. They are anchored to the Z-disk at their $NH_2$-terminal end and extend from there to the M-stripe. Titin exhibits two structurally and functionally distinct regions. The elastic I-strip titin, which is composed of immunoglobulin-like domains, and the PEVK region, which consists mainly of the four amino acids proline (P), glutamic acid (E), valine (V), and lysine (K). At the COOH-terminal end, just upstream of the M-line, is the titin kinase domain. Both the elastic I-band titin and the PEVK domain vary in length in different muscles and muscle fibers, respectively. Titin, like actin and myosin, occurs in muscle type-specific isoforms.

One of the best known mechanical functions of titin is that of a molecular spring. The elastic I-band region of titin contains serially linked molecular elements that behave like entropic springs with different bending stiffness. During sarcomere stretching, these elements stretch sequentially. The elastic force generated by titin molecules during passive stretch is responsible for approximately 50% of the total passive tension in skeletal muscle. The remaining 50% is generated during stretching of the extracellular collagen network. Furthermore, passive stiffness as well as viscoelasticity in non-activated striated muscle can be partially attributed to titin. The mechanical properties just described depend on the specific titin isoform. Training, disease, etc. may cause transformation of isoforms in cardiac and skeletal muscle (similar to the transformation of MyHC isoforms in skeletal muscle), which may have functional effects.

However, titin not only plays an important role in the structural organization of the sarcomere. It also performs the function of an intracellular length and force sensor. In this function, it detects mechanical forces, especially when stretched, integrates the different signals in the style of a network node, and translates the integrated signal into a molecular response to adapt to the stress (e.g. by phosphorylating other proteins). Thus, the titin molecule is associated with over 20 different proteins that are involved in signaling cascades related to hypertrophy, protein folding, or protein degradation, among others. Conversely, the titin molecule can be phosphorylated by intracellular kinases. Activation of such kinases occurs through signals arriving at the muscle fiber cell membrane and being transmitted to the kinases. Phosphorylation of titin not only changes the mechanical properties (stiffness) of the molecule during passive stretching, but also its role in signal transduction.

Assuming that under normal conditions a muscle strives to regulate the number of sarcomeres in series so that sarcomere lengths are optimally adjusted for typical ROM (varying with use/training), fascicle length is a surrogate for the number of sarcomeres in series. The longer the fascicles, the more serial sarcomeres. Another functional surrogate, as mentioned above, is the angular position at which the measured torque is highest. For example, if the specific joint angle increases with training, this probably indicates length growth, despite all the difficulties of the measurement method (see Sect. 2.8, discussion on the force-length curve).

Using ultrasound, it has been demonstrated in various human studies that resistance training can lead to a marked increase in fascicle length, both in young (Blazevich et al. 2007; Seynnes et al. 2007) and old individuals (Reeves et al. 2004). Analogous to the animal model, the question arises as to which stimulus is responsible in these cases of length adaptation. Is it stretch when the muscle is activated and/or force production when the muscle length is great (or greater than usual)? Anthony Blazevich and colleagues investigated this question. They trained young men and women for 10 weeks on a dynamometer. Resistance training was performed three times per week, with at least one day off between each training session. During these sessions, the study participants performed either a series of positive (i.e., miometric) or negative (i.e., pliometric) knee extensions.

Subjects were instructed to perform the movements explosively and with maximum effort. However, the device was set so that the angular velocity was constant and rather slow at $30°s^{-1}$ (i.e., it took approximately 3 s to traverse a knee joint angle of 90°). Very importantly, all study participants trained through a knee joint ROM of 95–100° regardless of force production mode (miometric or pliometric). This ROM is substantially greater than that for walking (~25°), jogging (~55°), or jumping (two-legged jump with countermovement: ~80°), but only slightly greater than the usual ROM for stair climbing (~88° for a staircase with steps 25.5 cm high; Blazevich et al. 2007). In any case, the muscles of the study participants were used over a greater muscle length than usual during training.

One result of the study (in addition to the expected increase in peak torque and muscle cross-section) was that the fascicle length of the vastus lateralis increased by approx. 3.1 (pliometric training) and 6.3% (miometric training) in the 10 weeks, depending on the group (Blazevich et al. 2007). Based on a mean fascicle length of approximately 7.6 cm (with a muscle length of approximately 25 cm), this corresponded to an increase in fascicle length of approximately 0.25–0.5 cm. The difference between the two groups was not statistically significant. For comparison: In the extreme example of bone distraction (see Sect. 10.2.3), the fascicle length increased by more than 100% in 3 months (from approx. 9 to 19 cm). Proportionally to the measured increase in fascicle length, the degree of angle in the knee joint at which peak torque was reached also increased. Thus, if the percentage increase in fascicle length was approximately 5%, the peak torque also occurred at an angular position in the knee joint that was shifted by 5% (in the direction of flexion, i.e. stretching of the vastus lateralis muscle).

Based on the result that both groups were able to increase the fascicle length of the vastus lateralis muscle, the researchers concluded that ROM (i.e., the length excursion of the muscle during exercise performance) was more critical than the force production mode (in this case, mio- or pliometric) for increasing fascicle length. Although further studies are needed to definitively address this question, data from animal and human studies suggest that exercise ROM, or the length of the muscle during force production, may play an important role in length adaptation. It is important to understand that "long" actually means "longer than usual". So, for example, if you regularly climb stairs (~88° ROM in the knee joint per step, see above) and then participate in a resistance training study with a ROM of 90°, then length adaptation in the vastus lateralis muscle is not expected (what's the point?). However, if you typically only stress this muscle to a ROM of 80° maximum (as in the two-legged jump with a countermovement), then you would be expected to experience an increase in fascicle length during the resistance training study (with 90° ROM).

Caution should therefore be exercised when interpreting study results and making generalizations: Fascicle length and thus number of sarcomeres in series may indeed increase in adult humans with training. However, whether and to what extent this can happen seems to depend on the "interfering signal". If you regularly produce force in training at a greater than usual muscle length (with a greater than usual ROM), the chances are good, at least for the vastus lateralis muscle, that length adaptation will occur. Conversely, studies that have failed to demonstrate an increase in fascicle length and/or angle-torque relationship with resistance training are not *a priori* evidence that length adaptation will fail to occur. If the selected training ROM is (too) small relative to the usual ROM of the study participants or if the relative stretch is too low, length adaptation is not to be expected.

Another aspect in this context that must also be taken into account is that the changes in the length of the muscle-tendon unit during training do not necessarily correspond to the changes in the length of the muscle. For example, in the case of the bipedal jump with a countermovement, we have seen that during the lowering phase the length of the muscle-tendon unit of the quadriceps femoris increases, with the length of the fascicle decreasing and the length of the tendon increasing (see Sect. 1.4). Therefore, in certain areas of the ROM, force production may be miometric, although the muscle-tendon unit behaves pliometrically. This could also be a reason why length adaptation was not demonstrated in all studies in which pliometrically oriented resistance training was completed. Fascicle length adaptation has also been associated with movement speed in resistance training. However, given that the adaptations described in the study by Blazevich et al. (2007) were achieved with a relatively slow movement speed (3 s for a ROM of 90°), the importance of movement speed seems to be of secondary importance.

In summary, the research results obtained in humans indicate that for training-induced length adaptation in adult humans, muscle fibers must produce force at a long length, i.e. in a stretched state, and/or pliometrically during training. "Long" in this context means "longer than usual", where "usual" again depends on the activity or training habits of the individual. The actual length change of activated muscle fibers seems to be more decisive than the length change of the muscle-tendon unit: even during mio- or isometric action of the muscle-tendon unit, individual muscle fibers can behave pliometrically. This data is compatible with the *popping sarcomere theory* discussed in Sect. 7.4, according to which it is not the magnitude of the external force but the extent of sarcomere stretching during pliometric force production by the muscle fiber that is responsible for the occurrence of microtrauma. The molecular and cellular processes thus set in motion could specifically lead to longitudinal hypertrophy.

The aspect of the specificity of hypertrophy is noteworthy. In both radial and longitudinal hypertrophy, the muscle produces more protein than it breaks down; in the former case, the protein or sarcomeres are incorporated in parallel, in the latter case serially. Since longitudinal hypertrophy can theoretically occur without concomitant radial hypertrophy, the acquisition and translation of the mechanical stimulus into structural adaptation must be very specific. While there is good evidence of length growth for the vastus lateralis muscle in humans (both young adults and seniors), it is unclear whether and to what extent such changes are possible in other muscles or muscle types. In addition, the results obtained in adults cannot be easily transferred to children, in whom, firstly, the length growth of the bones in interaction with the muscles is not yet complete and, secondly, other adaptations may occur due to the different malleability or adaptability of the tissues involved (compare the above-mentioned tendon lengthening instead of longitudinal hypertrophy in young animals during chronic passive stretching).

**Practical Guide to Length Adaptation Through Training**
How often the muscle should be stretched to a long length during force production, i.e. how many repetitions are required and/or how long the resistance should be held in the stretched position and/or how high the resistance must be in the process in order to trigger the adaptations described, is largely unknown. In the study by Blazevich et al. (2007) described above, 24–36 repetitions were performed per training session (three times per week for 10

weeks). Considering that the duration of one repetition was approximately 3.3 s (for a ROM of 100°), only a fraction of this duration (approximately 0.4 s) was spent per repetition on angular degrees above 88° (corresponding to the stretch the muscle experiences when climbing stairs; 100° = full knee flexion and thus stretching of the vastus lateralis muscle). Multiplying the number of repetitions by the duration at a ROM above 88° gives a total duration of tension at an unusually long muscle length of 9.6 (24 repetitions times 0.4 s per repetition) or 14.4 s (36 repetitions times 0.4 s per repetition).

These values can be used as a guide for resistance training: Per workout, active stretching with as much muscle length as possible (it must be longer than usual) for a total of about 12 s per muscle or per muscle function should be sufficient to induce length adaptation. You can elegantly incorporate active stretching by holding tension isometrically for 2 s while performing the exercise in the inverse position between flexion and extension. For example, if you can do 6 reps, that's at least 12 s in the stretched position. Alternatively, you can simply choose an appropriate training resistance, move into the fully stretched position, and hold the resistance until exhaustion, but for a minimum of 12 s. Incidentally, isometric muscle use at the reversal points described above also has the advantage of taking the momentum out of your movements (see Sect. 1.13) (Box 10.3).

---

**Box 10.3: Muscle Lengthening in Adults Through (Strength) Training?**

A common doctrine is that resistance training generally leads to shortened muscles and that the trained muscles must therefore be stretched immediately after the exercise performed or at the end of the program. This doctrine is scientifically untenable: firstly, because it would first be necessary to clarify what is specifically meant by a "shortened muscle". The fascicle or muscle fiber length, or the muscle length (it's not the same for pennated muscles)? And relative to what length should the muscle be shortened? Second, because with passive stretching under normal conditions, there is no serial addition of sarcomeres and thus no longitudinal hypertrophy. Third, because the opposite is more likely to be true, assuming you stress your muscles during training even at fullest stretch.

Resistance training has been shown to increase fascicle length (and thus the number of sarcomeres in series) in certain muscles in adult humans, for example the vastus lateralis muscle. An effective stimulus for length adaptation appears to be force production at relatively long muscle length. "Relatively long" in this context means "at a greater length than usual". Or more precisely, in practice you cannot directly control the muscle fiber or fascicle length, only the joint angle or *range of motion* (ROM). "Relatively long" therefore means that the ROM is greater than usual, which in turn is associated with greater muscle length.

> As discussed in Sect. 2.8.3, muscles adapt the number of serial sarcomeres to the load in such a way that their sarcomeres operate at optimal length, i.e. at or near the plateau of the length-force relationship. If you now stress muscles in resistance training at a greater muscle length (over a greater ROM) than is usually the case in your everyday life, you can expect longitudinal hypertrophy and an increase in mobility. However, the extent of length adaptation possible depends on the initial length. The shorter (relatively speaking) the muscle fibers are at the start of training, the greater the effects achieved are likely to be. In general, however, the effects achieved on fascicle length are rather modest and range from approx. 3–10% with three resistance training sessions per week over 5–10 weeks, depending on the initial length or ROM. In terms of absolute fascicle length (approx. 7 cm) in the vastus lateralis muscle, this means an increase in the range of a few millimeters. It is unclear to what extent the scientific evidence of longitudinal hypertrophy in the vastus lateralis muscle can be generalised to other muscles or muscle groups in the body.
>
> Whether the muscle-tendon unit is mio-, iso- or pliometrically active in the stretched position seems to be less important for triggering the adaptation than the effective length of the muscle fibers producing the force. In terms of length adaptation or building and maintaining flexibility, you can elegantly incorporate stretching under tension into your training. For example, if you are training the biceps muscle, focus on the reversal point between extension and flexion in the elbow joint. In the position of extension or maximum stretch of the biceps muscle, hold the tension isometrically for 2 s before slowly starting the new repetition from this position. Thus, for 6 repetitions performed, you will arrive at a minimum of 12 s of tension duration in the stretched position, which is roughly consistent with the tension duration achieved in the studies described. Alternatively, you can simply choose an appropriate training resistance, move into the fully stretched position, and hold the resistance until exhaustion, but for at least 12 s. Finally, you can also perform negative training (see Sect. 1.6 and Box. 1.2), in which you lower a high training resistance (about 140% of the usual load) in a controlled manner and slowly (at least during the first few repetitions). More specifically, you are *trying to* prevent the load from lowering. However, as the external torque exceeds the internal torque, the muscle is stretched during force production (see Box 1.2).

## 10.3 Radial Growth of Muscle (Radial Hypertrophy or Atrophy) in Humans

If the sarcomeres are built up or incorporated in parallel instead of serially and at the same time the number of sarcomeres in series does not decrease, this is called radial hypertrophy (see Box 8.4). Radial hypertrophy, or so-called thickness growth or muscle cross-sectional area increase, is the more familiar concept compared with longitudinal hypertrophy. Muscle cross-sectional area can also increase by parallel addition of sarcomeres if the number of serial sarcomeres decreases at the same time, but hypertrophy (understood as volume increase) is then not necessarily the result. It is a generally accepted fact that thicker muscles and more strength is the logical consequence of resistance training. But is this really the case or is it not rather wishful thinking? In fact, there is a great deal of variability between individuals in terms of the degree of adaptation to resistance training and in terms of both muscle (fiber) cross-section and peak force. But more on this later. Suffice it to say here that the percentage increases in muscle fiber and/or muscle cross-section tend to be greater than those for fascicle length. For example, in young untrained men who exercised their anterior thigh muscles three times per week (e.g., Monday, Wednesday, and Friday) for 4 months using three different exercises (leg extension, leg press, squat) of 3 sets each of 8–12 repetitions, a cross-sectional increase of approximately 22% and 37% on average was measured for type 1 and type 2 muscle fibers, respectively (Bickel et al. 2011). In another large-scale study of untrained individuals, the increase in biceps muscle cross-sectional area after three months of resistance training was approximately 20% (men) and 18% (women). The majority of the muscle protein that is built up during several weeks of resistance training in adults is therefore used to form parallel sarcomeres.

## 10.4 Summary

Every skeletal muscle consists of thousands of cylindrical muscle cells, the muscle fibers. If we consider the simple case of a spindle-shaped muscle, e.g. the biceps muscle, all the muscle fibers run parallel to each other in the longitudinal direction. The fibers in this case therefore run along the axis along which the muscle force is also transmitted to the tendons and bones. Each muscle fiber in turn contains thousands of thin, thread-like protein structures, the myofibrils. You can think of these myofibrils as long trains, each train consisting of a great many wagons (protein complexes) coupled together. The more myofibrils (trains) that run side by side, the larger the cross-sectional area of the corresponding muscle fibers, or the "thicker" the muscle fibers. The more carriages that are coupled lengthwise, the longer the myofibrils and therefore the longer the muscle fibers. The more carriages there are in a muscle fiber, the greater its cell mass or volume (cylinder volume = cross-sectional area of the cylinder multiplied by its height or length). Resistance training in combination with a reasonable protein intake leads to an increase in muscle fiber volume via an increase in protein mass, i.e. symbolically speaking to an increase in the number of carriages inside the muscle fiber. The increase in muscle fiber volume or mass is called muscle fiber hypertrophy. It should be noted that muscle fiber hypertrophy can occur through an increase in the number of myofibrils (trains) within a fiber and/or through an increase in the number of carriages (increase in length of myofibrils). In other words, the carriages (protein complexes) can be installed either parallel to each other and/or one behind the other. The former leads to an increase in cross-section, while the latter leads to an increase in length of the muscle fibers. What normally remains unchanged in adults is the number of muscle fibers. Normally, therefore, training in adults causes no muscle fiber hyperplasia (increase in the number of muscle fibers), or none at all, at least as far as short- to medium-term observation periods are concerned. Muscle hypertrophy, i.e. the increase in volume or mass of an entire muscle, therefore represents the summed muscle fiber hypertrophy in that muscle. The terms "muscle growth" or "increase in muscle mass" are commonly understood to mean only the cross-sectional increase in muscle. However, as just explained, the process of muscle (fiber) hypertrophy includes both thickness growth and length growth. Of course, carriages are also degraded, e.g., by lack of exercise, bedriddenness, disease, etc. In this case, there is a decrease in fiber cross-sectional areas and lengths, which in turn is called muscle fiber atrophy or muscle atrophy.

# 11

# How Is Skeletal Muscle Protein Synthesized and Broken Down?

## 11.1 Building Muscle Protein Mass

In the course of the increase in muscle cross-section or volume, the muscle (protein) mass also increases. But how does muscle growth actually work? Which training stimuli are crucial for radial hypertrophy? What do you have to pay attention to during training? It's not as if you train for a few weeks and suddenly, from one day to the next, out of the blue, you gain 20% muscle mass (contrary to what some experts say, that training-induced muscle growth happens in spurts). The metabolic basis for changes in muscle mass is the net muscle protein balance (NBIL). Muscle proteins, like all other proteins in our bodies, are constantly being synthesized and broken down – even now as you read this text.

The balance between synthesis and breakdown determines the protein content and thus the protein mass in the muscle in the long term. More precisely, changes in muscle mass are due to a change in the balance between the *muscle protein synthesis rate* (MPS) and the *muscle protein breakdown rate* (MPB) of myofibrillar protein. The mass of myofibrillar proteins in relation to the total protein mass of the muscle is much greater than that of mitochondrial or sarcoplasmic proteins, for example (see Box 8.3). Regardless of the time period (seconds to years), the instantaneous amount of muscle protein is thus the result of all changes in the NBIL up to that point (Fig. 11.1).

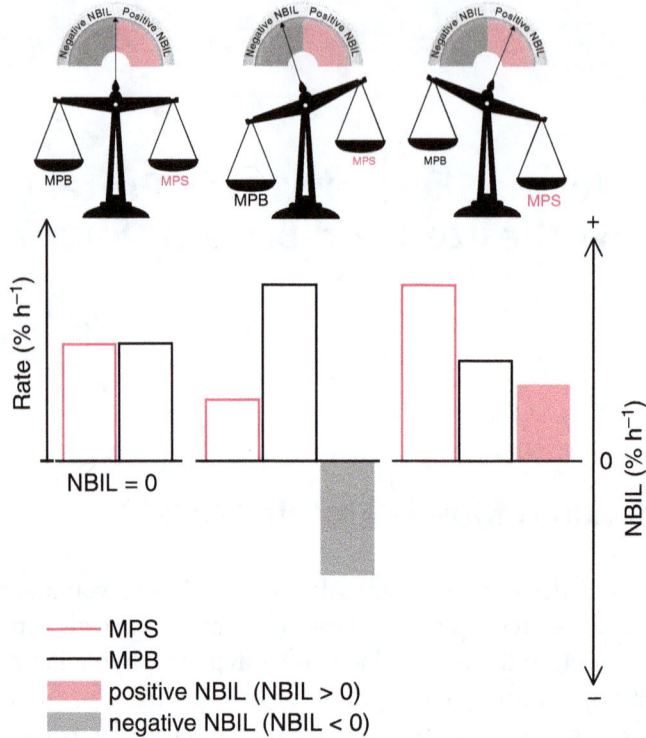

**Fig. 11.1** Net muscle protein balance (NBIL). The NBIL is calculated from the difference between the MPS and the MPB. If the MPS is equal to the MPB in a defined time interval, the NBIL is zero (NBIL = 0), i.e. the muscle protein mass remains unchanged. If the MPS is smaller than the MPB in a defined time interval, then net protein is degraded, the NBIL is then negative by definition (NBIL <0). Conversely, if the MPB is smaller than the MPS, protein mass increases and the NBIL is positive (NBIL >0). Thus, during periods with positive NBIL, muscle protein mass is built up, and during periods with negative NBIL, it is broken down. MPS, muscle protein synthesis rate; MPB, muscle protein breakdown rate

## 11.2 The Relationship Between MPS and MPB

If the MPS is greater than the MPB, there is net protein accumulation and the NBIL is positive by definition. Conversely, if the rate of degradation is greater than the rate of accumulation, there is a decrease in protein mass and the NBIL is negative. Therefore, during temporal periods of positive NBIL, protein mass is synthesized, and during periods of negative NBIL, it is degraded. As we saw in Box 8.3 and Sect. 8.8, more protein can be synthesized per unit time if, first, the translation rate or translation efficiency of mRNA into protein increases and/or, second, more mRNA molecules are available for translation. Since proteins are composed of amino acids, the amount of protein in a protein fraction (e.g., myofibrillar, mitochondrial, sarcoplasmic, etc.) can only increase if more amino acids reach the muscle fiber via the blood or if a remodeling occurs within the muscle fiber (e.g., a partial degradation of protein to amino acids in one protein fraction and use of these amino acids to partially synthesize proteins of another fraction).

Exclusive changes in MPB can never cause a shift from the catabolic (i.e. degrading) to the anabolic (i.e. synthesizing) state. This is because some of the amino acids released by protein degradation are oxidized (i.e., broken down) or transaminated (converted to other amino acids) and thus are no longer available for reincorporation into proteins. On the other hand, MPB is always associated with MPS up to a certain point, because the amino acids released during degradation contribute in part to the pool of intracellular amino acids. The rate at which free amino acids appear inside muscle fibers either through intracellular protein degradation (MPB) or through transport from the blood (i.e., the rate at which the intracellular pool of free amino acids increases) is critical to the increase in MPS.

## 11.3 How Your Muscles Hypertrophy and Atrophy Hourly

If we now look at the daily course of MPS and MPB in a healthy adult and untrained person, we can observe that both values fluctuate regularly starting from their basal value. The fluctuations are in opposite directions, i.e. the MPS is at its highest when the MPB is at its lowest and vice versa. Moreover, the excursions from the individual mean are greater for the MPS than for the MPB (Fig. 11.2). In fact, in healthy untrained individuals, regardless of age and sex, the MPB is a relatively constant quantity that is subject to obligatory fluctuations during the day, but which are smaller compared to the fluctuations of the MPS. Each time the MPS increases during the day and takes on values greater than the MPB (i.e., the NBIL is positive), muscle mass increases by a very small (i.e., macroscopically unmeasurable, much less visible) amount. If the MPS decreases to values lower than those of the MPB, muscle mass decreases infinitesimally (Fig. 11.2). In healthy humans, therefore, fluctuations in NBIL are primarily determined by fluctuations in MPS. In the next chapter I will discuss the reasons for the obligatory fluctuations of MPS and MPB.

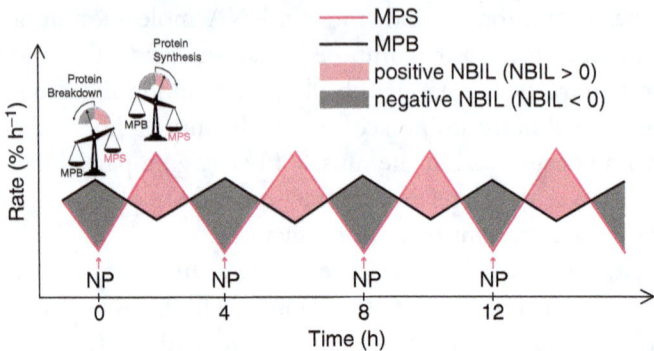

**Fig. 11.2** Variations in the rate of synthesis and breakdown of muscle protein over the course of the day. The rate indicates how much protein is synthesized or broken down in percentage per hour. Note that the MPS shows larger swings than the MPB. At the intersection of the MPS and MPB curves, the instantaneous NBIL is zero. In healthy untrained adults, stimulation of MPS in early and middle adulthood is primarily due to dietary protein or essential amino acid intake. Dietary protein or the essential amino acids it contains provide an anabolic stimulus to skeletal muscle. MPS, muscle protein synthesis rate; MPB, muscle protein breakdown rate; NBIL, net muscle protein balance; NP, dietary protein

## 11.4 Summary

You probably have an account at the bank or post office. If you deposit more money than you withdraw in a certain period of time, money accumulates in your account. The account balance is positive. If you withdraw more money than you deposit in the same period, you lose money. The account balance is then negative. If your goal is to accumulate money, you need to make sure that your net account balance is positive in the long run. Muscle growth works similarly: our muscles are largely made up of proteins (money). These muscle proteins are constantly being synthesized and broken down. Skeletal muscle is thus permanently being remodeled.

To build muscle protein mass, the so-called net protein balance – i.e. the difference between muscle protein build-up ("deposits") and breakdown ("withdrawals") – must be greater than zero over a period of weeks, months, years. You can achieve a positive net protein balance by either increasing muscle protein synthesis relative to breakdown and/or inhibiting muscle protein breakdown relative to synthesis. More specifically, it's about the difference in speed at which proteins are synthesized and broken down. In adult healthy humans, the increase in the rate at which muscle protein is synthesized is primarily why there is a positive net protein balance. This increase in the speed at which protein is synthesized is in turn brought about by two anabolic (building) stimuli, namely strength training and dietary protein. Invest in your health – pay into your muscle account regularly!

# 12

# Dietary Protein as an Anabolic Stimulus

## 12.1 Whole-Body Protein Metabolism Is Not Equal to Muscle Protein Metabolism

The proteins in our body are constantly being rebuilt, i.e. they are constantly being synthesized and broken down. This simultaneous synthesis and breakdown of protein forms the basis for the qualitative and quantitative maintenance of body protein, because "old" and/or damaged proteins must be continuously replaced by new ones in order to ensure protein functions. Protein synthesis and breakdown are influenced by various factors such as age, physical activity or exercise level, gender, hormonal status, disease, and diet. Long-term changes in body protein mass occur due to a chronic imbalance between synthesis and breakdown. Long-term changes in body protein mass are often measured by changes in *lean body mass*, which is determined by *dual energy X-ray absorptiometry* (DXA). However, lean body mass includes everything that is not fat and bone and should therefore not be equated with muscle mass.

With regard to body protein mass, and specifically in the context of muscle protein mass, a basic understanding of the regulation of the rate of synthesis and breakdown of protein in humans is essential. It is important to distinguish between total body protein metabolism and protein metabolism of individual tissues. For example, skeletal muscle contributes only about 25–30% of total body protein synthesis. In addition, skeletal muscle protein turnover at rest is relatively slow at approximately 0.6%/h (i.e., approximately 1.5%/d) compared to protein turnover in the blood (approximately

1–30%/h) or intestine (1–2%/h). Measurements of whole-body protein turnover are therefore poorly representative of skeletal muscle protein anabolism and thus must be interpreted with caution. Thus, acute diet-induced changes in whole-body protein turnover often primarily reflect the much faster protein turnover of intestinal and blood proteins rather than skeletal muscle protein turnover.

Irrespective of the anatomical or subcellular location of the protein fraction under consideration, the ingestion of dietary protein followed by hyperaminoacidemia leads to a transient increase in protein synthesis. This leads transiently, i.e. for about 3–4 h, to a positive net protein balance and thus to the accretion of protein. Conversely, during periods of fasting, relative hypoaminoacidemia with reduced protein synthesis prevails, during which protein breakdown is relatively increased (negative net protein balance with protein loss). Consequently, the (obligatory) alternation between phases of food intake (protein intake) and fasting in the range of a few hours leads to corresponding fluctuations in protein synthesis and breakdown. During body growth, pregnancy and exercise-induced muscle hypertrophy, the body continuously accumulates protein, i.e. it is in a chronic anabolic state. On the contrary, diseases, physical inactivity and the biological process of aging can lead to a chronic catabolic state.

## 12.2 The Anabolic Effect of Dietary Protein on Muscle Metabolism

We can now transfer the observations on whole-body protein metabolism to skeletal muscle: In untrained or muscularly not particularly active humans, the primary cause for the fluctuations of the *muscle protein synthesis rate* (MPS) and the *muscle protein breakdown rate* (MPB) lies in the food intake (more precisely in the protein intake). In other words, the times of the opposing maximum spikes in MPS and MPB coincide with the times of dietary protein intake (Fig. 11.2). When you eat a protein-containing meal, the protein is digested to amino acids and the amino acid concentration in the blood increases as a result (hyperaminoacidemia). Via the open capillaries (see also Sects. 6.6 and 12.8) the amino acids then reach the muscles and finally the muscle fibers, through whose cell membrane the amino acids are transported into the cell interior and used to synthesize the muscle proteins. Crucial for the stimulation of MPS are the essential amino acids, i.e. the amino acids which our organism cannot produce itself and which must therefore be supplied (in contrast to the non-essential amino acids). However, the effectiveness of this process - that is, the absorption of amino acids in the digestive tract, their transport in the blood to the muscle fibers, their import into the muscle fibers, and the synthesis of muscle protein - depends on many factors such as age, training (condition), perfusion (blood flow), protein quality and quantity, and so on (Fig. 12.1, see following sections in this chapter). Moreover, our capacity to digest and absorb dietary protein far exceeds the capacity of our skeletal muscles to use the amino acids made available by

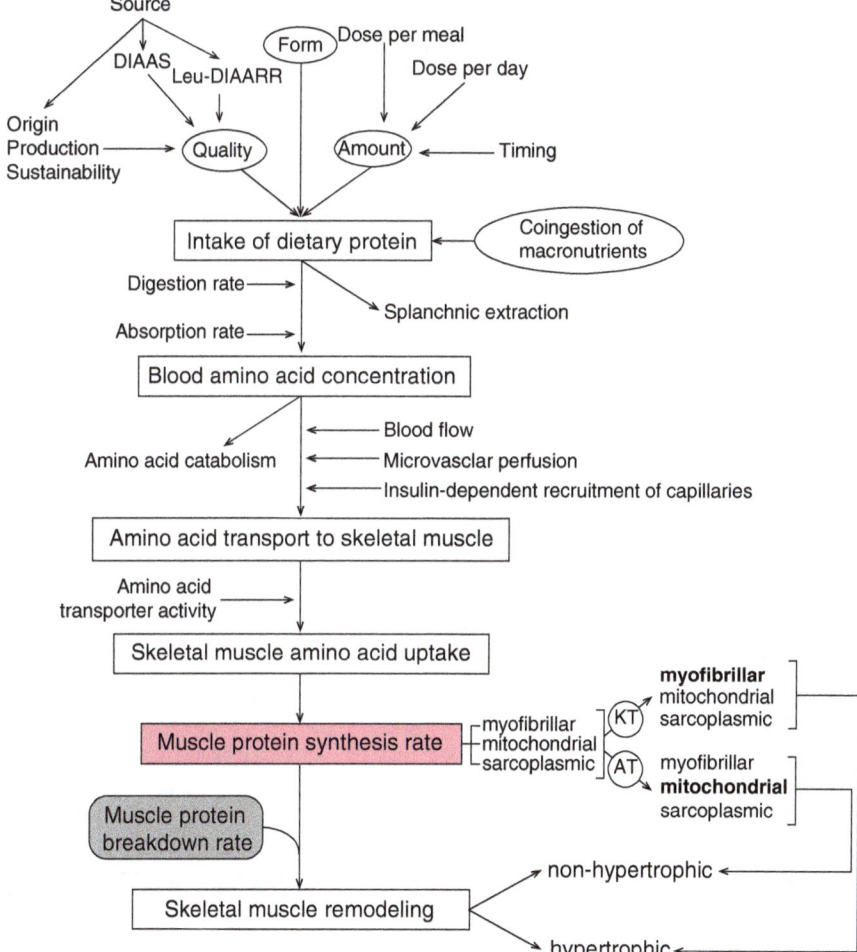

**Fig. 12.1** Factors that can influence amino acid availability and use. ET, endurance training; DIAARR (digestible indispensable amino acid reference ratio, see Sect. 12.3.2); DIAAS, *digestible indispensable amino acid score* (see Sect. 12.3); Leu, leucine (see Sect. 12.3); RT, resistance training

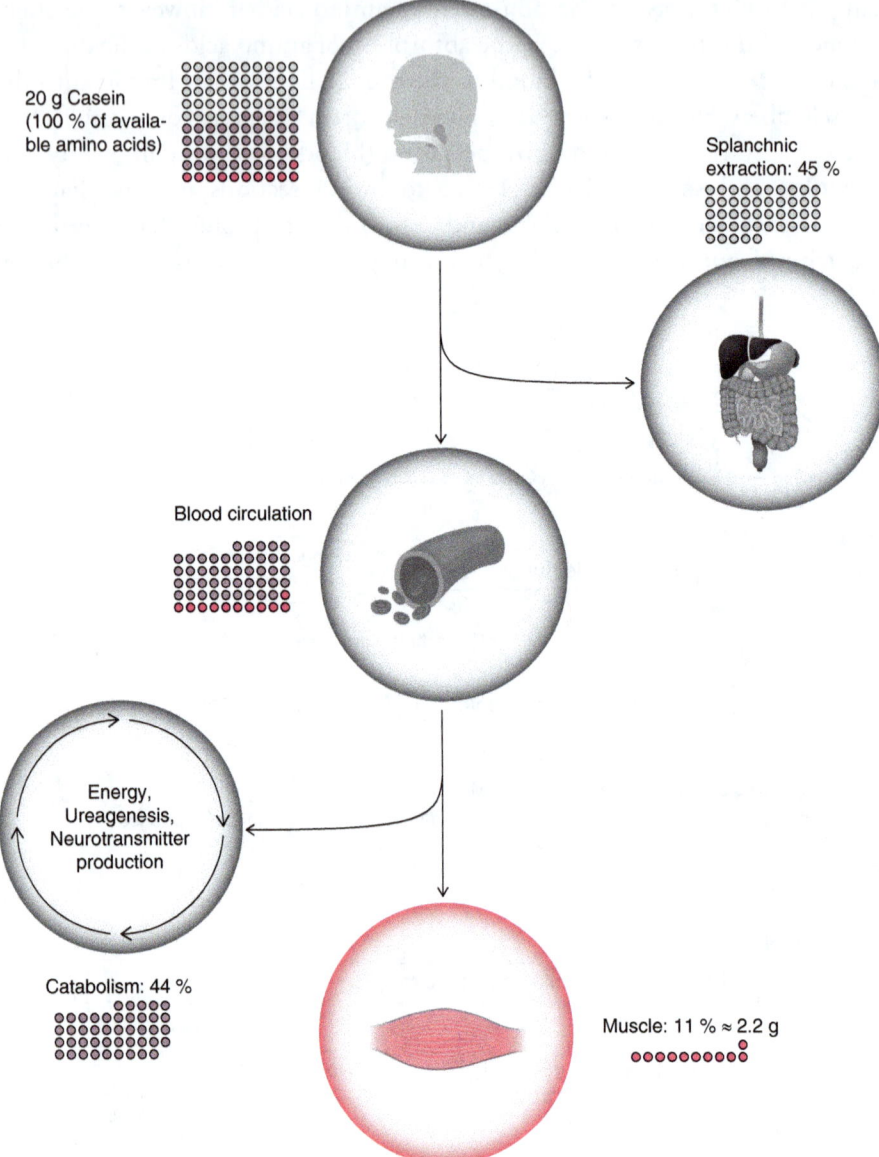

**Fig. 12.2** Proportionate use of dietary protein, or the amino acids contained therein, for *de novo protein synthesis* in human skeletal muscle

digestion for the purpose of muscle growth (Fig. 12.2). Groen et al. (2015) showed that, overall, only 55% of the amino acids absorbed from dietary protein enter the blood plasma and consequently cause an increase in amino acid concentration. The remaining 45% of amino acids are extracted by the splanchnic tissues. For example, the intestine is a metabolically highly active organ that uses amino acids for energy conversion processes and local protein synthesis in the intestine. Although skeletal muscle is the largest amino acid depot in the body, under resting conditions (i.e., not after exercise) only about 20% of the amino acids that become available in the blood are incorporated into muscle tissue. The remaining 80% are broken down and serve as substrates for a number of metabolic processes in the context of, for example, energy provision, urea production and, to a small extent, the production of neurotransmitters. In other words, only about 2.2 g or 11 % of the amino acids contained in 20 g of casein are used for *de novo* protein synthesis in skeletal muscle (Groen et al. 2015).

Accordingly, with a protein-containing meal, the MPS is stimulated, i.e. it increases. At the same time, MPB decreases slightly. The reason for this is that the consumption of a typical mixed meal is generally associated not only with the intake of dietary protein and amino acids, but also carbohydrates and fats. While virtually nothing is known about the effect of fats on MPS, carbohydrate intake leads to an increase in blood insulin concentration. Insulin has an inhibitory effect on MPB, but generally no direct stimulatory effect on MPS. Essential amino acids have a similar effect in that they cause a small hyperinsulinemia, i.e. a relatively small increase (compared to carbohydrates) in blood insulin concentration. However, if the amount of protein (or essential amino acids) consumed is sufficiently high, the amino acids alone are sufficient to increase the insulin concentration to a level that maximally inhibits MPB, i.e. no simultaneous intake of carbohydrates is necessary.

The reverse is true during diurnal periods of fasting (e.g., after nighttime fasting). It is obvious to all that the maintenance of protein mass in essential tissues and organs such as skin, brain, heart and liver is of central importance for our survival. Even in a fasting state, when amino acids are not available from food, these essential tissues and organs depend on a steady supply of amino acids from the blood. These amino acids serve as precursors for the synthesis of new proteins to compensate for the protein breakdown that occurs naturally in all tissues. In the fasting state, muscle (or muscle protein) serves as the main reservoir to compensate for the decrease in blood amino acid levels due to consumption by other tissues and organs (see Sect. 19.1). The amino acids from the blood that are supplied by the muscle also serve as precursors for hepatic gluconeogenesis (sugar formation in the liver). This is important for maintaining blood glucose concentrations in the blood. The protein mass of essential tissues and organs and the blood glucose concentration in the fasting state can therefore be kept relatively constant (see Sect. 19.1), but only if there is sufficient muscle mass to provide the required amino acids. In the fasting state, therefore, MPB rises obligatorily to support amino acid and glucose concentrations in the blood. At the same time, due to relative hypoaminoacidemia, MPS decreases. The result is a negative NBIL – muscle protein is broken down, muscle mass decreases.

## 12.3 Protein Quality Counts!

In terms of building and maintaining whole body protein mass, and specifically muscle protein mass, the quality of dietary protein ingested plays an important role. To assess protein quality, at least four factors can, or should, be considered:

**DIAAS (Digestible Indispensable Amino Acid Score)**
This is the latest index recommended by the *Food and Agriculture Organization of the United Nations* (FAO) for assessing the quality of a dietary protein source. The DIAAS reflects both the *indispensable* or *essential amino acid* content and the actual digestibility of a particular protein source relative to a reference protein, or *amino acid scoring pattern* (AASP). The AASP is based on the relative daily amino acid requirements of infants, children, adolescents and adults or on naturally occurring protein sources. However, for regulatory reasons, FAO recommends the use of only two AASPs: for baby foods, the AASP of breast milk is used, while for all other food sources and populations, the daily relative amino acid requirement of 0.5 to 3 year old children serves as the AASP.

The DIAAS is calculated for each essential amino acid as follows: DIAAS (%) = 100 × [(milligrams of essential amino acid in 1 g of dietary protein (test protein) multiplied by the coefficient for actual ileal digestibility of the same essential amino acid in the test protein)/(milligrams of the same essential amino acid in 1 g of reference protein) (amino acid reference sample)]. The essential amino acid(s) with the lowest DIAAS value are considered limiting (or interrupting) with respect to protein synthesis. Thus, "DIAAS" is always understood to mean the lowest determined DIAAS value. In other words, DIAAS (%) = lowest calculated value from [100 × (digestible essential amino acid content in 1 g dietary protein (in milligrams)/milligram of the same essential amino acid in 1 g reference protein or AASP)]. The value in square brackets corresponds to the ratio between the digestibility-corrected standardized content of a given essential amino acid in dietary protein to the digestibility-corrected standardized content of the same amino acid in reference protein (AASP). This ratio is called *digestible indispensable amino acid reference ratio* (DIAARR). According to FAO, food sources with a DIAAS greater than or equal to 100% are considered excellent quality protein sources, while those with a DIAAS between 75% and 99% are considered good quality protein sources. For food sources with a DIAAS lower than 75, the FAO recommends that no protein-related claims should be allowed.

The DIAAS replaces the previously used PDCAAS (*Protein Digestibility Corrected Amino Acid Score*), which has several shortcomings. The most important difference between the DIAAS and PDCAAS is that the DIAAS is based on the actual ileal digestibility of the essential amino acids in a protein source, whereas the PDCAAS only takes into account the (fecal) crude protein digestibility. Since it is very difficult to determine ileal digestibility experimentally directly in humans, *in vitro models* or animal experiments with pigs and rats are used instead. The pig is considered to be a suitable model organism with regard to the transferability of the results to humans.

As can be seen in Table 12.1, DIAAS is largely dependent on the protein source. For example, individually, milk-based protein sources (i.e. animal protein) have a higher DIAAS than plant-based sources (Table 12.1). The higher the DIAAS value, the higher the quality of the protein source. According to the FAO, DIAAS values below 75 % are considered food sources with insufficient protein quality. Of the protein sources listed, milk protein concentrate clearly has the highest protein quality according to the DIAAS quality criterion, while most plant proteins have a low DIAAS value (Table 12.1). Three

Table 12.1 DIAAS values for different protein sources

| Protein source | DIAAS (%) | First limiting AS |
|---|---|---|
| Milk protein concentrate (*milk protein concentrate*, MPC) | 120 | Met + Cys |
| Whey protein concentrate (*whey protein concentrate*, WPC) | 107 | His |
| Whey protein isolate (*whey protein isolate*, WPI) | 100 | His |
| Soy protein isolate (English: *soy protein isolate*, SPI) | 84 | Met + Cys |
| Pea protein concentrate (*pea protein concentrate*, PPC) | 62 | Met + Cys |
| Rice protein concentrate (*rice protein concentrate*, RPC) | 37 | Lys |

All data are taken from Mathai et al. (2017). The DIAAS values were calculated from the actual ileal digestibility of essential amino acids in growing pigs and the *amino acid scoring pattern* (AASP) for 0.5-3-year-old children

*AS* amino acid, *DIAAS*, lowest digestible indispensable amino acid score, *Cys* cysteine, *His* histidine, *Lys* lysine, *Met* methionine

reasons are given for the lower quality of plant proteins (van Vliet et al. 2015). Firstly, the digestibility of plant protein sources appears to be lower than that of animal protein sources, depending on the method of preparation, due to "antinutritional" factors. "Antinutritional" factors refer to ingredients that interfere with the digestibility and/or absorption of available proteins. However, this aspect is eliminated once purified preparations of plant protein such as isolates or concentrates are ingested. Secondly, plant proteins contain approx. 30–40% essential amino acids per 1 g protein mass. For animal proteins, this proportion is 40–50%. Finally, the relative content of certain essential amino acids such as lysine, methionine and leucine in plant proteins is disproportionately low compared to other essential amino acids. These qualitative aspects are compounded by the fact that the percentage protein content of plants is much lower compared to animal protein sources.

In many parts of the world, especially in Africa, Asia and South America, wild-caught insects have been on the traditional menu for thousands of years as suppliers of dietary protein. For ecological and economic reasons, edible insects have recently also attracted interest as a possible source of protein in Europe and North America. Insects or food creations based on them, such as insect bars, pasta, burgers, etc., can now be found at major distributors. Whether edible insects and/or insect products will meet with long-term acceptance in this country remains to be seen. From the point of view of muscle physiology, the question is rather how insect protein is to be assessed from a qualitative point of view in relation to milk, meat and egg protein as well as vegetable protein.

For insect protein, DIAAS and Leu-DIAARR values are not yet available, let alone data on the acute effect on MPS and/or NBIL. However, on a dry matter basis, it appears that the protein content of edible insects from the wild is relatively high, ranging from 40% (termites, beetles) to 60% (cockroaches, crickets, grasshoppers), and thus comparable to the protein content of conventional protein sources such as meat, eggs, milk or soybeans (Churchward-Venne et al. 2017). Since the calculation of crude protein content is based on nitrogen content and the exoskeleton (i.e., the external support structure) of insects is made of chitin, a nitrogen-containing polysaccharide, the true protein content of insects is likely to be a bit lower than assumed. It is also suspected that the insoluble chitin may also negatively affect the digestibility of insect protein.

It should be noted that for wild-caught insects, unlike farmed insects, the variability in protein content within the same species can be very high. The same applies to the content of essential amino acids per gram of protein. In general, however, several wild-caught insect species have reasonable levels of essential amino acids. Specifically with respect to leucine content, certain wild-caught insects, such as beetles, hymenoptera, termites and grasshoppers, contain more milligrams of leucine per gram of protein than is the case with soy protein isolate, but similar to micellar casein.

For insect species that are bred specifically for use in human nutrition, the variability in protein content is less because many environmental factors can be standardized during breeding. The protein content of farmed insects is about the same as for wild-caught insects and is thus comparable to the protein content of classical Western European animal protein sources. However, farmed insects have a significantly lower content of essential amino acids per gram of protein than wild-caught insects, meat, eggs, milk or soybeans (Churchward-Venne et al. 2017).

In summary, insects have a protein content similar to that of other animal protein sources or soybeans. With regard to the content of essential amino acids per gram of protein, farmed insects currently perform worse than wild-caught insects, but the variability in protein content is smaller. Finally, scientific data on the ileal digestibility of insect protein are largely lacking. Thus, at the present time, the protein quality of insect protein cannot yet be assessed according to the criteria relevant for humans and recommended by the FAO (see DIAAS). Scientific data on the effect of insect protein on MPS and/or NBIL are completely lacking to date.

## DIAARR

An important finding related to protein quality is that the essential amino acid leucine (Leu) is not only a building block for protein synthesis, but is considered the essential amino acid in skeletal muscle that triggers protein synthesis. This concept is known as the *"leucine threshold"*. It essentially states that the increase in MPS is triggered by a rapid increase in the concentration of leucine in the blood, and consequently in the intracellular concentration of leucine in the muscle fibers. Therefore, a high Leu-DIAARR value represents a separate, important quality attribute. The leucine threshold for maximizing MPS in young adults is approximately 2 g per meal or protein intake. Previously, it was assumed that older individuals generally have a higher leucine threshold (approximately 3 g) compared to younger individuals, meaning that a greater amount of leucine is required both at rest and after resistance training to maximally stimulate MPS after ingestion (see Sect. 19.6). However, recent results suggest that this is not generally true, at least for healthy older individuals who are physically active (Moro et al. 2018). Thus, leucine-enriched protein supplements are not *a priori* more useful than unmodified animal and/or plant protein sources of high protein quality.

**Table 12.2** Leu-DIAARR values for different protein sources

| Protein source | Leu-DIAARR |
|---|---|
| Whey protein isolate (*whey protein isolate*, WPI) | 2.57 |
| Whey protein concentrate (*whey protein concentrate*, WPC) | 1.93 |
| Milk protein concentrate (*milk protein concentrate*, MPC) | 1.77 |
| Pea protein concentrate (*pea protein concentrate*, PPC) | 1.37 |
| Soy protein concentrate (English: *soy protein concentrate*, SPC) | 1.29 |
| Rice protein concentrate (*rice protein concentrate*, RPC) | 1.11 |

All data are from Rutherfurd et al. (2015). DIAARR values were calculated from the actual ileal digestibility of essential amino acids in growing rats and the *amino acid scoring pattern* (AASP) for 0.5 to 3 year old children

*DIAARR* digestible indispensable amino acid reference ratio, *Leu* leucine

While Leu-DIAARR values are not yet available for insect proteins, the corresponding values for milk-based protein sources are higher than for vegetable protein sources (Table 12.2). The combination of DIAAS and Leu-DIAARR contributes significantly to the quality of a dietary protein and the highest possible values are therefore desirable for both indices. This makes protein intake generally more efficient and, depending on the amount consumed (see Sect. 12.4), more effective.

**Stimulation of MPS vs. Stimulation of Whole-Body Protein Metabolism**
In general, there is still little scientific data available on the differential effects of different types of protein (isolated or mixed) on (myofibrillar) MPS and/or NBIL, especially with regard to longer observation periods (greater than 6 h). As far as isolated protein sources are concerned, the protein fractions casein and whey contained in milk have been compared. In this regard, individual studies show that the increase in mixed MPS after whey protein ingestion is greater compared to casein in the first hours after ingestion when the amount of essential amino acids (approximately 10 g each) is matched (e.g. Tang et al. 2009). As possible reasons for the observed differences, the authors mentioned on the one hand the different digestibility and the slightly different content of leucine (in this study for the whey protein 2.3 g leucine per 10 g essential amino acids compared to 1.8 g per 10 g for casein). However, other studies show no net difference between the two protein types in terms of increasing myofibrillar MPS for the first 6 h after ingestion (Reitelseder et al. 2011). As might be expected, the results in this study also tend to indicate that whey

protein stimulates MPS more than casein during the first 3 h after protein ingestion, but that the opposite is true during the second 3 h of observation.

Whey protein has also been compared to soy protein, a plant-based protein, in terms of its effect on mixed MPS. Whey protein intake is associated with a greater increase in mixed MPS than soy protein, both at rest and after resistance training (Tang et al. 2009). A long-term study (9 months of resistance training with whey or soy protein supplementation) appears to confirm this advantage of whey over soy based on the observed greater increase in lean mass with whey protein supplementation. Finally, comparing casein to soy, soy protein leads to a greater increase in mixed MPS at rest as well as after resistance training in the first 3 h after ingestion (Tang et al. 2009).

In summary, due to the sparse data available (1–2 studies for each comparison), no general conclusions can be drawn at present. Furthermore, many other plant proteins and also insect proteins need to be tested with regard to their effect on myofibrillar MPS and/or NBIL.

However, when protein anabolism is considered at the level of the body rather than the muscle, a different picture emerges. For example, Boirie et al. (1997) showed that protein anabolism measured over 7 h was more strongly stimulated by a controlled administration of casein compared with whey protein (with identical leucine content). Whey protein produced a transient increase in whole-body protein synthesis and leucine oxidation at rest (Boirie et al. 1997). Conversely, casein had a moderate effect on whole-body protein synthesis but inhibited protein breakdown (Boirie et al. 1997). Whole-body protein metabolism studies thus suggest that different protein sources may have different effects on protein synthesis and degradation. However, measurements of whole-body protein metabolism must be interpreted with caution (see Sect. 12.1). In contrast to the rapidly digested whey protein, the longer digestion time of micellar casein is likely to stimulate splanchnic (i.e. visceral) protein synthesis more strongly, as reflected in the stronger whole-body response (Dangin et al. 2001). Soy proteins have also been postulated to be more efficiently incorporated into splanchnic proteins than into muscle proteins (Fouillet et al. 2002), which, together with the difference in leucine content, may explain the lower acute anabolic effect on skeletal muscle.

In principle, it is conceivable that the above-mentioned possible disadvantages of plant proteins (see DIAAS) can be compensated for by (a) consuming more plant protein, (b) additionally enriching the plant protein source with essential amino acids, (c) cultivating plants that have a better amino acid profile, and (d) combining protein sources that differ in their amino acid profile.

However, to date, experimental studies on the effectiveness of such measures on MPS and/or NBIL are lacking.

## Origin/Production of the Protein Product, Environmental Footprint and Unknown Health Effects of Long-Term Consumption

In general, to assess the goodness of a food, not only its positive ingredients should be considered, but also those that are useless or even harmful. It is not enough to associate meat, milk, eggs, soy, insects or shakes and bars with protein, because depending on the protein source, origin, production and processing, they may contain significant amounts of undesirable substances such as chemicals, hormones, pesticides, pickling salts, etc., which are unlikely to benefit your health in the long term. On top of that, with highly processed products, there are a lot of additives that preserve, emulsify, color, provide flavor, and so on. These are all things that you don't necessarily want in your body, especially if you are taking the product several times a day over a long period of time. It goes without saying that the above ingredients are totally useless in terms of the actual purpose of taking the protein product, which is to increase the rate of muscle protein synthesis and promote body protein turnover. The quality of a protein product is therefore not only defined by what is contained in it, but also to the same extent by what is not contained in it. Of course, the same applies to nutrition in general. If there are useless and/or potentially harmful additives in the product, it will lower the quality of the product. From a health perspective, it does you no good in the long run if the protein content and amino acid composition of a protein powder or bar are top notch, but the additives contained in it, either individually or in combination, could negatively affect your health in the long run.

Just as resistance training only needs you and training resistance, supporting the training effect only needs you and natural dietary proteins. As a minimum quality, natural, certified organic products are certainly not a bad choice. Organic products don't provide any added benefit in terms of increasing MPS in the first place. They are also not without doubt in terms of ecological footprint. Organic products do, however, offer some protection from undesirable ingredients because the guiding principle in organic farming is to operate "in harmony with nature". This means that natural life processes should be promoted and nutrient cycles largely closed. On the websites of the organic labels, consumers are assured that the animals are kept in a particularly species-appropriate manner, that most of them are fed with the farm's own organic feed and that, in the event of illness, they first benefit from gentle treatment methods. Additives such as synthetic sweeteners and the use of genetic engineering are avoided. Organic certified products also have in common that their production, raw materials, recipes, processing, transport and storage are checked by independent control and certification bodies.

However, the organic standards vary internationally and depending on the organic label, the holistic approach to sustainability is lived or interpreted with varying degrees of strictness. So you must be aware that even with an organic protein product, such as an organic protein powder, you have no absolute guarantee about the quality of all the ingredients it contains. However, by choosing a 100% natural (i.e. without any additives that alter taste, colour or consistency) organic protein source, you have done everything proportionate and reasonable in your power to avoid undesirable ingredients.

## 12.4 The Protein Quantity Counts as Well!

There is a dose-response relationship between the amount of essential amino acids or protein ingested and the increase in MPS. It was shown that in young men the mixed MPS increases with increasing protein dose up to approx. 20 g egg protein in the style of a saturation function and then reaches a plateau (Moore et al. 2009). From the intake of 20 g egg protein upwards, there was no further increase in MPS (Fig. 12.3). On the contrary, after reaching the necessary but sufficient amount to maximally stimulate the mixed MPS (approximately 20 g), amino acid oxidation and the formation of urea increased, meaning that the body was trying to break down excess protein. The authors speculated that with chronic overdose, there might be a reduced increase in MPS (at rest and after exercise) at the same protein dose (Moore et al. 2009).

These results are consistent with the finding from a previous study that the dose-response relationship in young men at rest (i.e., without having exercised prior to ingestion) saturates at an intake of 10 g of essential amino acids (Cuthbertson et al. 2005). The agreement is not surprising in that animal protein (e.g., whey protein, milk, casein, beef, and eggs) typically contains approximately 44–52% essential amino acids (as a percentage of total protein mass), i.e., for every 20 g of animal protein, approximately 10 g (50% of 20 g) are essential amino acids. By comparison, in human skeletal muscle protein, the percentage of essential amino acids relative to total protein mass is approximately 45%.

Witard et al. (2014) were able to confirm that the same dose-response relationship also exists between the ingested amount of whey protein and the increase in myofibrillar MPS in young men at rest (Fig. 12.4). In contrast to

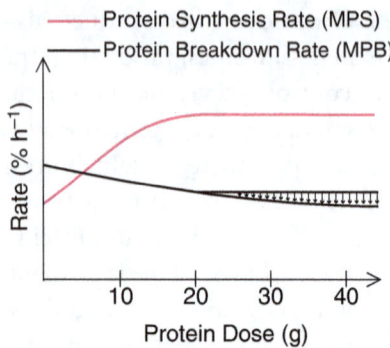

**Fig. 12.3** Dose-response relationship between the ingested amount of animal protein and the synthesis and breakdown rate of muscle protein in young men. MPS increases with increasing protein dose (amount of protein) and reaches a plateau at approximately 20 g of animal protein per intake time point. Higher protein intakes than 20 g do not result in further increases in MPS. The MPB decreases slightly with increasing protein dose until a plateau is reached here as well. However, it is possible that ingested protein amounts of >20 g also positively influence MPB, so that the rate of degradation continues to decrease, as indicated by the arrows (an additional anabolic effect, i.e. the net muscle protein balance is more positive than without the effect). However, this hypothetical effect has not (yet) been substantiated experimentally. *MPS* muscle protein synthesis rate, *MPB* muscle protein breakdown rate

young men, in whom ingestion of 40 g of whey protein compared to 20 g provided no additional benefit in terms of increasing myofibrillar MPS, seniors required this higher dose to achieve a comparably similar myofibrillar MPS. Yang et al. (2012) showed that under resting conditions in seniors, administration of 40 g whey protein compared with 20 g resulted in an additional significant increase in myofibrillar MPS of approximately 21% on average (Fig. 12.4). It has been postulated that the higher necessary and sufficient protein dose per intake time point for maximal stimulation of myofibrillar MPS in seniors is probably a manifestation of so-called "anabolic resistance in old age" (see Sect. 19.6). However, as already mentioned in Sect. 12.3.2, the latest study results indicate that "anabolic resistance" is non-existent in healthy, physically active elderly people.

One difficulty inherent in the protein doses in healthy adult males quoted so far is that they are absolute and not relative. This means that the figures do not take into account the fact that body and muscle mass can vary massively from individual to individual. Therefore, absolute protein recommendations are subject to error in individual cases. Information on protein intake per intake time and total per day should therefore be normalised to 1 kg body or muscle mass. It would be good to normalize to muscle mass (or lean mass), because skeletal muscle represents the largest amino acid reservoir in the

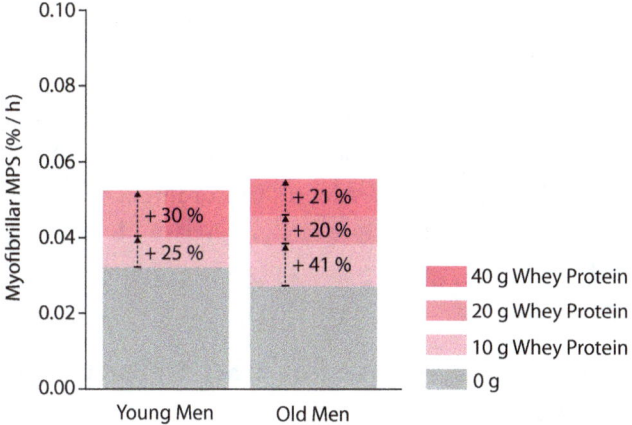

**Fig. 12.4** Dose-response relationship between the ingested amount of whey protein and the increase in myofibrillar muscle protein synthesis rate (MPS) in the thigh muscles of adult young men and seniors under resting conditions. (Adapted from Witard et al. 2014; Yang et al. 2012)

human body. However, lean mass, let alone muscle mass, is not experimentally accessible to the vast majority of individuals. Therefore, for reasons of practicability, only the normalization to body mass is widely used.

In a retrospective analysis of 6 studies with a total of 65 young men and 43 seniors, the relative protein dose (grams of protein per kilogram of body mass) at which the maximum stimulatory effect on myofibrillar MPS is achieved at rest (i.e. no training for at least 48 h) was calculated (Moore et al. 2015). The dietary protein administered was protein shakes, prepared with whey protein powder and water in 5 studies and egg white powder and water in one study. For the MPS, only the period of 3–4 h after time of ingestion was considered. Thus, strictly speaking, the analyses and interpretations of Moore et al. (2015) refer practically only to the effect of whey protein shakes in the first 3–4 h after ingestion. They found that the necessary and sufficient amount of whey protein for maximal stimulation of myofibrillar MPS in young men was 0.24 g/kg on average, with the upper limit of the 95 percent confidence interval being 0.30 g/kg. To this, the authors added an arbitrary "safety margin" of 0.10 g/kg to account for possible quality differences between animal and plant protein sources. On this basis, they formulated their recommendation that young men should take 0.40 g/kg per intake time point (32 g for an athlete with 80 kg body mass) for maximal stimulation of myofibrillar MPS. For seniors, the authors calculated a corresponding mean value of 0.40 g/kg. The upper limit of the 95 percent confidence interval was 0.59 g/kg. Even if these values should be correct and the myofibrillar MPS cannot be increased any further with higher doses above a certain amount of protein, this should not be interpreted to mean that the maximum anabolic effect has been reached. In the opinion of other well-known research colleagues, there is no practical upper limit to the anabolic effect of the dietary proteins or amino acids contained in mixed meals (unlike protein shakes) (see Sect. 12.6).

See Sect. 14.7 for the current scientific recommendations on total daily dietary protein intake and how these relate to the single dose recommendations.

## 12.5 Why Eating Alone Isn't Sufficient to Bulk Up Muscles

The anabolic response to ingesting dietary protein is only temporary. Otherwise, as an adult, always assuming that the MPB does not change much, you could become more muscular by eating protein alone! This is of course not the case. As a non-active or less active, healthy person, all you can do is prevent yourself from losing muscle protein early on by eating a proper dietary protein intake. The reaction sequence to the supply of the saturation amount of protein in humans is approximately as follows: After a latency phase (i.e. a time delay) of approx. 30 min, the myofibrillar MPS rises sharply, reaches approx. two to three times the initial value after approx. 1.5 h, and is already back at the initial value after 2–3 h. The MPS then increases again.

This is also the case when the availability of circulating amino acids in the blood remains high. The muscle therefore becomes refractory after approx. 1.5 h, i.e. insensitive to the circulating amino acids in the blood (called *muscle full effect*). The term *muscle full* was chosen in reference to the developmental biology hypothesis of Joe Millward, according to which the absolute extent of muscle fiber hypertrophy was limited by the inelastic collagen in the endomysium (the so-called *bag full hypothesis*). As evidence for the temporary insensitivity of MPS to circulating amino acids, the following was shown: When amino acids were infused directly into the blood and their concentration in the blood was maintained at levels that occur after food intake, it took 1.5 h for the MPS to reach its highest level. After another 2 h, the MPS had dropped back to baseline and remained there for the remaining 6 h of observation. It should be noted that the drop to the initial value and the subsequent persistence at this level took place despite high amino acid concentrations in the blood (Bohé et al. 2001).

## 12.6 The Concept of Full Muscle

Based on the observation of the *muscle full effect,* the view emerged that it would be better to distribute protein intake over several intake times that are several hours apart, instead of ingesting the recommended daily amount of protein as a single dose, for example. Proponents of this thesis include Moore et al. (2012a), who investigated the effect of different intake schedules on whole-body protein metabolism during 12 h after a resistance training session. Participants in this study received 80 g of whey protein isolate over a 12 h period, either 8 × 10 g at 1.5 h intervals, 4 × 20 g at 3 h intervals, or 2 × 40 g at 6 h intervals. From the results, the study investigators concluded, first, that the pattern of dietary protein administration, rather than just the total amount ingested daily, may have an impact on protein metabolism, and second, that individuals seeking to optimize whole-body NBIL are likely to benefit more from repeatedly consuming protein servings of approximately 20 g at regular intervals of approximately 3 h (Moore et al. 2012a). In a follow-up study, the same administration patterns in the 12 h immediately following a resistance training session were examined for their effect on increasing myofibrillar MPS. Again, the administration of 4 × 20 g at 3 h intervals was found to be superior to the other administration patterns (Areta et al. 2013). Finally, Mamerow et al. (2014) demonstrated that, in the context of complete meals, evenly dividing the amount of protein (33 % each) between 3 meals in adult men and women aged approximately 37 years over 24 h resulted in higher mixed MPS compared with uneven division (approximately 11, 17, and 72 % for morning, lunch, and dinner, respectively).

It must be mentioned, however, that in the scientific literature the information on the "optimal" time interval is not always consistent. There is also the opinion that 20–25 g of protein, administered every 4–5 h, is optimal (hence the general recommendation of 3–5 h). The *muscle full concept* is not without controversy, despite a broad base of scientific evidence. Indeed, the concept is based on the fundamental observation that increases in plasma amino acid concentration are directly related to stimulation of MPS, up to a point where further increases in plasma amino acid concentration do not result in further increases in MPS. As long as the rate of influx (the rate of transport across the cell membrane) of amino acids from blood plasma into muscle fibers is moderate relative to the MPS, the intracellular amino acid concentration remains relatively constant. When the peak MPS is reached, the intracellular amino acid concentration increases as long as the plasma amino acid concentration also continues to increase.

According to the critics, however, this does not automatically mean that the maximum anabolic response is reached at this point. On the contrary, they argue that the anabolic response can be further increased at this point, not via further stimulation of the MPS, but via an inhibition or limitation of the MPB induced by the high intracellular amino acid concentration (Deutz and Wolfe 2013). The hypothesis of the critics of the *muscle full concept* is therefore that after reaching the maximum MPS, a further increase in the intracellular amino acid concentration could represent the signal for limiting the MPB. Since NBIL represents the difference between MPS and MPB, inhibition of MPB would mean an increase in the anabolic response while MPS remains constant (Fig. 12.3).

Consistent with Deutz and Wolfe's (2013) hypothesis, Wolfe and colleagues demonstrated the following in a series of studies:

1. In the context of complete (or balanced) meals containing protein, carbohydrate, and fat, ingestion of 70 g protein (beef) compared with 40 g in approximately 30-year-old men and women at rest and after weight training did not result in any additional increase in mixed MPS, as expected. However, administration of 70 g resulted in significantly greater whole-body NBIL in all situations. This effect was primarily due to a significant and large decrease in whole-body protein breakdown rate (PB). Secondarily, a small but significant increase in whole-body protein synthesis rate (PS) also contributed to the increase in NBIL (Kim et al. 2016). The authors concluded that the maximal stimulation of mixed MPS achieved at 40 g did not limit the total anabolic response to the administration of a larger amount of dietary protein (here 70 g).
2. In contrast to the results of Mamerow et al. (2014), there were no differences in the mixed MPS (over 22 h) and total body NBIL (over 16 h) in men and women aged 52–75 years between an even (33, 33, and 33% for morning, lunch, and dinner, respectively) and uneven (15, 20, 65%) distribution of protein amount in this study (1.1 g protein per kilogram body mass per day) across the three main meals (Kim et al. 2015).
3. When these two different protein intake regimens were implemented daily (always in the context of complete meals) in two groups of 51-69 year-old men and women over an 8-week period, *notably* without resistance training, there were also no measurable group differences in changes for mixed MPS, total body NBIL, lean mass, or surrogate markers of muscle force after 8 weeks (Kim et al. 2018).

Based on these experimental results and theoretical calculations, these authors currently argue that the dose-response relationship between the amount of dietary protein ingested and the maximal anabolic response is linear over a wide range of protein intake. It is further unlikely that one can positively influence lean mass by changing the relative proportion (evenly or unevenly distributed) of the amount of protein in the three main meals unless the total amount of dietary protein consumed is also significantly increased at the same time.

Accordingly, one criticism of the *muscle full concept* is that the extent of muscle and whole-body protein anabolism should not simply be equated with the increase in MPS, but that MPB, PS and PB (and thus NBIL) should also be taken into account. MPB is methodologically more difficult to access than MPS, which is part of the reason that MPB has generally not been measured, or rarely measured, in experiments on the effect of dietary protein on the muscle anabolic response. In humans, when considering the balance between MPS and MPB from hour to hour, MPS fluctuates approximately three to five times more than MPB during transitions between food intake, postprandial, and postabsorptive states, accounting for training-induced fluctuations (Glynn et al. 2010). In light of this, muscle mass in humans, at least as far as healthy (or asymptomatic) individuals are concerned, appears to be primarily regulated by MPS. Thus, although the increase in MPS after ingestion of dietary protein and/or after resistance training should not be used as a synonym for the anabolic response, for the time being, until new, better methods for measuring MPB are available, there remains no alternative but to base dietary recommendations for optimizing muscle adaptations on MPS response data.

## 12.7 Amino Acids, Protein Shakes or Meals?

It is important to remember that most dose-response relationships have been studied following administration of pure amino acids, isolated protein (e.g., whey protein, soy, and casein), or specific foods (milk or meat), but not mixed, complete meals. In fact, consumption of a typical mixed meal is associated not only with protein intake, but also carbohydrate and fat intake. Virtually nothing is yet known about the effect of dietary fats on protein-induced increases in MPS. A single study demonstrated that the increase in MPS was greater after ingestion of whole milk (8.2 g fat, 8.0 g protein, 11.4 g carbohydrate; 2625 MJ or 627 kcal) than with fat-free milk or a neutral fat-free drink of equivalent energy content. The reason for the greater increase in MPS with whole milk is not clear, but may be related to greater muscle blood flow in this study.

Unlike for the simultaneous intake of fat and protein, the role of carbohydrates in the regulation of human protein metabolism has been investigated in numerous studies. The intake of carbohydrates is associated with the increase of insulin concentration in the blood. Insulin is an anabolic hormone that has a strong inhibitory effect on MPB and thus can positively influence NBIL. Nevertheless, without concomitant amino acid (or protein) intake, carbohydrate intake does not result in a positive NBIL (e.g., Miller et al. 2003). In addition, most studies show that concurrent carbohydrate and protein intake does not increase MPS more or inhibit MPB more compared to protein intake alone. In one study, Staples et al. (2011) administered 25 g of whey protein (in the form of a protein shake) to young men, either alone or together with 50 g of carbohydrate in the form of maltodextrin. Although insulin release was approximately five times greater for the combined intake of maltodextrin and whey protein than for the intake of protein alone, MPS, MPB, and blood flow did not differ under either condition.

## 12.8 Are Carbohydrates Necessary in a Protein Shake?

The results described above suggest that the increase in amino acid and insulin concentrations in blood plasma following the ingestion of 25 g of whey protein alone was sufficient to maximize any effect of insulin on MPS. You read that correctly: Whey protein intake alone results in a slight increase in blood insulin concentration. Incidentally, this is also the case with soy, but not casein, for the same energy and nitrogen content. However, the increase in insulin concentration is far less than when protein and maltodextrin are consumed simultaneously. The observation that after combined protein/carbohydrate intake, MPB was not inhibited more than with protein alone, despite a much higher insulin concentration, is consistent with results from other studies on the subject. Thus, in a study of the dose-response relationship between insulin concentration in blood plasma and MPS or MPB, it was shown, firstly, that an insulin concentration of only 5 µU ml$^{-1}$ (which corresponds approximately to the insulin concentration measured in the fasting state, for example in the morning after getting up) is necessary to maximize the effect of amino acids on MPS, and secondly, that the inhibition of MPB is maximal at an insulin concentration of 30 µU ml$^{-1}$ and higher insulin concentrations are not more effective (Greenhaff et al. 2008).

Based on the data in the Staples et al. (2011) study, the insulin concentration required for maximal increase in MPS and maximal inhibition of MPB can be further narrowed: In the study of young men, 25 g of whey protein was sufficient to achieve a peak concentration of approximately 19 µU ml$^{-1}$ and an average concentration of approximately 11 µU ml$^{-1}$ for insulin. Thus, the MPS could be maximally stimulated and the MPB maximally inhibited. Accordingly, if you consume a protein shake containing the sufficient and necessary amount of protein to increase MPS according to the *muscle full hypothesis* (0.3 g protein per kilogram body mass per time point of ingestion), then the associated increase in insulin concentration in the blood is sufficient to maximally inhibit MPB, i.e. under these conditions no additional and simultaneous intake of carbohydrates is necessary to maximize the anabolic effect.

Although carbohydrates are not of fundamental importance for the changes in NBIL if enough protein is consumed, it should be noted here that carbohydrates naturally play an important role in the resynthesis of muscle glycogen. The concentration of muscle glycogen decreases during resistance training and must be regenerated to maintain performance or to be able to train. It is conceivable that supplemental carbohydrate intake could play a more important role if you are ingesting an insufficient amount of protein (for maximal stimulation of MPS). Locally infused insulin without concomitant dietary amino acid intake may increase blood flow, amino acid transport, and intracellular availability of amino acids and thus MPS. Thus, the effect of insulin or concomitantly ingested carbohydrates may theoretically be permissive (if the amount of protein is adequate) or stimulatory (if the amount of protein is too low), depending on the amount of protein ingested (or on the concentration of amino acids in the blood). Finally, it is also conceivable that depending on the individual (age, training condition), the vasodilatory effect of insulin and thus the blood flow in the muscle could be influenced to different degrees. The more blood capillaries are recruited or perfused in the muscle, the more nutrients or amino acids are transported to a given muscle fiber and the greater the potential stimulatory effect on MPS.

## 12.9 Why Not Take Isolated Amino Acids?

Direct oral intake of isolated amino acids is not beneficial, as whey protein intake appears to result in greater protein anabolism than the corresponding fraction of pure essential or nonessential amino acids, at least as far as older individuals are concerned (Katsanos et al. 2008; Paddon-Jones et al. 2006). This suggests that the mechanisms underlying the greater effect of whey protein (compared to pure essential or non-essential amino acids) are not exclusively due to its amino acid content and composition. However, it is quite conceivable that administration of pure amino acid mixtures may be more beneficial if, first, the individual's digestion is impaired and/or, second, the protein ingested is more difficult to digest (e.g., non-ground meat). For example, protein anabolism is greater when the same amount of meat is eaten as ground meat instead of in one piece. Remember, however, that for the estimation of the anabolic effect, the MPS and the MPB should always be taken into account and that therefore the observed study results for isolated protein sources do not necessarily and in every case have to correspond to those for mixed meals (*nota bene* with more than 20 g of protein).

## 12.10 Summary

If you want to build a wall, you need not only the necessary tools, but also the right building blocks, e.g. materials such as bricks, cement, mortar etc. Each building block must also be present in the right quantity, i.e. in a balanced proportion to the other building blocks. It is of no use if you have 100 kg of mortar but only 2 kg of bricks. The brick you have the least of will determine how big or strong the wall can be. So which material supplier do you choose? Assuming that you want to achieve as much as possible with as little effort as possible, the choice is likely to fall on the supplier who can provide you with all the building blocks in the right quantities and in the right proportions. When it comes to building muscle, it's much the same. It takes the right amount of dietary protein, and the amount required and sufficient to stimulate the MPS to the maximum depends on the protein quality.

There are at least four factors to consider when assessing protein quality and therefore the products you consume: (1) DIAAS is an index of protein quality and reflects both the essential amino acid content and the ileal digestibility of a particular protein source relative to a reference protein, or amino acid scoring pattern. The latter in particular can be influenced by antinutritional factors and is a particular concern for natural plant protein sources and insect proteins. (2) leu-DIAARR: This is the ratio of the digestibility-corrected standardized content of the essential amino acid leucine in dietary protein to the digestibility-corrected standardized content of leucine in reference protein. The essential amino acid leucine is considered to play a special role in protein metabolism in skeletal muscle in that it is not only a building block for protein synthesis, but is considered to be the amino acid that triggers protein synthesis. (3) another quality factor is the specific ability of a protein source to increase myofibrillar MPS. However, in general, there is still little scientific data on the differential effects of different protein types (isolated or mixed) on myofibrillar MPS and/or NBIL, especially regarding longer observation periods (greater than 6 h). (4) superfluous and/or potentially harmful additional ingredients that have nothing whatsoever to do with the actually desired effect, namely the increase in MPS. These additives include natural and artificial sweeteners, colourings, flavourings, etc.

Dairy proteins have the highest scores in terms of DIAAS and Leu-DIAARR compared to other protein sources. However, if the amount of protein consumed is correct, it should hardly matter whether a whey concentrate or isolate is used, regardless of whether someone considers themselves a "hobby athlete" or a "competitive athlete". In other words, interindividual differences in the magnitude of the adaptive response (e.g., muscle hypertrophy and muscle force gains) to resistance training are very unlikely to be attributable to whether someone uses whey concentrate or isolate.

Plant proteins generally have lower DIAAS and Leu-DIAAR values than animal proteins. Therefore, in terms of the effect on protein metabolism, they have less effect for a given amount of protein ingested. In other words, the stimulation of muscle protein metabolism with 20 g of wheat protein is smaller than with 20 g of whey protein, for example. The possible disadvantage of vegetable proteins can be compensated by (a) consuming more vegetable protein: In order to theoretically achieve the same effect on MPS as with 27 g of pure whey protein, one would have to consume approx. 2.9 kg of potatoes, 265 g of corn, 500 g of rice, 180 g of peas, 100 g of soy or 300 g of wheat for comparison, (b) the vegetable protein source is additionally enriched with essential amino acids, (c) vegetable protein sources that differ in their amino acid profile are combined. Figuratively speaking, in this case the building blocks would have to be obtained from different suppliers. You should pay particular attention to this important aspect if your diet does not include the consumption of dairy products and/or meat.

Insects have a protein content similar to that of other animal protein sources or soybeans. In terms of the content of essential amino acids per gram of protein, farmed insects currently perform worse than wild-caught insects, but the variability in protein content is smaller. As scientific data on the ileal digestibility of insect protein are still largely lacking, the protein quality of insect protein cannot yet be assessed according to the criteria relevant for humans and recommended by the FAO. Scientific data on the effect of insect protein on MPS and/or NBIL are completely lacking to date.

Regardless of the protein source, but especially when it comes to protein products that you take often and over a long period of time (e.g. protein powders for shakes, bars, etc.) you should especially make sure that the product is free of useless (in terms of MPS) or potentially harmful ingredients. Your muscles do not need artificial or natural sweeteners, flavors, thickeners and other additives to grow, only high-quality protein. Therefore, it is generally recommended to choose products with organic certification as a starting point. This guarantees a certain minimum quality (with the reservations described in the text).

There appears to be a dose-response relationship between the amount of protein ingested as a single dose and the stimulation of myofibrillar MPS that resembles a saturation curve. In young adult males, myofibrillar MPS increases linearly with single doses up to approximately 0.24 g/kg body mass whey protein in shake form and fails to increase further thereafter with higher doses up to 40 g whey protein. In seniors, the plateau in the dose-response relationship appears to be reached on average only at about 0.4 g/kg body mass. The fact that a higher protein dose is required for a similarly strong anabolic response in seniors compared to young adult men has previously been interpreted as possible anabolic resistance in old age. However, recent results show that in healthy active elderly individuals there is no anabolic resistance and therefore no problem with protein and/or training dose. This means that possible anabolic resistance in old age may have more to do with the health and training status of the individual than with age *per se*. In any case, however, it is important to understand that the maximal increase in myofibrillar MPS after administration of a protein shake is not the same as the maximal anabolic response. For the latter, one must consider MPB and thus muscular and/or total body NBIL. Current data suggest that after reaching maximal MPS response, the anabolic response continues to increase in the context of a complete meal with protein doses up to 70 g from animal protein sources.

# 13

# Resistance Exercise as an Anabolic Stimulus

## 13.1 The Acute Anabolic Muscle Response to Resistance Exercise

Similar to dietary protein intake, resistance exercise by itself can increase myofibrillar MPS. The extent of this increase varies from individual to individual and also depends to a large extent on age. There are studies that speak of a two- to fivefold increase in the baseline value (Kumar et al. 2009a). On average, however, an exercise-induced increase in myofibrillar MPS of approximately 50 percentage points from the resting value is observed in young men (Fig. 13.1). In young men, the relative increase in myofibrillar MPS in the first few hours after resistance exercise is about the same as after ingestion of 20–40 g of animal protein (see Chap. 12; Fig. 12.4). In analogy to the reduced increase in myofibrillar MPS after ingestion of a certain amount of dietary protein, and in agreement with the theory of anabolic resistance in old age (see Sect. 19.4), the strength of the MPS response tends to be weaker on average in seniors than in young adults for the same resistance exercise stimulus (Fig. 13.1, for comparison: Fig. 12.4). However, recent research results challenge this view (Moro et al. 2018; see Sects. 12.3 and 12.10).

However, unlike protein intake, this anabolic effect of training lasts longer. In one study, myofibrillar MPS was examined at rest and 6, 24, 48, and 72 h after resistance exercise (Miller et al. 2005). The result was that myofibrillar MPS was significantly increased up to 72 h after resistance exercise, with the peak value measured 24 h after resistance exercise. However, MPB also increases unless protein and/or carbohydrates are consumed in sufficient

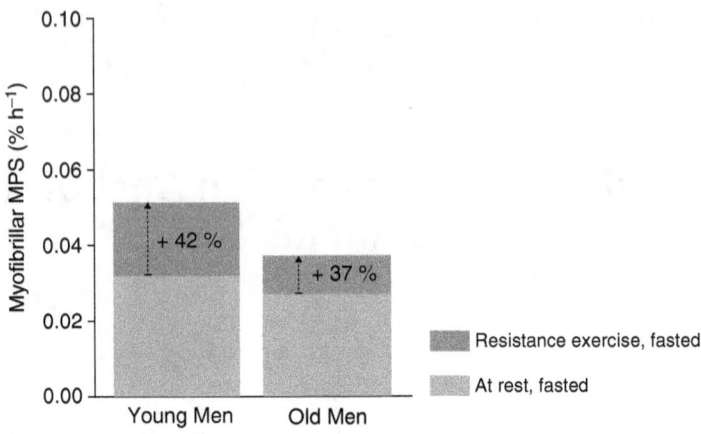

**Fig. 13.1** Increase in myofibrillar muscle protein synthesis (MPS) rate in thigh muscles in the first few hours after resistance exercise of the same muscle group without protein intake in adult young men and seniors. (Adapted from Witard et al. 2014; Yang et al. 2012)

amounts or at all (Phillips et al. 1997). Thus, if a person performs a demanding resistance exercise programme in a fasting state, i.e. starting from a negative NBIL, and does not consume any protein/carbohydrates (or too little of them), the NBIL becomes more positive but remains negative in absolute terms (Fig. 13.2). In the long run, muscle mass would thus decrease. You will therefore not be able to build or rebuild your muscles if you do not take in essential amino acids. However, by taking in the necessary and sufficient amount of protein at sensible intervals and in the right quality in combination with resistance exercise, you will achieve the positive NBIL that is absolutely necessary for muscle hypertrophy (see Chap. 15).

## 13.2 Bridging the Gap Between Muscle Protein Synthesis and Motor Unit Recruitment

Because of the size principle that applies to a defined motor task and the motor units that can be recruited to it (i.e., each neuromuscular compartment), MyHC type 2 fibers are activated only with increasing force, fatigue, or movement speed (see Chap. 9). As you may recall, ballistic movement execution or high movement speed is associated with a phasic (transient) activity pattern of high threshold motor units. Based on these neuromuscular or neurophysiological bases, I predicted back in 2006 (Toigo 2006a, b; Toigo and Boutellier 2006) that the magnitude of the MPS increase or the anabolic stimulus through resistance exercise must primarily depend on two variables:

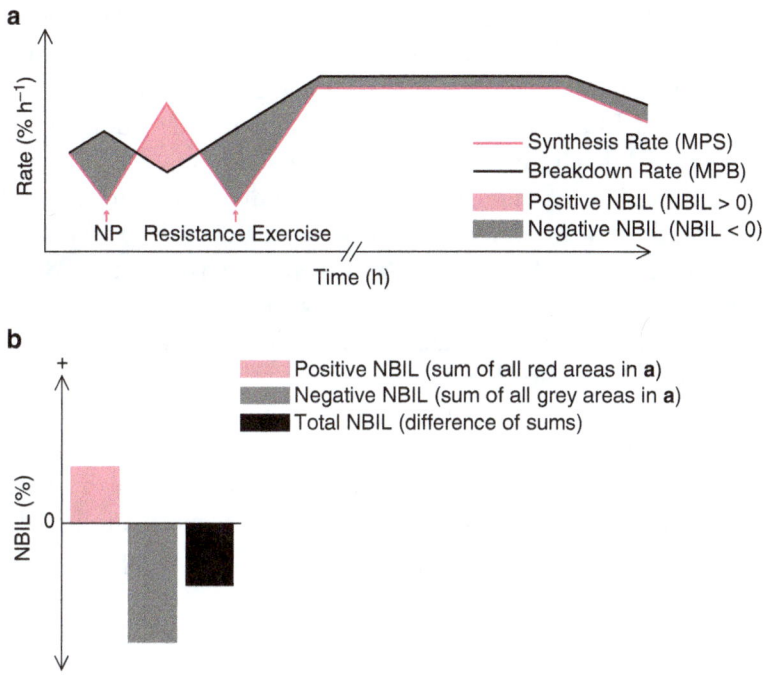

**Fig. 13.2** Effect of a single resistance exercise session on the rate of synthesis and breakdown of myofibrillar muscle protein. (**a**) No or too little dietary protein is consumed in the hours and days following the training session. Resistance exercise alone results in a marked increase in MPS. The increased MPS can last for different lengths of time – days or just hours – depending on the type (intensity, duration, etc.) of training. At the same time, however, MPB also increases and is higher than MPS over the entire duration – days or hours. (**b**) The result is that NBIL, considered over hours and days, is negative (NBIL <0). *MPS* muscle protein synthesis rate, *MPB* muscle protein breakdown rate, *NBIL* net muscle protein balance, *NP* dietary protein

on the one hand, on the extent of the recruitment of motor units and thus on the number and type of activated muscle fibers and, on the other hand, on the duration during which the muscle fibers produces force (time under tension (TUT), see Sect. 13.7) – in other words: on the magnitude and duration of the motor drive (see Sects. 9.9, 13.5 and Box 9.3).

## 13.3 How Does Training Intensity Affect Muscle Protein Synthesis?

Meanwhile, this prediction that the magnitude of MPS increase or anabolic stimulus by resistance exercise depends on the magnitude and duration of motor drive has been experimentally confirmed several times. Let us first consider the influence of training load on the increase in MPS. How do you experimentally clarify the question of whether resistance exercise with different loads – for example, 20% or 70% of the load that can only be moved once over the defined ROM (*one-repetition maximum* or 1RM) despite maximal effort – leads to different increases in MPS? If you now assume that, for example, the thigh muscles of study participants are individually stressed on the leg extension machine with either 20% (for one thigh) or 70% (for the other) and the same number of repetitions and then the change in MPS on both sides is compared, then you are unfortunately wrong.

The reason that this study design does not allow us to answer the question of whether the different loads are the reason for the different increase in MPS is simple. If you perform the same number of repetitions in both cases, the external mechanical work done is different (see Sect. 1.10). If you measure MPS responses that differ from each other, you will not be able to tell whether they are due to differences in loads (or forces) or in the mechanical work done. Incidentally, the same principle applies to the ominous comparison between single-set and multi-set training. If you repeat the same exercise (an exercise usually consists of multiple repetitions of the same movement) multiple times (and thus perform multiple sets of repetitions), the mechanical work done is greater than if you perform the exercise identically but only once. Consequently, you can no longer tell apart whether any differences in training adaptation are due to multiple execution or simply to greater mechanical work. I'll go into more detail later on the question of whether single-set and multi-set training are better for muscle growth.

## 13.4 The Dose-Response Relationship Between Training Load and the Acute Increase in Muscle Protein Synthesis

Kumar et al. (2009b) examined the dose-response relationship between exercise load during a knee extension (expressed as % of 1RM) and acute stimulation of MPS (in the vastus lateralis muscle) in young and older men, matched for external mechanical work. It was found that for the same external mechanical work, loads ≤40% of 1RM did not result in a significant increase in MPS, that between 40 and 60% of 1RM MPS increased linearly with increasing load, and that above 60% of 1RM MPS reached a plateau (i.e., above 60% of 1RM MPS did not increase significantly further despite further increases in load up to 90% of 1RM). However, if the same exercise is now performed at

30 or 90% of 1RM to the point of voluntary failure of the motor task (as opposed to performing it with the same external mechanical work), there are no differences between the two intensities with respect to the increase in MPS (Fig. 13.3).

These results are consistent with the statements in Sects. 9.3, 9.8 and 9.9 and Box. 9.3 that for high threshold motor unit recruitment, the increase in motor drive is more important than the external mechanical result it produces. Accordingly, if you exercise at a lower force or training load relative to the force value of full recruitment (e.g. 85–95% of peak voluntary force for larger muscles), you can still activate all muscle fibers that can be used for the motor task: Provided, however, you hold or move resistance until you can't anymore, that is, until exhaustion. In this case, the motor units with a high

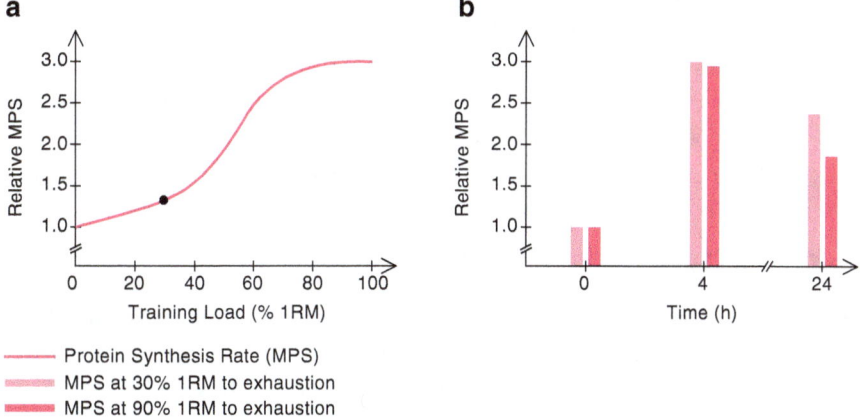

**Fig. 13.3** Effect of training load on relative MPS. (**a**) Dose-response relationship between the magnitude of the training load, expressed as a % of the one-repetition maximum (the load that can be moved only once through the defined range of motion despite maximal effort) and relative MPS. Note that this plot is for the case where the external mechanical work is held constant for the different training intensities (e.g., the external mechanical work for 3 sets at 20% of the 1RM à 27 repetitions each per set is equivalent to the external mechanical work of 6 sets at 90% of the 1RM à 3 repetitions each per set). In this case, therefore, training is not performed to exhaustion. The black dot symbolizes the relative MPS for a training load of 30% of the 1RM. (**b**) Relative MPS 4 and 24 h after a resistance exercise session for two cases considered: a low training load of 30% of the 1RM and a high training load of 90% of the 1RM. In both cases, training is performed to exhaustion. The graph shows that a moderate training load produces the same increase in MPS as a high training load, provided that training is performed to exhaustion. Thus, higher training loads do not *a priori* result in a greater increase in MPS. *MPS* muscle protein synthesis rate, *1RM* one-repetition maximum

threshold value are increasingly recruited via the discussed mechanism of fatigue (see Sect. 9.12).

## 13.5 What Influence Does the Muscular Time Under Tension Have on the Anabolism of the Muscle?

Burd et al. (2011a) investigated this question. The experimental model was basically the same as mentioned above. The researchers trained young men on the knee extension machine with a load of 30% of the 1RM (which was equivalent to approximately 30 kg in the study) and 3 sets with 2 min rest between each set. You had the subjects perform the knee extensions with one leg until voluntary exhaustion, that is, until no complete repetition (i.e., over the full ROM) was possible despite maximal effort. They used 6 s for the miometric movement phase and 6 s for the pliometric movement phase, i.e. 12 s for 1 repetition (slow rhythm). The researchers recorded the number of repetitions that could be performed in this way and had the subjects perform the same number of repetitions with the other leg, but with a movement rhythm of 1 s each for the miometric and pliometric phases (fast rhythm). They then determined the myofibrillar MPS in each case as a measure of the strength of the anabolic stimulus and compared them.

Mind you, the external mechanical work was the same for both stimuli, because the external force was the same in both cases and the same number of repetitions were performed with the same ROM, i.e. via the same pathway (approximately 12, 7 and 6 repetitions for sets 1–3). However, the resulting muscular TUT was significantly different: for each set, the TUT was approximately eight times greater for the slow compared to the fast rhythm (set 1: 198 s to 25 s; set 2: 119 s to 14 s; set 3: 90 s to 11 s). The total or summed TUT was approximately 407 s for the slow rhythm and approximately 50 s for the fast rhythm (Burd et al. 2011a). Since the same external mechanical work was performed in both cases, this means that the external mechanical power (remember: power = work/time; see Sect. 1.11) was much lower for the slow rhythm than for the fast one. Under which conditions do you estimate the anabolic response of the thigh muscle was greater?

Myofibrillar MPS was approximately 40% higher 24–30 h after training with slow rhythm than after training with fast rhythm. This correlated with the greater muscle activation (higher motor drive) measured during training with slow relative to fast rhythm. The authors' conclusion was that muscular

TUT during exercise has a significant effect on muscle anabolism (Burd et al. 2011). However, it remains unclear what TUT is optimal to stimulate MPS and whether the TUT must be accumulated without breaks or may be intermittent.

## 13.6 Which Is More Effective: Single-Set or Multi-set Training? A Pointless Question

In the following I will try to derive or work out indications for a reasonable TUT. Remember that all considerations are made with regard to the acute anabolic effect or the increase in MPS. So the following considerations are relevant if the training goal is muscle hypertrophy. I emphasize this only because larger muscles do not always lead to more external force and because, conversely, peak voluntary force can be increased even without an increase in muscle mass (see Chap. 22). It should also be borne in mind that in this section the TUT mentioned so far only describes the time between the onset of lifting the training resistance and setting it down. In Sects. 13.7 and 13.8 you will learn why the "effective time under tension" (ETUT) is a more relevant parameter than simply the TUT.

In a previous study in young men, Burd et al. (2010) sought to clarify whether multi-set training (in this case, 3 sets with 2 min rest in between, 3SET) had a greater acute effect on MPS than single-set training (performing a single set of a single exercise, 1SET). They applied the usual experimental protocol: One set was performed with one leg and 3 sets were performed with the other on the knee extension machine. All sets were performed at a training load of 70% of the 1RM (approximately 65 kg in this study) until voluntary exhaustion (see above). The movement rhythm for both interventions was the fast rhythm (1 s each for the mio and pliometric phases). When performing 1SET, study participants were able to perform approximately 14 repetitions for a total TUT of approximately 34 s. When performing 3SET, they managed approximately 14, 11, and 9 repetitions and a TUT of approximately 33, 27, and 24 s for sets 1 to 3, respectively (total TUT approximately 84 s).

You know by now from my comment above (see Sect. 13.3) that this study design is not valid for addressing the question of whether performing multiple sets 2 min apart is more beneficial in terms of increasing MPS, because in this design, both the work performed and the total TUT were varied in the comparison between 1SET and 3SET. Therefore, you cannot separate these effects. In other words, you cannot clearly attribute the observed effect on MPS to either the greater total TUT or the greater external mechanical work (training volume). Either way, the result was that both 1SET and 3SET, measured 5 h after training, had led to a significant increase in myofibrillar MPS, but the effect of 3SET relative to 1SET was stronger. Moreover, 29 h after 1SET training, myofibrillar MPS was indistinguishable from baseline at rest, whereas it was still slightly elevated for 3SET.

A similar pattern with respect to the increase in MPS emerges when you compare the effect of 4 sets at 90% of 1RM to exhaustion (5 repetitions performed with a fast rhythm per set on average, i.e. 16.3 s of TUT per set on average and approximately 64 s of total TUT) with the effect of 4 sets at 30% of 1RM to exhaustion (24 repetitions performed with a fast rhythm per set on average, i.e. 43.3 s of TUT per set on average and approximately 172 s of total TUT). Four hours after training, myofibrillar MPS is significantly increased in both training variants (no difference between 90 and 30%) while 24 h after training, myofibrillar MPS is only increased in the variant with 30% of 1RM and thus with the longer total TUT.

## 13.7 The Key to Muscle Growth

In summary, it can therefore be stated that in the studies described above, a longer summed TUT (in the examples given, approx. 64, 84, 172 or 407 s) until voluntary exhaustion was associated with a longer-lasting acute increase in myofibrillar MPS and, in this respect, had a more anabolic effect than a total duration of tension of ≤60 s. I now postulate that the actual stimulus for robust stimulation of the MPS is not primarily the *time to task failure (so far denoted as TUT)*, but the FF-recruitment time integral, more or less independent of the method by which it was generated. The FF-recruitment-time integral corresponds to the area under the recruitment-time curve for the sections with complete recruitment (S + FR + FF; grey areas in Fig. 13.4, each delimited by a white dashed line on the left and right, see examples below). In Sect. 6.8, we saw that during high-intensity resistance exercise on the knee extension machine, 80% of the total amount of ATP required is generated by the breakdown of PCr and anaerobic glycolysis during the first 30 s. The contribution of these systems to the total ATP requirement decreases with time. Thereafter, the contribution of these systems decreases with increasing exercise time or TUT. Between 30 and 120 s it is still approx. 45% and from 120 s until the time of exercise termination it is still approx. 30% (see Sect. 6.8). Since the enzyme systems for the regeneration of ATP via myofibrillar CK and anaerobic glycolysis are more pronounced or more efficient in type 2

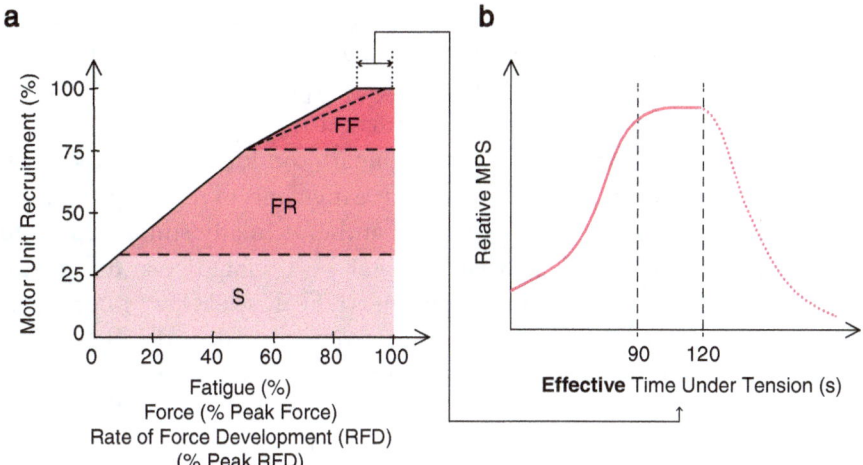

**Fig. 13.4** Examples of how you can influence the size of the FF-recruitment-time integral and thus the potential hypertrophy effect in practice via the recruitment factors "fatigue", "force" and "rate of force development". The FF-recruitment-time integral corresponds to the area under the recruitment-time curve for the sections with complete recruitment, or high or highest recruitment (S + FR + FF; gray areas delimited by a white dashed line on the left and right, respectively). See text for details. *FF* fast fatigable (see Fig. 4.2a); *FR* fast fatigue resistant (see Fig. 4.2b); *S* slow (see Fig. 4.2c)

fibers than in type 1 fibers (see Sects. 6.4 and 6.5), these results signal that metabolic fatigue of high threshold motor units (especially of the FF type) is reached after approximately 120 s. Finally, observations at the level of individual motor units also provide us with important information about the TUT during exercise. In Sect. 4.6 I described the original experiments of Burke et al. (1971) in which the properties of motor units in the cat gastrocnemius muscle were studied. In these experiments, the researchers also studied the susceptibility to fatigue of the different types of motor units and found, upon tetanic stimulation, that the FF-type motor units were still able to produce about 20% of the initial force after a TUT of 1 min and only 10% of the initial force after 2 min (i.e., a force loss of 80–90% within 1–2 min). In contrast, the S-type motor units showed virtually no fatigue, because even after 1 h the force was virtually unchanged. The FR-type motor units still produced 90% of the initial force after 2 min, but thereafter this decreased over time and was still about 10% after 1 h (Burke et al. 1973).

A few years later, Garnett et al. (1979) attempted to reproduce or test the results of Burke et al. (1973) on the human gastrocnemius muscle. Similar to the results from the cat experiments, they too found that fatigability was greatest for FF-type motor units. The relationship between TUT and force decay was also comparable in terms of magnitude. After a TUT of 150 s, FF-type motor units still produced approximately 0–63% of the initial force. In contrast, the loss of force for the S and FR types after 150 s was less than 15 and more than 20%, respectively (Garnett et al. 1979).

Based on this integrative and interdisciplinary consideration of experimental data from human experiments (acute measurements of muscle protein and energy metabolism and the fatigability of intramuscularly stimulated motor units), it is possible to deduce what the total TUT should be at full recruitment, i.e. the "effective time under tension" (ETUT, see below) to optimally stimulate the MPS. This duration is approximately 90–120 s (Fig. 13.5). Please bear in mind, however, that these estimates, which are based on scientific data, are only an approximation of the true, unknown value. They should therefore be taken as a guide and relate to a defined exercise or muscle function, i.e. the ETUT within an exercise.

However, they illustrate a fact that is fundamental in training for muscle hypertrophy: If the training load is (too) high and thus the duration of tension is (too) short to metabolically fatigue the high threshold or FF-type motor units, then multiple sets are likely necessary to robustly stimulate the MPS (longer than 1–2 h). Conversely, there is no scientifically logical reason to assume that anabolic stimulation should be greater *a priori in* the case of multiple set execution than in the case of single-set training.

The vehemence with which "experts" advocate the seemingly different concepts of single and multi-set training has ideological overtones. From a scientific point of view, the question of the number of sets does not make sense, because a muscle does not respond *a priori to* the label you attach to your training, but to what it experiences mechanically and metabolically. This is clear from the considerations outlined above. Therefore, the terms "single-set

**Fig. 13.5** (continued) and rate of force development. The shape of the curve is the same as in Fig. 9.6, except for the area of FF-type motor unit recruitment (the dashed line at the top is the same as in Fig. 9.6). The reason for the deviation is that in this figure all influencing factors (fatigue, force, speed) are combined. (**b**) ETUT with complete recruitment of the FF-type motor units (see plateau phase in a). There is a hypothetical dose-response relationship between ETUT to exhaustion of high threshold motor units and relative MPS. If the ETUT is too short, there is no significant effect on hypertrophy. If the ETUT is too long and thus the energy stress (the increase in the [AMP]/[ATP] ratio) is too high, then the increase in MPS is inhibited. The optimal range (maximum of the curve) is estimated to be a summed ETUT (understood to exhaustion) of 90–120 s per exercise or muscle function. Note that the labeling of the motor units (S, FR, and FF) in this schematic is emblematic of their threshold of excitation-from low (S), meaning low threshold, to high (FF), meaning high threshold. *S* slow, *FR* fast fatigue resistant, *FF* fast fatigable, *MPS* muscle protein synthesis rate

13 Resistance Exercise as an Anabolic Stimulus 187

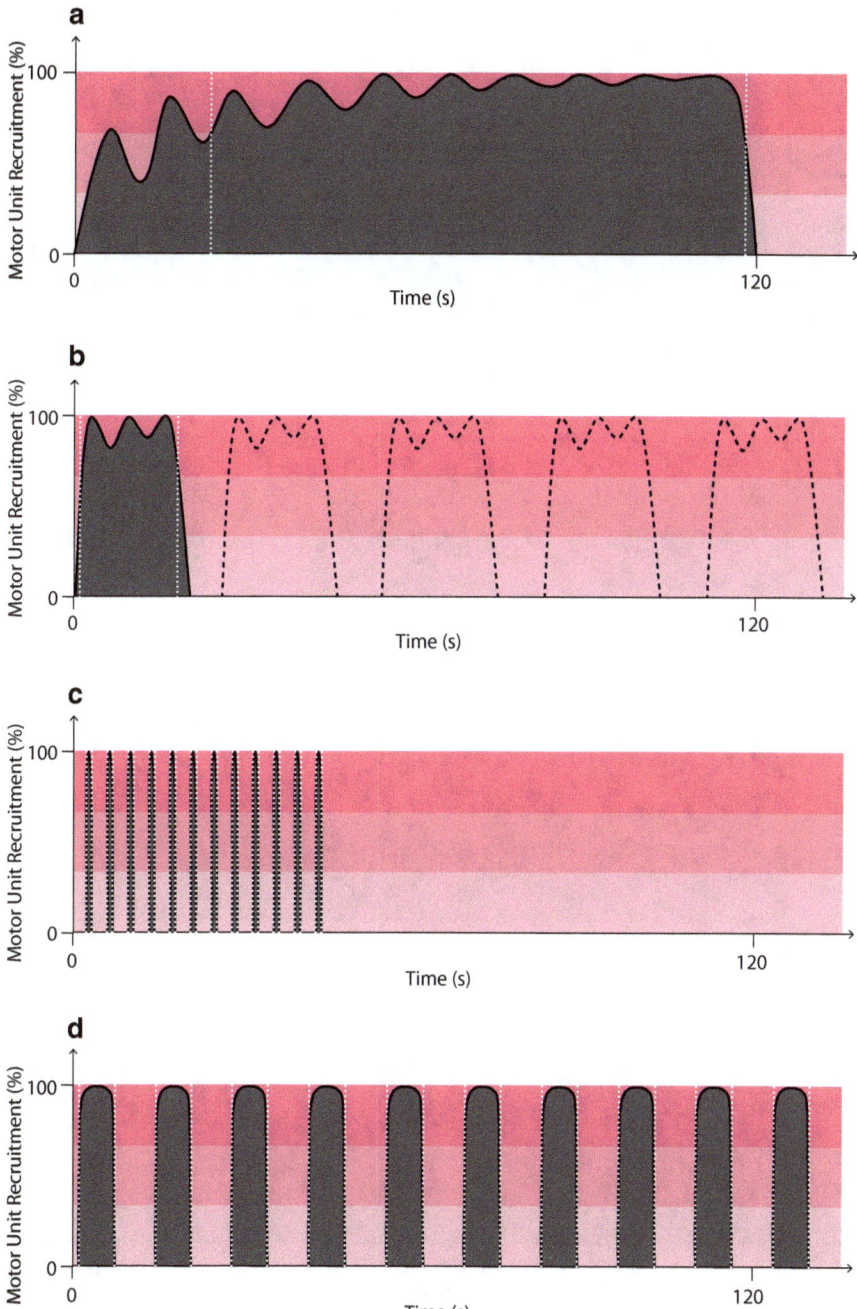

**Fig. 13.5** Hypothetical effect of effective time under tension (ETUT) of high-threshold motor units on MPS. (**a**) Dependence of motor unit recruitment on force level, fatigue,

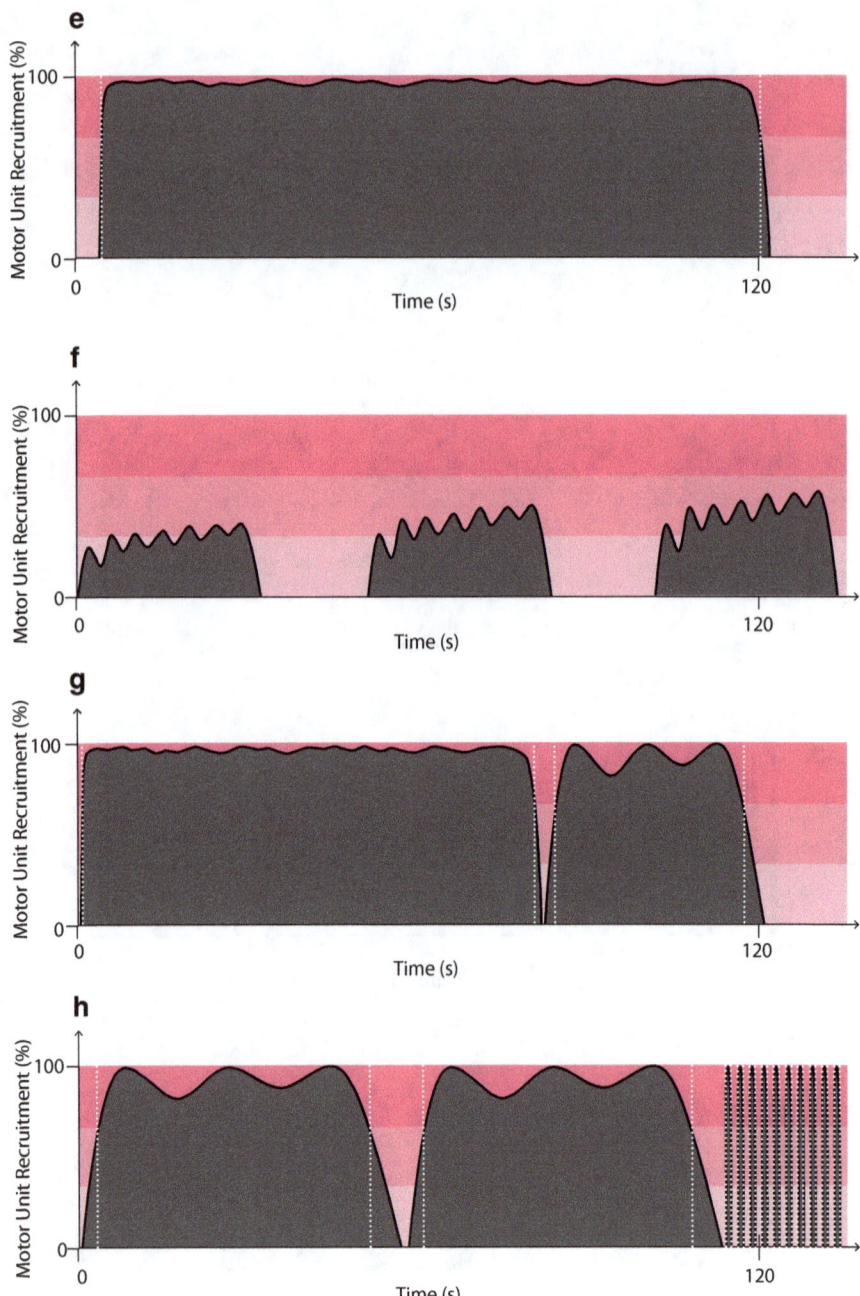

**Fig. 13.5** (continued)

training" and "multi-set training" are definitely not sufficient or suitable to define these mechanical and metabolic processes during training. So-called meta-analyses, which statistically process and summarize the results of several original studies, do not remedy this situation either, because, among other things, information on the TUT, speed of movement, external mechanical force/work/power, etc. is always missing, so that it is never clear what the object of the comparison actually is. As mentioned above, in humans the effects of repeating the same exercise several times can hardly be isolated from other possible influencing variables. Thus, the answer to the recurring question of whether single-set or multi-set training is more effective is: "It depends on how the exercise is performed." *A priori*, neither one nor the other has a greater effect on muscle growth. However, unless you are a *high responder* (see Sect. 21.1), classic single-set training may unnecessarily put obstacles in the way of developing your individual muscle hypertrophy and muscle force potential (see Sect. 14.6).

Similar to the terms of single-set and multi-set training, the buzzwords *high intensity* and *high volume* are also scientifically, i.e. mechanistically, undefined in relation to resistance exercise. Neither the sender nor the receiver are normally clear about what is actually meant by "high", "intensity" and "volume" in neuromuscular and molecular/cell biological terms. They now know better: "intensity" is to be understood in resistance exercise at the level of the recruitment-time integral and the correlation between the FF recruitment-time integral and the increase in MPS/NBIL.

Below are a few examples of how you can use the recruitment factors "fatigue", "force" and "rate of force development" to influence the size of the FF recruitment time integral and thus the potential hypertrophy effect.

1. If, in an unfatigued state, you select a load for an exercise that corresponds to ≤85% of the 1RM, not all motor units that can be recruited for the corresponding motor task are recruited at the start of the exercise. If you now perform one repetition after the other continuously (i.e. without removing the load) and slowly, fatigue increases over time. If fatigue increases over time, recruitment and frequency also increase (Fig. 13.4a). However, the shape of the recruitment-time curve is wave-like increasing, because within each repetition the force of the muscle varies depending on its length (cf. Figs. 2.1b, 2.4, 3.1a and 3.2a) and the force development mode (miometric, isometric, pliometric; Fig. 5.2): Depending on muscle length (joint angle) and force development mode, the muscle has to exert different amounts of force to cope with the external load, i.e. to move or hold it. Since the internal muscle force varies within a repetition, *even* if the exter-

nal load is the same, the frequency and recruitment of motor units also vary within a repetition. Over time, however, mean recruitment increases with fatigue until the load can no longer be overcome or maintained and the exercise has to be stopped (Fig. 13.4a). Remember: The "effective time under tension" (ETUT) describes the TUT at full recruitment when the exercise is performed to (or just before) exhaustion. In Fig. 13.4, the ETUT each correspond to the time between reaching and leaving full recruitment (indicated by white vertical dashed lines).

2. With a training load of approximately ≥85–95% of the 1RM, all motor units are recruited from the start. However, as muscle force decreases more and more with each repetition, the external torque is soon greater than the internal torque and you can no longer move the resistance (Fig. 13.4b). This does not mean that the FF-type motor units are exhausted – they just cannot generate as much force as would be required to overcome the external torque!

   Thus, if the training load is so high (≥85–95% of the 1RM) that you do not exceed 20 s per set despite maximal effort, this means that the FF-type motor units have only experienced a TUT of 20 s at best (Fig. 13.4b). This is less than what would be required to exhaust the FF-specific energy systems. In such cases, you must repeat the exercise or lower the resistance and continue until a sufficiently high TUT has been achieved (Fig. 13.4b). Consider the above example: even when the 20-s set was repeated three times (total TUT of FF-type motor units approximately 60 s), myofibrillar MPS was briefly elevated but quickly dropped and was indistinguishable from baseline 24 h after exercise. This relationship may also explain why, historically, so-called intramuscular coordination (IK) training has been used when muscle force gains but not hypertrophy is desired (see Chap. 22). Apart from the fact that the term 'intramuscular coordination' has no basis in natural science (see Box. 9.1), this involves exercisers applying repetitions at a high training load and relatively high speed, resulting in a continuous TUT that is (too) low to robustly increase myofibrillar MPS. This is noteworthy given that recruitment is complete due to high load, and further demonstrates that TUT to exhaustion may be more crucial than training load level. In terms of neural adaptations, there is little difference between short and long duration of tension as long as the exercises are performed to exhaustion. In both cases, the described adaptations occur in the increase of the instantaneous firing rate and thus more muscle (fiber) force (see Chap. 22).

3. While in the example of Fig. 13.4a the primary recruitment factor is fatigue and in Fig. 13.4b it is force, in the example of Fig. 13.4c it is the

rate of force development. As described (cf. Chap. 9; Fig. 9.7), when force development is very rapid, the motor units are recruited only phasically, or they remain recruited only tonically when the final force is greater than the tonic recruitment threshold (see Chap. 9). Thus, the TUT for the high threshold (FF) motor units, and thus the type 2 fibers, is in principle low due to the phasic recruitment or derecruitment pattern (see Sect. 9.11). This is evident in Fig. 13.4c from the fact that for each of the twelve repetitions shown, the blue areas between the white dashed lines, and thus both the FF recruitment-time integral for one repetition and the summed FF recruitment-time integral, are very small. As a consequence, the increase in MPS (see Sect. 13.5) is expected to be comparatively smaller if you perform a given number of repetitions very fast instead of slowly. The data of Burd et al. (2011a) show that for the same number of repetitions and the same external mechanical work (i.e., also the same external force), the acute anabolic effect on the trained muscle is greater with a longer TUT (i.e., with a slower exercise rhythm) than with a shorter TUT (i.e., with a faster exercise rhythm). However, it is theoretically quite conceivable that the MPS can still be effectively and sustainably increased by performing very many individual fast repetitions.

4. A thorough understanding of my concept of the FF-recruitment-time-integral and its connection with the MPS and NBIL allows you to bring the many "training systems" used in practice down to the lowest common neuromuscular, or biological, denominator and to assess them. For example, the "rest-pause" training system, in all its possible manifestations, is nothing more than another possible form of application within the concept of the FF-recruitment-time integral (Fig. 13.4d), because each individual repetition can be conceived of as a "set." But more importantly, by understanding the basics presented here, you can emancipate yourself from the unmanageable amount of "training systems" circulating, if that is what you want.

5. Taking this idea further, the logical conclusion would be that a robust increase in myofibrillar MPS could also be expected from an isometric muscle action performed to complete exhaustion in a given joint angular position, provided that the ETUT is sufficiently high (Fig. 13.4e). Thus, a recruitment-time integral that is conducive to muscle hypertrophy can, in principle, also be achieved by placing the muscle being trained in the maximum possible shortened position against a high load (miometric force development, see Sect. 1.5) and holding it in this position for as long as is somehow possible (isometric force development, see Sect. 1.5). Of course, as time goes on you will become fatigued, so that despite maximum volun-

tary effort you will not be able to hold the load in the position you have assumed. However, you will still struggle with full effort against the lowering of the load, i.e. you will try to slow down the lowering of the load (very slow pliometric force generation, see Sect. 1.5) until the load forces you back to the starting position. The load should be selected so that approximately 120 s elapse between the time the load is lifted and the time it touches down (Fig. 13.4e). Applied to the leg extension machine, this means that you bring a high load into full extension in a controlled manner and hold it there for as long as possible. At some point the load will "force" you back to the starting position. However, at all times you are trying to prevent this by pushing against it with your fullest effort. So you try to stop the load during the whole braking movement. Of course you lose this duel against the load, but you gain a good training stimulus for increasing muscle mass and muscle force!

The angle position chosen could have an influence on the direction of hypertrophy (longitudinal and/or radial). If you choose an angular position in which the muscle is stretched (i.e. used for longer than usual), the adaptive stimulus for longitudinal hypertrophy is included (see Sect. 10.2.6).

6. The fact that so-called "multi-set training" does not produce better results than "single-set training" in terms of the recruitment-time integral on principle is illustrated in Fig. 13.4f: If the combination of the magnitude of the load, fatigue and/or rate of force development is not right and/or if the quality of exercise execution is not right (i.e. if the load does not "arrive" at the muscles to be trained), nothing is of any use.

Incidentally, it is a mental error to refer to multi-set training as the repeated performance of the same exercise within a training session (with rests between sets), although this is unfortunately common in science as well as in the fitness, weight training and bodybuilding world. Rather, by performing different exercises for the same muscle (see Sect. 9.14 on task-specific motor unit recruitment), a large proportion of muscle fibers may experience an addition of the ETUT of the different exercises. This is because individual motor units can be used for several anatomical functions (see Sect. 9.14). In the broadest sense, therefore, you may well be performing multi-set training even if you perform each exercise only once but train or perform exercises for different anatomical functions for the same muscle.

7. The different strategies for recruiting motor units (level of force, fatigue and rate of force development) can also be combined well, for example in the context of "drop sets" or similar (cf. Fig. 13.4g, h).

## 13.8 The Difference Between Time Under Tension, Effective Time Under Tension and Number of Repetitions

The term "time under tension", commonly abbreviated as TUT, is well and truly reduced to the time between the lifting of the training resistance or load and setting it down However, we have seen that the FF-recruitment time integral experienced by the muscle is a determinant of myofibrillar MPS stimulation and, extrapolated from this, muscle hypertrophy. This is in principle independent of the strategy used to generate full recruitment. As can be seen from the experiments described above, the TUT in the narrower sense thus refers to the duration during which a particular motor unit or muscle fiber produces (maximum) force before its function is impaired (see Sect. 13.7).

If you perform externally visible movements or train dynamically during resistance exercise, then I recommend that you keep the resistance isometric for 2 s when reversing from the pliometric to the miometric muscle action (i.e. when the muscle-tendon unit is fully stretched) (cf. Box. 10.3). The training resistance should then be chosen so that you can do this at least six times, giving a TUT of about 12 s in the stretched position (see Sect. 10.2.6). The same applies to the reversal from miometric to pliometric muscle action (i.e. with the muscle-tendon unit fully shortened). As mentioned earlier, this form of training not only has advantages in terms of stimulating longitudinal hypertrophy, but also contributes to increased muscle fiber TUT due to deceleration (see Sect. 1.13). As an arbitrary practical example, let's assume that you have chosen a training load that you can anatomically move perfectly throughout the ROM and that allows you a time to force or position failure of 100 s. Let's further assume that, based on the considerations above, you move the training load in such a way that you use 2 s each for the isometric phases at the reversal points and 3–4 s for the miometric and pliometric phases. This way, you need about 10–12 s per repetition, bringing your total to about 7–9 repetitions. No, I didn't miscalculate. If you perform the exercise to voluntary exhaustion, that is, to the point where you can no longer move the training resistance for a few seconds despite maximum effort or it pushes you back to the starting position, then the miometric movement phases will automatically slow down towards the end. Near the end, push or pull for a few seconds without the resistance moving. In this case, the effective number of repetitions is less than the theoretically calculated number (i.e. about 8–10). Thus, when you perform an exercise to exhaustion, the time proportion of the different force generation modes (isometrically shortened, miometric, isometrically stretched, pliometric) changes within each repetition: the overcoming (miometric) phase necessarily becomes longer as you become more fatigued and find it increasingly difficult to overcome the load in the allotted time, while the braking (pliometric) phase tends to become shorter towards the end. In fact, as you fatigue, you find it increasingly difficult to brake the load in the allotted time. Thus, when performing an exercise as exemplified above and shown as one of many possible implementation variations to the FF recruitment-time integral in Fig. 13.4a, a given movement rhythm can actually only be accurately maintained during the first few repetitions. Incidentally, this also applies to the execution of "explosive" or fast movements: As soon as fatigue exceeds a certain level, you slow down in the miometric movement phase and/or you can no longer maintain the original.

While the TUT per repetition in the miometric phase of a movement increases with increasing fatigue, it tends to decrease in the pliometric phase. The latter can be observed in a more pronounced form during negative training: the rate of the change in length (in this case, the stretch) increases with each repetition, even though you are trying to brake the load with maximum voluntary effort. This is clearly illustrated by the example of the purely pliometric pull-ups, which you may remember (see Box 1.2): Each time you bring yourself to the starting position with the help of the leg muscles, the muscle force in the back and arm muscles being trained drops temporarily. A negative set is therefore made up of individual pliometric muscle actions (and the time intervals you need to get to the starting position). Despite maximal voluntary effort, the (effective) TUT decreases from repetition to repetition over time: for example, 10 s (1st repetition), 10 s (2nd repetition), 9 s (3rd repetition), 9 s (4th repetition), then with each repetition 1 s less TUT until the exercise is stopped. In other words, the higher the training resistance (dumbbell, machine, or your body) for a given muscle force, or the more fatigued your muscle for a given external load, the faster the braking movement. During the last repetitions, the training resistance, for example the dumbbell, will fall to earth unbraked, so to speak. Therefore, special care must be taken during negative training.

From the sum of these considerations it becomes clear that the number of repetitions alone is not a reliable indicator for the TUT, and certainly not for the ETUT. Training recommendations that only include the load level and the number of repetitions are insufficient to adequately describe the training stimulus in resistance exercise for this reason, among others.

## 13.9 Is Pliometric (Eccentric) More Effective than Miometric (Concentric)?

Pliometric muscle activity or negative training is generally associated with greater hypertrophy effects (Roig et al. 2009). It is therefore surprising that in a study of the acute temporal change of myofibrillar MPS following either mio- or pliometric exercise, no difference was measured between the two types of activity (Cuthbertson et al. 2006). Indeed, it appears that when the amount of total external work is matched between the two training modalities, the same amount of hypertrophy results regardless of modality, at least when considered over a 9-week training period. Moore et al. (2012b) demonstrated this using an experiment in which they trained the arm flexor muscles of young male study participants in a purely mio- or pliometric fashion on a dynamometer. The velocity of movement of the lever arm was fixed (i.e. isokinetic) at 45 angular degrees per second. The TUT per repetition over a ROM of 90° (between 10° and 100° elbow flexion) was therefore approximately 2 s for each repetition. During this process, the study participants always attempted to push against the lever arm with maximum muscle force.

The subjects exercised miometrically with one arm and pliometrically with the other. However, at maximum voluntary effort, the resulting torque is greater for the pliometric relative to the miometric effort (see Sect. 1.6 and Box 1.2). Thus, the amount of external mechanical work would also be greater in the pliometric relative to the miometric case for the same ROM and number of repetitions. Therefore, for the miometric-training upper arm, the number of repetitions was increased such that the total external mechanical work performed was the same as for the pliometric-training upper arm. After a training period of 9 weeks with 2 training sessions per week, the result was that both upper arms (pliometrically or miometrically trained) had gained approximately 5% in muscle cross-sectional area (Moore et al. 2012b). In this sense, pliometrically oriented training appears to be more time efficient rather than more effective compared to miometric training.

## 13.10 Skeletal Muscles Also Have a "Feeling of Satiety"

Similar to the muscle *full response of* the muscle to dietary protein or essential amino acids, the anabolic response of the muscle to training is of limited duration. Figuratively speaking, the muscle shuts down protein synthesis once it has been fed or filled with training stimuli (analogous to essential amino acids). So more is not better – on the contrary. Immediately after training, the increase in MPS occurs with a certain time delay (latency period), which is related to the strength of the mechanical (microtrauma, see Sects. 7.3, 7.4 and 7.5) and/or energetic ([AMP]/[ATP] ratio; see Sect. 15.2) stress. The greater the mechanical and/or energetic stress, the longer the latency.

It would be interesting to see if latency is related to the degree of microtrauma induced. We have seen in Sect. 8.1 that microtrauma in skeletal muscle leads to highly orchestrated degeneration and regeneration processes. It is precisely the inflammatory reaction that initially takes place that could inhibit MPS, because it is known that systemic inflammatory processes can impair MPS. It is also known from animal experiments in mice and rats that MPS is suppressed *during* muscle loading. It was found in these experiments that the magnitude of suppression depended on the number of electrical nerve stimulations. The extent and duration of MPS suppression during exercise could therefore be a determinant of how long the latency period is before MPS increases after exercise.

## 13.11 What Is the Optimum Time Interval with Which to Train a Particular Muscle?

It depends on how you have been training. We have seen above that the myofibrillar MPS remains elevated for different lengths of time depending on the total TUT. Documented is an increase up to 72 h, in certain cases the MPS can be back to baseline level after 2 h already. Ideally, the time intervals would be set to maximize the integral of myofibrillar MPS over time, that is, the area under the MPS curve over time. Therefore, it cannot be ruled out that more frequent training, for example 1 set every 3–5 h may be as effective or perhaps even more effective than the more classical form of one to two training sessions per week with a higher total TUT. However, you would have to apply this training paradigm to every muscle, which makes it very unlikely to be practical after all. If you still have the opportunity to try this type of training, I'd love to hear your feedback! Please also read the comments on this question in Sect. 15.3.

## 13.12 Misconception of Supercompensation

Who hasn't heard of the vivid but ominous concept of supercompensation? Essentially, it is based on the assertion that biological systems react to stress with an exaggerated response. Physiological bone adaptation to mechanical stimuli, for example, does not work in this way (see Sect. 19.2). The aim of regulation in this case is not, as is generally wrongly assumed, to make the bone as heavy as possible, but as strong as necessary.

A supercompensation curve is shown in a diagram with x- and y-axis, whereby the axes are rather seldom labelled with concrete measured quantities (see Sect. 1.7). Often the axes are not labelled at all. Common labels for the y-axis include "system status", "performance capability", etc. But what is actually meant by these vague labels? Does the performance capacity stand for power, force, torque, running speed? Does system status stand for the speed of protein synthesis, the amount or phosphorylation of proteins, the number of specific mRNA molecules, or perhaps for the concentrations of hormones, metabolites and substrates (especially muscle glycogen) in blood or muscle? The x-axis often indicates time as a general quantity.

As a model for the general adaptation mechanism of a biological system, the concept is therefore no good. The reason why signal transduction cascades and metabolic processes are activated and/or deactivated is not that "something" *must* have decreased beforehand (because that is what the model postulates). In the most extreme case, you don't even need to exercise for exceptionally large and strong muscles! How? Single point mutations in the gene sequence can have such an effect that muscle mass in different species is increased several times over, even in the untrained state (see Sect. 21.2). In future, therefore, in addition to the usual pharmacological interventions, we will have to discuss gene doping and *exercise mimetics* in particular. The latter are small molecules that can, for example, trigger adaptation processes in the muscles that are similar to those of training.

It should be clear by now that adaptation of the neuromuscular system is a concerted interaction of different molecules, cells, tissues and organs. Thus, adaptation is inherently integrative with respect to a time scale (microseconds to years) and an order of magnitude (nanometers to meters). The concept of supercompensation fails to represent this complexity or conveys a false, (too) trivial picture. Finally, the term "supercompensation" is inherently contradictory. "Compensation" means something like "balance" and "super" in this context means "over". Now, you may be able to overcompensate slightly, but then you are no longer talking about compensation but growth. So the term "supercompensation" is about as meaningless as "supramaximal strength" or "supramaximal training". If a value is maximal, then by definition no value can exist that is higher (i.e. supra).

## 13.13 Summary

A tiring debate that has prevailed for decades revolves around the question of whether "single-set training" or "multi-set training" is better for muscle growth. Generally, "single-set training" is understood to mean performing exactly one series of repetitions for each exercise completed in resistance exercise. Accordingly, "multi-set training" involves performing several such series of repetitions. A primary goal of resistance exercise is to stress the muscle mechanically and metabolically in such a way that the muscle-building processes are stimulated over a long period of time. From a scientific point of view, therefore, the question cannot be answered in any other way than: "It depends on how the exercise is performed!". The number of sets is not a priori a stimulus to which the muscles respond with growth and it is therefore of secondary importance. The same applies to the number of repetitions. Depending on the design, a single repetition can also be considered a "set". Much more important than the number of sets and repetitions is the FF-recruitment-time integral for the muscles to be trained. The FF-recruitment-time integral corresponds to the area under the recruitment-time curve, for the time periods with complete recruitment of all motor units available for the specific movement function. A FF recruitment-time integral conducive to muscle hypertrophy can be realized by combining two cardinal factors. The first factor is the recruitment of all available motor units. In principle, the first factor can be realized by several recruitment strategies and/or combinations of them: The amount of force applied, the fatigue (or the degree of fatigue reached), and/or the rate of force generation. The second factor is a sufficiently high TUT in the state of full recruitment (i.e. a sufficiently high ETUT), and this is independent of the recruitment strategy used. *Notably*, TUT, when understood as the duration of time between lifting and setting down the training load, is not necessarily synonymous with the much more crucial ETUT, which describes the TUT at full recruitment (until exhaustion, or force decay, or fatigue). Both factors combined are mechanistically related to the strength of excitation of the MPS and thus to the NBIL. The latter provides the compelling metabolic basis for muscle hypertrophy.

Broadly speaking, to meet these factors for your training in practice, the following can be recommended as an example or guide: For each exercise, aim for a transient force drop of at least about 50% within approximately 90–120 s of ETUT. For example, if you start the first repetition with a load of 100 kg and a precisely defined movement rhythm, you should no longer be able to perform more than 2–3 repetitions with 50 kg in the original movement rhythm immediately (i.e. within 1–2 s) after forcing the load down after a total of 90–120 s of ETUT. The "better" you can train, i.e. the more targeted and isolated you can fatigue the muscles, the greater the temporary drop can be (70% is quite possible). Whether you accomplish this with single (maximal) reps, drop sets, continuous dynamic reps, isometric actions, etc., or combinations thereof, is probably of secondary importance to triggering radial hypertrophy. However, I recommend that you vary your recruitment strategy. For longitudinal hypertrophy, it is also advisable to pay due attention to force generation at long muscle lengths (i.e. in the stretched position). Apart from training safety and quality (targeted "delivery" of the load to the target muscle), a slow rhythm of movement allows you to optimise the ETUT, which can make your training more time-efficient. Perform several different exercises per muscle or muscle group, i.e. train a muscle in all its movement functions if possible. These factors, which you can specifically influence during training, hold the key to muscle growth.

# 14

# The Synergistic Relationship Between Resistance Exercise and Dietary Protein Intake

## 14.1 The Synergistic Effect Between Resistance Exercise and Dietary Protein

We have seen that a single resistance exercise session without additional intake of dietary protein is able to increase MPS for a few hours to more than 72 h, depending on the stimulus, but NBIL remains negative after resistance exercise because MPB also increases with resistance exercise (Fig. 13.2). The increase in MPS, measured after a single resistance exercise session and averaged, is greater in young men compared to seniors (Fig. 13.1). Further, you have learned that there is a dose-response relationship between the FF recruitment time integral, denominated «effective time under tensio» (ETUT) to exhaustion (i.e., to significant force decay) and the increase in (myofibrillar) MPS after resistance exercise, and that recruitment of FF motor units can be accomplished by several strategies (Figs. 13.4 and 13.5).

Dietary protein alone, i.e. not in combination with resistance exercise, leads to a transient positive NBIL and thus has a similar effect on MPS as resistance exercise alone (Fig. 11.2). However, an important difference between the two anabolic stimuli is that after the single protein supplement, MPS is increased for only a few hours, whereas after a single resistance exercise session, the effect on MPS can extend to several days. Similar to resistance exercise, a dose-response relationship exists for dietary protein between the amount of protein ingested per meal or protein intake and the increase in (myofibrillar) MPS, with the saturation dose for maximal stimulation of myofibrillar MPS being reached at an average of approximately 20 g of whey protein in young men (Fig. 12.4). In seniors, the required dose appears to be almost twice as high on average (Fig. 12.4). After ingestion of this maximum stimulating dose, a refractory phase of a few hours occurs as described, during which the MPS remains indifferent to a constantly high or further increasing amino acid concentration in the blood. Please remember at this point that the increase in MPS should not be equated with the "anabolic effect" (see Sect. 12.6). There is also a dose-response relationship between the amount of protein ingested, the inhibition of (M)PB, the increase in PS and thus the (whole body) NBIL (see Sect. 12.6 and Fig. 12.3). It is generally agreed that theoretically there is a maximal anabolic response to dietary protein intake. However, how much dietary protein would be necessary to elicit this maximal anabolic response is a matter of controversy.

If we now compare the relative increase in MPS after a single ingestion of whey protein with the effect of a single resistance exercise session on MPS, it appears that during the first hours after the ingestion of 20 g of whey protein, both young men (approx. +63 percentage points) and seniors (approx. +69 percentage points) experience a greater average increase in MPS than immediately after a resistance exercise session (approx. +42 vs. +37 percentage points, cf. Fig. 12.4 with Fig. 13.1). After a single administration of 40 g of whey protein, the MPS of seniors even increases by an average of approx. 104 percentage points (compared to +37 percentage points after a resistance exercise session).

What happens when you combine the two anabolic stimuli, resistance exercise and dietary protein? Is the increase in myofibrillar MPS greater when protein is ingested close in time to resistance exercise? Is the increase in MPS greater after administration of dietary protein at rest (i.e. not timed to a workout) if you have strength trained the day before? In short, what is the interaction between resistance exercise and dietary protein? The importance of this question automatically follows from the observation that resistance exercise alone (i.e., without protein or essential amino acid intake) does not result in a positive NBIL despite a marked increase in MPS. If a deficiency in essential amino acids were persistent, it would result in a maladaptation, meaning the exerciser would lose muscle mass over time. It follows that a muscle cannot be built or remodeled without sufficient protein being supplied.

Let's get this out of the way right away: The amount of protein per intake time that can produce a maximum MPS response at rest is approximately the same as the amount of protein that is sufficient to also produce the maximum potentiation effect when combined with resistance exercise. In contrast to protein intake alone, you do not need to change anything in terms of the amount of protein supplied per intake time if you are resistance exercise.

Resistance exercise leads to a preconditioning of the muscle: The muscle becomes more sensitive or receptive to dietary amino acids. In other words, resistance exercise increases the *muscle full target value* (see Sects. 12.5 and 13.1), i.e. compared with the intake of protein alone, the MPS is only switched off at a higher value. Accordingly, an intake of protein that is timely relative to resistance exercise leads to a potentiation of the MPS, both in terms of peak value and duration (Fig. 14.1). In young men, myofibrillar MPS is shown to increase approximately 2.5-fold in the first hours after a resistance exercise session when 20–40 g of whey protein (dissolved in water, i.e. as a shake) is ingested following leg training (compared to the effect of resistance exercise alone, Fig. 14.2). Even with the combination of resistance exercise and dietary protein, however, it can be seen that in young men the maximum relative effect on myofibrillar MPS is achieved on average with 20 g whey protein (+19% relative to the value achieved after administration of 10 g, Fig. 14.2). In contrast, in the seniors the maximum relative synergistic effect on the MPS is seen with 40 g whey protein (+40% relative to the value achieved after administration of 20 g, Fig. 14.2). Overall, myofibrillar MPS in the first hours after a resistance exercise session in seniors increases on average about 5.5 times more when a shake with 40 g whey protein is taken following leg training (compared to the effect of resistance exercise alone, Fig. 14.2). However, these results should be viewed critically, as recent studies have failed to demonstrate anabolic resistance in healthy, physically active elderly people (Moro et al. 2018).

Little research has been done to determine whether protein supplementation following a full-body workout (or at least a workout of multiple muscle groups in the same session) reduces the increase in MPS in a defined muscle compared to training the same muscle in isolation. For example, is the increase in MPS in the biceps brachii muscle smaller after a whole-body program followed by protein intake than after biceps training alone and intake of the same amount of protein? The data of West et al. (2009) suggest that at least when training a small muscle group (biceps brachii muscle) together with a large muscle group (quadriceps femoris muscle), the increase in myofibrillar MPS in the small muscle is not impaired compared to training the same muscle in isolation (without training other muscles in the same training session) in young men (with the same administration of 25 g protein immediately after training). However, it cannot be excluded that the amount of protein supplied when training very many muscle groups, all competing for amino acids from the blood, may be a limiting factor for the increase in MPS in individual muscles. It could therefore be that in the case of whole-body training, the amount of protein necessary and sufficient for maximum stimulation

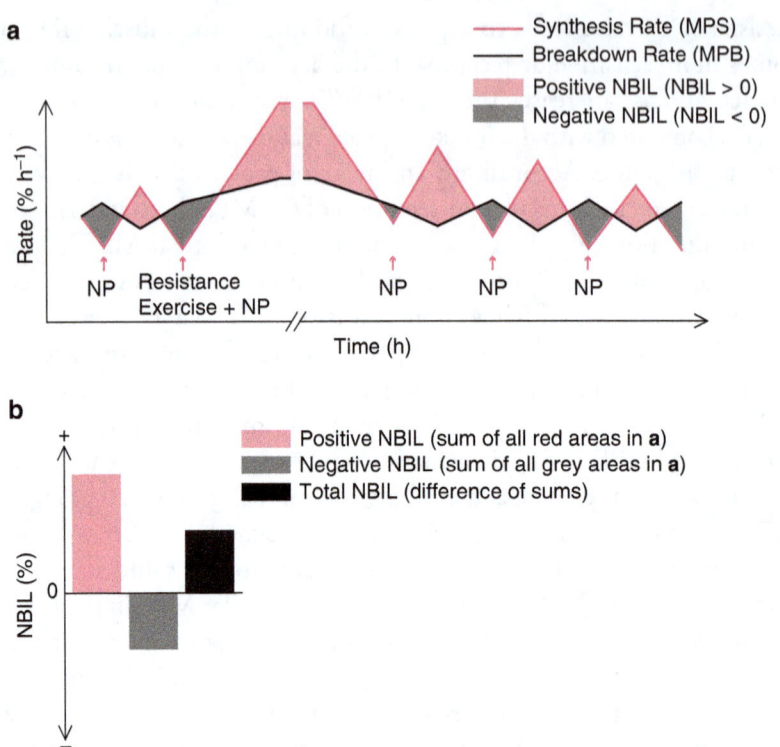

**Fig. 14.1** Synergistic effect between resistance exercise and protein intake. (**a**) If high-quality and properly dosed dietary protein (NP) is ingested immediately after a single resistance exercise session, MPS increases much more than for NP or resistance exercise considered separately. In addition, MPB increases less compared to resistance exercise alone (i.e., resistance exercise without ingestion of NP). Note that resistance exercise makes the trained muscles more sensitive to NP, as evidenced by the fact that even hours and days after resistance exercise, the MPS for a defined amount of NP is higher than when the same amount of NP is taken in the untrained state. (**b**) The result is that the net muscle protein balance (NBIL) viewed over hours and days is positive (NBIL >0). If the resistance exercise stimuli are now applied repeatedly at appropriate intervals (depending on the training stimulus or the increase and decrease in MPS dependent on it), macroscopic muscle growth will occur due to the repeated positive NBIL. *MPS* muscle protein build-up rate, *MPB* muscle protein breakdown rate, *NBIL* net muscle protein balance, *NP* dietary protein

of the myofibrillar MPS of all trained muscles is greater per time point of intake (possibly with a longer refractory phase for this).

A recently published study of young, strength-trained men suggests that this limitation may indeed occur after training multiple, large muscle groups. In these young men, myofibrillar MPS of the vastus lateralis increased more after resistance exercise when they received 40 g of protein compared to 20 g

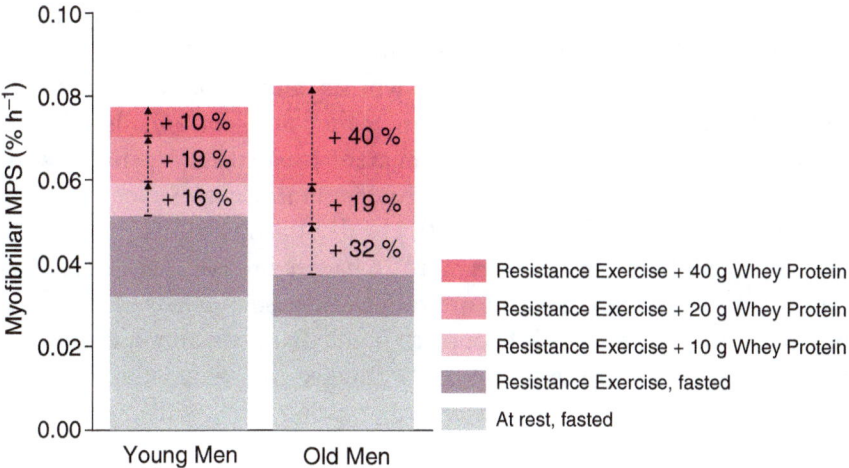

**Fig. 14.2** Dose-response relationship between the amount of whey protein ingested following thigh muscle resistance exercise and the increase in myofibrillar muscle protein synthesis (MPS) rate in the same muscle group in adult young men and seniors. (Adapted from Witard et al. 2014; Yang et al. 2012)

of protein. In this case, the smaller protein dose (20 g) did not appear to be sufficient to maximally stimulate MPS in all trained muscles (MacNaughton et al. 2016). However, this result has not been replicated to date and other studies with better designs suggest the opposite (see Sect. 16.3).

## 14.2 Protein Intake: Best Before, During or After Resistance Exercise?

When should protein be administered relative to the timing of resistance exercise to maximize MPS and thus training adaptations? This question has received much scientific attention (e.g. Cribb and Hayes 2006). After all, there are basically three options: before, during, and after resistance exercise. In all studies in which protein intake occurred immediately after training, it has been shown that there is a synergistic effect of resistance exercise and dietary protein with respect to MPS. In contrast, few studies in general have been conducted in which either protein or amino acids were administered immediately prior to training. In addition, the results have been inconsistent. Studies on the effect of ingesting protein during training are virtually nonexistent.

Based on these data, one scientific camp is therefore of the opinion that the intake of protein (more generally: of nutrients) immediately after resistance exercise makes the most sense. Other scientists, on the contrary, find that the timing of intake is essentially irrelevant, as the *muscle full effect* is delayed by at least 24 h after a workout. This statement is based on experimental data that have shown that the increased sensitivity of muscle to dietary amino acids lasts for at least 24 h. Burd et al. (2011b) demonstrated that the MPS to a given amount of protein increases more 24 h after a resistance exercise session than when the identical amount of protein is ingested independent of training. Thus, proponents of this hypothesis argue that nutrient availability *per se* is more crucial than the exact timing of intake. This would also explain the observation that effective hypertrophy is possible even with protein intake that is not optimal in the short term.

I'll go a step further and take a more nuanced view. There are two things you need to consider when choosing the timing. First, as discussed in Sect. 15.2, MPS is suppressed *during* force production. High amino acid availability is of no use then, as the muscle is not receptive to it. Secondly, the increase in MPS after force production or resistance exercise only starts after a latency period, which can vary in length depending on the type of training (energetic and/or mechanical stress) (see Sects. 15.2 and 15.3).

It follows that the muscle is "blind" to the amino acids circulating in the blood during resistance exercise, not only acutely during force production, but also in the pauses between any sets (latency period). The notion that you flood the system with amino acids before training and then the muscle sucks up the amino acids in the breaks between sets like a swimmer gasping for air is not true. The longer your workout, meaning the more sets you perform, the less sense it makes to consume protein or amino acids immediately before or during your workout.

If you work a muscle group with an infinite number of sets during training, the MPS remains suppressed during the whole time (also during the breaks between the sets) and the risk increases that the anabolic stimulus is inhibited. This can happen, for example, if the increase in MPS is inhibited by the high energy stress or if the mechanical stress becomes so great that it exceeds the regenerative capacity (see Sects. 7.3 and 15.2). In addition, high-volume training may increase latency, which can make optimal timing more difficult in terms of resistance exercise-protein interaction.

When ingesting 20 g of whey protein (in aqueous solution) on an empty stomach, the blood concentration of essential amino acids (in general) and leucine (in particular) in young men reaches its peak value after approx. 30 min and then decreases again over the next 2–3 h. However, 90–120 min after ingestion, the concentration is already statistically indistinguishable from baseline. Can you recall the response of myofibrillar MPS to 20 g dietary protein (see Sect. 12.5)? Approximately 30 min after ingestion, the myofibrillar MPS rises sharply, reaches approx. two to three times the initial value after approx. 1.5 h and falls back to the initial value after 2 h. This time course is congruent with the development of the amino acid concentration in the blood described at the beginning.

One can therefore speculate that it would be optimal to time the intake of protein to training such that the amino acid concentration in the blood is highest after the training-induced latency period has elapsed. The problem is that the training-induced latency is dependent on training, and you essentially don't know this dose-response relationship yet. So the way you perform resistance exercise not only determines how much and sustained the MPS increases after training, but also influences the extent to which dietary amino acids can act synergistically.

So far, so good. Unfortunately, however, there are at least two flaws. First, all studies to date that have examined the dose-response relationship between MPS and the amount of protein administered have examined measurements in study participants after resistance exercise in the fasting state (i.e., after overnight fasting). However, this does not correspond to the training behavior of most exercisers, who tend to complete their training 2–3 h after a meal. The practical relevance of the described studies on the dose-response relationship was therefore questionable until now. Only recently, Witard et al. (2014) contributed to clarify this aspect and investigated in young men the acute increase in myofibrillar MPS for different amounts of whey protein approximately 3 h 45 min after a very high-protein (0.55 g protein per kilogram body mass) breakfast was administered, with or without preceding resistance exercise. It was found that myofibrillar MPS could be stimulated again to the same extent after the time interval of about 3 h 45 min as after the high-protein breakfast, but only if the necessary and sufficient amount of whey protein isolate (20 g) was ingested. The muscles of young men are therefore "responsive" again approx. 3 h 45 min after a protein-containing meal. This study result is consistent with the results on the effect of the administration pattern of dietary protein on MPS and/or NBIL (see Sect. 12.6).

Second, the vast majority of studies on the dose-response relationship between protein dose and MPS stimulation after resistance exercise have been done after training individual muscle groups (as opposed to whole body training). I am not aware of any study that has investigated, for example, whether the MPS response in the thigh muscle is different with or without protein intake and with protein intakes of different doses when several other muscle groups are trained before or after the thighs (see Sects. 14.1 and 16.3).

Overall, the picture is as follows: During energy-demanding force production, protein synthesis is not a priority for a muscle and is thus suppressed. Depending on the extent of the energetic and/or mechanical stress, the increase in MPS occurs more or less delayed. At the time, it would be ideal if amino acid availability in the blood were maximal, because essential amino acids have a synergistic effect on MPS. Without training, after administration of the necessary and sufficient amount of protein to maximally stimulate MPS, the muscle is refractory for about 3–4 h, that is, not receptive to amino acids from the blood. Resistance exercise, however, leads to the sensitization of the muscle to amino acids from the blood, so that an anabolic window is opened for several hours and possibly days after resistance exercise.

## 14.3 Does Resistance Exercise Affect Protein Digestion?

In the context of digestion rate and efficiency, it has recently been demonstrated that a single resistance exercise session can impair protein digestion and absorption (van Wijck et al. 2013). Young men completed a high-volume leg workout: 6 sets of 10 repetitions on a horizontal leg press followed by 6 sets of 12 repetitions on a leg extension machine. As is almost always the case, the actual training was inadequately described in this report (see Toigo and Boutellier 2006). The young men were all healthy and trained for approx. 5–10 h per week in several sports (but which ones exactly were not specified).

Immediately after training, the young men were given 250 ml of a drink containing 20 g of casein (intrinsically isotope-labelled casein). The digestion as well as the absorption of this protein was then measured and the values were compared with the values previously recorded at rest (i.e. without training). In addition, they tested whether small intestinal lesions occurred during these processes. The authors suspected that resistance exercise would lead to splanchnic (i.e. visceral) blood loss due to the rapid redistribution of blood from the abdominal region to the working muscles. In previous studies, the same authors demonstrated that such exercise-induced splanchnic blood loss can lead to small intestinal injuries. Here, they now wanted to test whether such injuries could impair protein absorption.

The result of the study was that this type of resistance exercise led to an increase in the marker for small intestinal injuries and, compared to resting conditions, it led to a lower increase in the concentration of essential amino acids in the blood, which was reduced throughout the observation period. The authors' conclusion was that this type of resistance exercise in young, polysport-trained men may result in small, transient intestinal injuries that may impair digestion and absorption of dietary protein.

The relevance of these results is not clear, however, because it is unknown whether these differences also lead to significant differences in MPS and whether it is not rather a general effect that occurs with unaccustomed training. I've often seen people get dizzy, even briefly pass out, lose color in their face, and/or vomit during their first hard workout. This all has to do with the rapid redistribution of blood in the body mentioned above, among other things. After a few training sessions, however, these effects no longer occur in most people, so it can be assumed that with increasing experience the body only redistributes as much blood as is necessary. Therefore, there is currently no evidence that protein intake should be delayed after training. This view is also shared by the authors of the study mentioned above.

## 14.4 Is Carbohydrate Intake Necessary Immediately After Resistance Exercise to Maximize MPS or Minimize MPB?

The answer to the question is no. The simultaneous intake of carbohydrates does not bring an additional increase in MPS nor an additional decrease in MPB compared to the intake of protein alone. The situation after weight training is therefore no different from the situation at rest, which we have already discussed in Sect. 12.8. Why do you need carbohydrates at all? A single session of resistance exercise can reduce glycogen content in the muscles used by 24–40% (see Sect. 6.5), with the greatest percentage reduction occurring in type 2 fibers. The extent to which the glycogen content of the muscle decreases depends on how much ATP has been produced with glycolytic regeneration (see Sect. 6.5). This in turn depends on which motor units were recruited during training and which force level was maintained for how long. In general, however, the more sets you complete or the longer your training, the greater the resulting decrease in muscle glycogen content is likely to be.

## 14.5 Is the Anabolic Response of the Muscle Weaker if You Train with Relatively Empty Muscle Glycogen Stores?

In the short term, the answer is no. It could be shown in young men that the reduction of the muscle glycogen content through diet and training to 50% of the initial value had no influence on the increase in MPS after resistance exercise (in both conditions 8 sets of leg extensions of 5 repetitions each at 80% of the 1RM; the information that is important for us, such as the time under tension, is again not known), neither in the fasting state nor after the administration of protein and carbohydrates (Camera et al. 2012). Thus, it doesn't matter whether you show up to training fasting or whether your muscle glycogen stores are full to the brim or half-empty when it comes to increasing MPS. Statements that you *need to* consume a lot of carbohydrates in order to record effective muscle hypertrophy are fairy tales.

Logically, a fairly empty muscle glycogen store can have a negative effect on your training, namely when the necessary training intensity can no longer be generated. More specifically, when the glycogen reserves in type 2 muscle fibers are too small to maintain the ETUT required for muscle hypertrophy at the tonic recruitment threshold (see Sect. 13.7). If you want to remain competitive in the long term, you should replenish your muscle glycogen stores after exercise. Replenishing stores, rather than increasing MPS or inhibiting MPB, therefore represents a possible reason why carbohydrate administration might be useful after resistance exercise.

Studies of bodybuilders show that, depending on the diet phase, an average of approx. 4–7 g of carbohydrates per kilogram of body mass are consumed per day. For optimal regeneration of glycogen stores after resistance exercise, 1 g of carbohydrate per kilogram of body mass per hour is recommended. This value can be reduced to 0.8 g if carbohydrates are ingested together with protein. However, unless you train hard for many hours a day several days a week, a diet that is normal for our society should be more than sufficient to replenish muscle glycogen stores after resistance exercise, especially if you dose the resistance exercise properly. However, for athletes with a packed competition agenda and high energy demands, more attention needs to be paid to this aspect (Box 14.1).

> **Box 14.1: Weight and Mass-Gainers**
>
> This type of supplement is a very high energy product that, if you are not malnourished or under-energized relative to your energy consumption, will have one main result: You will get fatter. In this respect, the term *mass-gainer* may have some truth to it. Body mass increases, but stupidly not due to an increase in muscle mass, as is usually desired by the buyer, but due to an increase in fat mass. Therefore, don't let the product label lead you to make the thinking error of equating body mass with muscle mass. So if you don't have ambitions as a sumo wrestler, you don't need excess energy intake. Your appearance is determined less by your total body mass and more by the ratio of muscle mass to fat mass (see Sect. 20.1).

## 14.6 Transfer from Acute to Long-Term Effects?

Analogous to the case of anabolic hormones (see Sect. 16.3), the acute increase in myofibrillar MPS in the vastus lateralis measured after the first resistance exercise session (followed by a 30 g milk protein shake) of a four-month resistance exercise program is also not correlated with muscle hypertrophy measured after four months in previously untrained young men (Mitchell et al. 2014). Consequently, the magnitude of the MPS increase after the first training session in combination with protein intake does not necessarily predict how much muscle hypertrophy will occur in the untrained when the same anabolic stimulus is applied multiple times over an extended period of time. In other words, those study participants with the greatest (or weakest) acute MPS increase were not those with the greatest (or lowest) hypertrophy response. While the fluctuations in MPS and MPB that immediately follow an anabolic stimulus serve as a mechanistic basis for muscle hypertrophy and are useful for assessing the relative acute effectiveness of a training stimulus or a particular dietary strategy, they are poorly suited to explain the long-term interindividual variability (see Chap. 21) in the hypertrophy response.

This was also shown in recent studies in which MPS was measured over a period of several weeks of training using advanced isotope methods (deuterium oxide, "heavy water") (Brook et al. 2015). The resulting data tentatively suggest that the MPS response to each standardized resistance exercise stimulus attenuates over time (Fig. 14.3). After only a few weeks, the increase in myofibrillar MPS to the same relative resistance exercise stimulus (i.e., as a percentage to the 1RM) is small or even absent in young, previously untrained males, causing the increase in average MPS to attenuate again (Fig. 14.3). This is currently interpreted to mean that in the early phase of a resistance

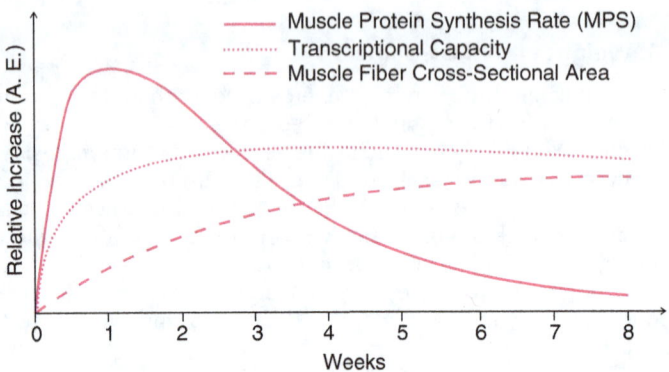

**Fig. 14.3** Possible attenuation of the muscle-building process with repeated, standardized strength-training stimuli over time. a. E., arbitrary units. (Adapted from Brook et al. 2015)

exercise program, the increase in MPS serves primarily to repair damaged muscle tissue and thus muscle remodeling. At the same time, transcriptional capacity increases (see Sect. 8.8). According to the current hypothesis, the increased MPS during this phase specifically serves the synthesis of myofibrillar protein (Fig. 14.3), which is manifested in the increase in the cross-sectional area of the trained muscle fibers. Due to the weakened anabolic response of the same muscle fibers to the same relative anabolic stimulus over time, the hypertrophy effect observed on average appears to peak after 2–3 months (approximately +8% muscle cross-sectional area for quadriceps muscles and approximately +16% for elbow flexors, see Sect. 21.3). However, the significance and generalisability of these study data is very limited. Apart from the fact that they would first have to be reproduced in several studies with different populations, they only apply to the specifically applied training program. However, this is precisely what presented a potentially fundamental difficulty. While an 1RM test was performed every 10 days followed by an increase in training load ("progressive resistance exercise"), the training frequency, training exercise, number of sets, and number of repetitions per training session remained unchanged (6 sets of unilateral knee extension on the knee extension machine with 8 repetitions each at 75% RM1; no information on movement rhythm, tension duration, and/or fatigue available). However, we know that, among other things, training frequency can become a determining factor in the maintenance of the hypertrophy effect with increasing training duration (see Sect. 15.3). You will also be aware that the hypertrophy of a particular muscle must be understood as the sum of the muscle fiber hypertrophy in the corresponding neuromuscular compartments (see Sects. 9.14 and 9.17):

Thus, even if the hypertrophy potential of the muscle fibers belonging to a particular neuromuscular compartment is exhausted, this does not necessarily mean that the hypertrophy potential of the corresponding muscle is also exhausted.

## 14.7 When Does Protein Supplementation Make Sense?

As I have argued in the previous sections, it is considered certain that dietary protein intake in combination with resistance exercise increases MPS and reduces MPB and thus enables or is required for a positive NBIL. Thus, it is also automatically assumed that protein supplementation would be necessary to maximize the hypertrophy response of muscles over the long term, that is, over several weeks, months, and years. Consequently, many people who train, whether in amateur or professional sports, also consume protein supplements to accompany their training. But the question remains: Do people who take protein supplements during or after training gain more muscle mass and strength on average over a longer period of time than those who do not?

The answer to this question is by no means as clear as one would assume at first glance. This is also reflected in the controversial scientific data situation. While some studies can demonstrate greater training effects with protein supplementation in the form of an increase in fat-free body mass (i.e. lean plus bone mass), cross-sectional area of muscle fibers and/or strength (or torque or power), other studies do not confirm these results. The possible reasons for the lack of additive effects with protein supplementation are many. For example, the duration of the training phase, training status (e.g., trained or untrained, however that was determined), the age and gender of the exercisers, the amount and type of protein supplemented, and the timing of protein intake may all have an impact on study outcomes. Another reason for a long-term lack of positive effect could be the adaptation to protein intake *per se*, i.e. that the positive acute effects become smaller or even disappear with increasing time.

Based on the available literature, it is therefore not easy to assess whether protein supplementation has an additional effect. There are now several meta-analyses that combine the results of many individual studies and evaluate them statistically. Meta-analyses can thus provide an insight into the tendency of the scientific data situation. A serious problem, however, is that such analyses by their very nature no longer address the important detailed questions and cannot uncover causal relationships. An advantage, on the other hand, is that when all the individual studies are pulled together and examined, those that do not meet basic scientific criteria can be filtered out.

In nutrition and training studies, this means, among other things, that the study must be placebo-controlled. The study participants receive either the supposedly active substance (e.g. protein) or a placebo (i.e. something that is indistinguishable from the active substance in terms of texture, taste, quantity, appearance, etc., but does not contain an active substance). In the best case, and if generally possible, the same subjects receive both the active substance and the placebo, but in a random order so that possible different effects can also be studied in the same subject.

In the first meta-analysis on the effect of protein supplementation on muscle and strength gain during a prolonged resistance exercise phase, 22 of originally 139 internationally published studies met the (quality) criteria defined for this meta-analysis (Cermak et al. 2012). Compared to placebo supplementation, protein supplementation resulted in a significantly greater increase in lean mass. The weighted mean additional benefit (difference) across all studies was approximately +0.69 kg. Those aged under 50 and over 50 benefited to a similar extent from protein supplementation: approx. +0.81 (under 50) and approx. +0.48 kg (over 50). Similarly, the effect was similar in trained and untrained subjects: approximately +0.98 (trained) and approximately +0.75 kg (untrained). In contrast to fat-free mass, protein supplementation had no effect on the loss of fat mass (weighted mean across all studies: approx. -0.10 kg).

Analogous to fat-free mass, protein supplementation led to a greater increase in 1RM on the leg press in exercisers compared to placebo (weighted mean difference across all trials: +13.5 kg). Again, the effect was similar in under 50- (approximately +14.4 kg) and over 50-year-olds (approximately +13.1 kg). Too few data sets were available for a comparison between trained and untrained subjects.

Compared with placebo, protein supplementation also resulted in a greater increase in the cross-sectional area of type 1 fibers (weighted mean difference: +212 µm$^2$) and type 2 fibers (weighted mean difference: +291 µm$^2$). However, subgroup analysis revealed that these values were solely due to the additional effect in the under-50 group. That is, in those exercising over 50 years of age, protein supplementation had no additional benefit on vastus lateralis fiber cross-sectional area. However, this result is not necessarily surprising in view of the possibly too low protein dosage (see below).

The authors' conclusion was that in younger and older healthy individuals, dietary supplementation of protein is effective in increasing skeletal muscle adaptations to approximately three months of resistance exercise. Thus, based on the data from the meta-analysis, it can be said that protein supplementation resulted in greater increases in lean body mass, muscle cross-sectional area, and 1RM in under 50-year-old men and women. Except for fiber cross-sectional area, these additional effects also occurred to a similar extent in those over 50 years of age. Thus, concerted protein supplementation may be considered useful in all adults to potentiate the effects of resistance exercise on surrogates for muscle mass and strength. This is probably all the more true as the 22 studies included in the meta-analysis did not have an optimal design with regard to either training or protein supplementation.

A recently published meta-analysis also examined the effect of protein supplementation on muscle and strength gains in men and women of different ages during a resistance exercise intervention (Morton et al. 2018). Of 155 articles on the topic, 49 met the defined quality criteria and were included in the analysis. Overall, this allowed for the analysis of data from 1863 study participants. The durations of resistance exercise interventions ranged from 6 weeks to one year. In contrast to placebo supplementation or no supplementation (control group), protein supplementation led to a significantly higher increase in lean mass. Resistance exercise without protein supplementation resulted in a mean increase in lean mass of approximately 1.1 kg. The additional benefit of protein supplementation was a weighted mean of 0.30 kg across all studies. This additional benefit was significantly greater in trained subjects (+1.05 kg) compared to untrained subjects (+0.15 kg). Similarly, there were differences with respect to the age of the study participants. In younger individuals (<45 years), the additional benefit of protein supplementation on increasing lean mass (+0.55 kg) was significantly greater compared to older study participants (+0.06 kg). However, it is important to note that the protein dose in older participants may be suboptimal in the studies investigated (see below). Protein supplementation also led to an additional increase in the decrease in fat mass of approx. -0.41 kg.

A comparable effect to the change in fat-free mass was observed with the increase in 1RM. Resistance exercise without protein supplementation resulted in an average increase in 1RM of 27.0 kg. Protein supplementation resulted in an additional increase in 1RM of 2.49 kg. For this variable, trained individuals also showed a higher additional benefit of protein supplementation (+4.27 kg) compared to untrained individuals (+0.99 kg).

In a subgroup of 10 studies, muscle biopsies were also taken to examine the effects on muscle fiber cross-sections. Here, the results of the different muscle fiber types were summarized and only a mean value was given. Resistance exercise alone resulted in an average increase in muscle fiber cross sections of

+808 μm². Protein supplementation resulted in a weighted mean additional increase of +310 μm².

However, it should be noted in this meta-analysis that there were very large differences in resistance exercise and supplementation protocols within the included studies. Some of these protocols do not correspond to the optimal training and nutrition recommendations outlined in this book. Therefore, the adaptations to training or the adaptations to the combination of resistance exercise and protein hardly correspond to the optimum that an exercising person can achieve.

In this respect, the results of this study seem to confirm the data of the first meta-analysis by Cermak et al. (2012). Another important factor in the new meta-analysis by Morton et al. (2018) was that the group with protein supplementation increased total daily protein intake by an average of 23 g during the training phase, while total daily protein intake remained constant in the control group. Based on this result, the study group investigated the influence of total daily protein intake on the increase in lean mass. It was found that the increase in lean mass with resistance exercise increased linearly with increasing total protein intake, but only up to a value of 1.62 g protein per kilogram body mass per day (95 percent confidence interval: 1.03–2.20 g/kg/d). Higher total daily protein intake was not associated with any additional benefit. Based on this, the study authors concluded that protein supplementation to increase lean mass and 1RM makes sense on average up to a total daily protein intake of 1.62 g per kilogram of body mass. If a person's daily protein intake is already higher, no further increase in fat-free mass or 1RM can be expected from protein supplementation.

Earlier, Reidy and Rasmussen (2016) came to a similar conclusion in their systematic and detailed analysis of all published scientific articles on the topic of resistance exercise and protein supplementation. Although they showed in their work that in some studies protein supplementation in combination with resistance exercise has a positive effect on lean mass, they also pointed out that this result is not confirmed or supported by the majority of the evaluated studies. Reidy and Rasmussen (2016) postulated on the basis of their meticulous analysis that protein supplementation has no additional benefit on muscle and strength growth if the daily protein intake is sufficient. Accordingly, protein supplementation could primarily benefit individuals whose daily protein intake is insufficient in terms of quantity, quality and possibly the timing of intake.

How should values of approx. 1.6 g/kg/d (average value) and 2.2 g/kg/d (upper limit of the 95 percent confidence interval) be interpreted in relation to the guideline values of the national nutrition societies for protein intake?

Most nutrition societies (e.g. Switzerland, Austria, Germany, USA and Canada) have a *recommended dietary allowance* (RDA) of 0.8 g/kg/d for adults. According to this recommendation, a person with a body mass of 80 kg should consume 64 g of protein per day. The value of 0.80 g/kg/d is applied irrespective of the age, sex and training and exercise load of the person and should theoretically cover the minimum protein requirement in healthy adults in approx. 97.5 out of 100 cases. This recommendation also does not take *protein quality* into account. However, recent scientific studies using more accurate measurement methods (*indicator amino acid oxidation* (IAAO) *method*) now suggest that the minimum protein requirement has been significantly underestimated, from childhood to old age.

Several research colleagues have taken the position, based on the most recent data, that for optimal health effects, 1.5–2.2 g/kg/d of high-quality protein (see Sect. 12.3 on protein quality) is a reasonable recommendation for adults (Pencharz et al. 2016). Others consider the optimal range for adults to be at least 1.2–1.6 g/kg/d. The new scientific recommendations for daily protein intake, which are, of *course,* aimed at maintaining and promoting health, are about 2 to 3 times higher than the total daily protein intake currently recommended by official bodies. If we take the upper values of these two ranges (1.6 and 2.2 g/kg/d, respectively), they correspond fairly closely to the above-mentioned mean threshold value of 1.6 g/kg/d and the upper limit of the 95 percent confidence interval of 2.2 g/kg/d for people who want to increase muscle mass and strength by means of resistance exercise. In this sense, the necessary amount of daily dietary protein for increasing muscle mass and strength through resistance exercise corresponds to the necessary amount for maintaining and promoting general health. Moreover, the values of 1.6 and 2.2 g/kg/d are also fairly consistent with the protein requirements recently determined by the IAAO method on a non-training day in young bodybuilders. For the estimated average protein requirement, a value of 1.7 g/kg/d was determined via the IAAO method, with the upper limit of the 95 percent confidence interval for the RDA being 2.2 g/kg/d (Bandegan et al. 2017).

As I have described in detail (see Sects. 12.4 and 12.6), some research colleagues are of the opinion that the total daily protein intake should be divided into several meals per day (at least 3–5 h apart). In Tables 14.1 and 14.2 you will find corresponding examples of the possible distribution of a total daily protein intake of 1.6 and 2.2 g/kg/d, respectively.

The recommendation for a pre-bedtime protein serving is based on several research papers on pre-sleep protein (e.g. Res et al. 2012). The authors of these studies suggested that at least 40 g of animal protein was necessary 1–3 h before bedtime to more sustainably stimulate MPS during nocturnal food/

**Table 14.1** Example of daily protein intake of 1.6 g/kg for a young adult person with 80 kg body mass

| Approximate time | Protein amount (absolute and relative) |
|---|---|
| Breakfast (meal) | 32 g (0.4 g/kg[b]) |
| Lunch (meal) | 32 g (0.4 g/kg[b]) |
| Afternoon, immediately after resistance exercise (protein shake) | 24 g (0.3 g/kg[a]) |
| Dinner (meal) | 40 g (0.5 g/kg[b]) |
| **Total** | **128 g (1.6 g/kg)** |

[a]Pure protein shakes based on high-quality milk proteins: min. 0.24 g/kg, max. 0.30 g/kg
[b]Complete meals: min. 0.4 g/kg (0.3 g/kg + "safety margin" of 0.1 g/kg for possible differences in protein source or protein quality), see also Tables 12.1 and 12.2

**Table 14.2** Example of daily protein intake of 2.2 g/kg for a young adult person with 80 kg body mass

| Approximate time | Protein amount (absolute and relative) |
|---|---|
| Breakfast (meal) | 40 g (0.5 g/kg[b]) |
| Lunch (meal) | 40 g (0.5 g/kg[b]) |
| Afternoon, immediately after resistance exercise (protein shake) | 24 g (0.3 g/kg[a]) |
| Dinner (meal) | 48 g (0.6 g/kg[b]) |
| 1–3 h before bedtime ("pre-sleep" protein shake) | 24 g (0.3 g/kg[a]) |
| **Total** | **176 g (2.2 g/kg)** |

[a]Pure protein shakes based on high-quality milk proteins: min. 0.24 g/kg, max. 0.3 g/kg
[b]Complete meals: min. 0.4 g/kg (0.3 g/kg + "safety margin" of 0.1 g/kg for possible differences in protein source or protein quality), see also Tables 12.1 and 12.2

protein abstinence in young men and possibly seniors, and to improve nocturnal nitrogen balance. For example, it has been shown that daily ingestion of a "pre-sleep" protein shake resulted in greater increases in muscle cross-sectional area and strength compared to a placebo drink over a 12-week period with 3 resistance exercise sessions per week in young men (Snijders et al. 2015). However, looking a little closer retrospectively, it appears that the two groups differed in terms of total daily protein intake. While the placebo group had a total protein intake of 1.3 g/kg/d, the group with the additional milk protein-based "pre-sleep" shake came in at 1.9 g/kg/d (Snijders et al. 2015). As you now know, recent publications suggest that up to a total protein dose of 1.6 g/kg/d on average and adequate protein quality, a given protein supplementation can lead to benefits in terms of muscle and strength gains during resistance exercise. It is thus unclear whether the better results for the "pre-sleep" group are due to the timing of protein intake, or whether they are not rather related to the fact that only in this group the total daily protein intake of 1.9 g/kg/d was above the threshold of 1.6 g/kg/d. In other words, it could also be argued that the group differences were due to the placebo group exercising below and the "pre-sleep" group exercising above the suggested threshold of 1.6 g/kg/d. This interpretation would be consistent with the view that timing of protein intake is rather a minor issue as long as the total daily protein intake is correct. More and better scientific studies are therefore needed to provide clarity in this regard.

Finally, it should be pointed out once again in all clarity that sufficient protein intake to the extent of the values discussed above can only help to create the fertile soil on which your resistance exercise can optimally flourish. Neither "magic" resistance exercise programs nor disproportionately high protein intakes can be used to override the genetic predisposition to the body's characteristics of muscle mass and strength and their adaptive strength to environmental stimuli (Box 14.2).

---

**Box 14.2: Does a Negative Energy Balance Necessarily Result in a Loss of Muscle Mass if Resistance Exercise Is Performed at the Same Time?**

The few studies that have been conducted on this topic focus on two populations: Elderly people who are severely overweight or obese according to BMI and undergoing dieting for fat reduction, and competitive bodybuilders who are in the competition preparation phase. In one study, 16 women aged 68 years with a BMI of approximately 29 kg m$^{-2}$ underwent a three-month, energy-reduced (by 2092 kJ or 500 kcal per day) diet. Protein intake was 1 g protein per kilogram body mass per day. Eight of 16 women remained sedentary during this period, while the remaining eight followed a strength-training program (Campbell et al. 2009). It was found that compared to the sedentary women, the women who strength trained during the diet lost similar amounts of fat (resistance exercise: approximately -4.7 kg, no resistance exercise: approximately -4.1 kg), suffered no water-related loss of lean mass (resistance exercise: approximately -0.3 kg; no resistance exercise: approximately -1.6 kg), and that only the resistance exercise group improved 1RM by 12–34% depending on the exercise (Campbell et al. 2009). In other words, there was no decrease in MPS (rather the opposite was true) and muscle protein mass in any group, but the diet did result in muscular hypohydration (i.e., lack of water in the muscle) in the no resistance exercise group.

In competitive bodybuilding, a very low percentage of body fat is a contributing factor to success in competition. Therefore, several weeks before competition, bodybuilders adjust both diet and training to reduce fat mass while maintaining or increasing muscle mass. Outside of the pre-competition phase, daily energy intake averages approximately 173 kJ (approximately 41 kcal) per kilogram of body mass per day for bodybuilders and approximately 125 kJ (approximately 30 kcal for women; Slater and Phillips 2011). In this context, the average carbohydrate intake is approximately 5.2 g (men) and 4.3 g (women) per kilogram of body mass per day, and the total daily intake of dietary fat is approximately 115 g (men) and 43 g (women). During the competition preparation phase, however, bodybuilders massively reduce their energy intake. For example, it was shown in a study that young bodybuilders who were using anabolic steroids at the time gradually reduced their daily energy intake during the 12-week preparation phase from an initial approx. 11.8 MJ (standard deviation [SD] 3.1) or approx. 2811 kcal (SD 747) to approx. 8.4 MJ (SD 2.4) or approx. 2041 kcal (SD 586) (Bamman et al. 1993). They lost an average of about 4.9 kg of fat mass (from 8.3 to 3.4 kg), while fat-free mass decreased from an average of 82.7 to 80.3 kg. Accordingly, during the preparation phase, body mass was reduced by approximately 7.3 kg and percentage body fat calculated from skinfold thicknesses decreased from an average of 9.1 to 4.1% (Bamman et al. 1993). There are other studies that also conclude that there need not be a loss of muscle mass in bodybuilders during the severe reduction in percent body fat. However, there are just as many other studies that tend to conclude that there may be a loss of muscle mass when attempting to reduce percent body fat to extremely low levels.

This suggests that the effect of a negative energy balance (*nota bene* in combination with resistance exercise) on muscle mass depends on several factors: extent and duration of energy restriction, relative proportion of carbohydrates and fat, protein intake (amount and timing), strength and endurance training (type, intensity, duration, frequency, etc.) and the substrate utilisation modulated by this (i.e. whether carbohydrates or fat are primarily oxidised during training and afterwards). In addition, there are certainly nutrigenetic factors, i.e. genetic factors that help determine which type of energy restriction (e.g. via a reduction in the proportion of carbohydrates or fat alone, or both combined) you respond to with greater fat loss. Finally, age can also play an important role (see Sect. 19.6). One thing is clear: a long-term negative energy balance due to dieting, without resistance exercise at the same time, leads to a loss of muscle mass. The negative effect is presumably due to the stimulation of MPB, but has not been shown to be due to the reduction of MPS (Villareal et al. 2012). In this context, resistance exercise could prevent an increase in muscle loss in the case of negative energy balance.

## 14.8 Summary

Dietary protein and resistance exercise act synergistically to increase MPS. Just as the magnifying function of a photocopier produces a larger image of the copy, resistance exercise magnifies the muscle-building effect of dietary protein, or the essential amino acids it contains. In this sense, resistance exercise leads to preconditioning of the muscle, making the muscle more sensitive or receptive to dietary amino acids. Consequently, in combination with resistance exercise, the ingestion of dietary protein leads to a greater and longer-lasting increase in MPS. Even in this case, however, a protein dose (ingested in the form of a protein shake) of approximately 0.24 g of whey protein per kilogram of body mass per time of ingestion is sufficient on average for young adult males to maximally stimulate MPS. If someone does not want to rely on the average value, it is correspondingly a maximum of 0.3 g of protein per kilogram of body mass.

During the training and shortly afterwards, the MPS is inhibited in the trained muscles. This effect lasts for a certain time and depends on the intensity of the training. For these reasons, the dietary protein should ideally be supplied in such a way that the time of highest amino acid availability in the blood coincides with the time of highest muscle sensitivity to amino acids. Not only must the muscle's susceptibility to the essential amino acids be considered, but also the length of time required to digest the dietary protein. For these reasons, the optimal timing of protein intake (before, during or after resistance exercise) depends on how you specifically train and the duration of the workout. In general, it is recommended that protein is consumed immediately after training.

If they consume a protein source that contains the sufficient and necessary amount of protein of the right quality, the MPS will be maximally stimulated. If these conditions are met, there is no additional benefit to carbohydrates in terms of increasing MPS. Carbohydrates can, of course, play an important role in replenishing muscle carbohydrate stores that have been partially depleted by training. However, relative to the magnitude of the immediate increase in MPS from a resistance exercise session, in the short term even a half-empty carbohydrate store does not impair the muscle-building effect of resistance exercise. When consuming the correct protein dose after training, the training effect on muscle building is the same as when training with a full carbohydrate store. If you eat a varied diet, train hard for no more than one to two hours a day and/or do heavy physical work in your daily life, there is hardly any additional need for carbohydrates. Accordingly, you can easily do without shakes that are enriched with carbohydrates.

The most current scientific data suggests that dietary protein supplementation can positively influence muscle and strength growth in healthy adult men and women, although this conclusion is not without controversy. The potential positive effect on increasing lean mass is achieved on average at a daily intake of approximately 1.6 g of protein per kilogram of body mass (i.e., 1.6 g/kg/d). The 95-percent confidence interval around the mean has a lower limit of 1.0 g/kg/d and an upper limit of 2.2 g/kg/d. This interval contains the true value of the population with 95 percent probability. Thus, on average, 1.6 g/kg/d and in almost all cases 2.2 g/kg/d are sufficient. However, these amounts only apply if the protein ingested is of adequate quality. In the case of a purely plant-based diet, the quantities can be expected to be generally higher due to the lower quality of plant proteins, even if different plant protein sources are combined.

Practical tips (importance in descending order):

1. Aim for a total protein intake per day based on your body mass of 1.6 up to 2.2 g/kg if you want to maximize (M)PS and (total body) NBIL with resistance exercise. These figures apply to adult men and women who are not concurrently under energy restriction (i.e. not on an energy-reduced "diet", see below). Although there were no gender differences in the underlying studies with only a limited amount of data from women, it must be pointed out that the experimental data for women lags far behind men and that there is definitely a need to catch up.
2. Spread this total dose over the day at 3–5 h intervals in individual protein doses and take a protein dose immediately following a resistance exercise session. If you consume protein shakes based on whey or egg protein powder, there is no evidence for the use of larger doses than 0.3 g/kg per intake time. In the context of complete meals, taking into account the total daily dose, there seems to be no upper limit for the anabolic effect in practice. For reasons of possible insufficient quality of the protein sources supplied, a minimum protein dose of 0.4 g/kg seems to be recommended for complete meals. Remember, however, that the timing of protein intake is controversial. Some research colleagues believe that the timing of protein intake is of secondary importance as long as the total daily protein intake is correct.
3. Taking into account the total daily protein intake (see point 1), take a protein dose 1–3 h before bedtime, if your daily schedule allows.
4. If you are on an energy-restricted diet, or have a negative energy balance, be sure to accompany the diet regime with resistance exercise to prevent the loss of lean mass. Daily protein intake recommendations in this regard range from 1.6 to 2.7 g/kg body mass. However, these intake recommendations clearly require broader experimental support.

Relax. According to scientific data, about 70% of muscle mass is inherited and 30% is influenced by environmental factors (see Sect. 21.1). The increase in muscle mass that you can achieve with training is also largely hereditary and is determined in its entirety by your individual response matrix (see Sect. 20.7). In order to have an exceptionally large muscle mass and/or strength, you therefore need, above all, suitable (epi-)genetic prerequisites, both for high initial values and for trainability. By training hard in combination with sensible (protein) nutrition you support the maximum development of your individual potential. However, you can't reinvent the latter (yet). Protein supplements will certainly not transform you from a *low responder to* a *high responder* (see Sect. 21.1). Or to put it in the words of the famous physiologist Per-Olof Åstrand: "The most important thing an aspiring athlete can do is to choose the right parents".

# 15

# Does Endurance Training Inhibit Muscle Growth?

## 15.1 Who Bites Whom: The Resistance Training the Endurance Training or Vice Versa?

During his postdoctoral studies, Robert Hickson thought he noticed that long runs with his mentor John Holloszy were literally "getting to him" (i.e., causing loss of muscle mass). The two agreed that this was the first issue Hickson should investigate once he was in an independent position. Thus, in 1980, Hickson published the much-cited first experimental evidence for the specificity of training adaptation (Hickson 1980). He had different groups of young adults (mainly men) complete either resistance training (RT), endurance training (ET), or both combined (with a few hours rest in between) over a 10-week period (RTET). He observed that during the first half of the training phase, the 1RM increased continuously in both the RT and RTET groups (but not ET). However, while 1RM continued to increase in the RT group thereafter, it remained unchanged in the RTET group and even decreased slightly again. The increase in thigh circumference was also greater for the RT group than for the RTET group, with no change in thigh circumference at all for the ET group (Hickson 1980).

Hickson's conclusion was that endurance training done in addition to resistance training interfered with the development of 1RM and thigh circumference (hence the term "interference effect"), meaning that the combination of timely resistance and endurance training inhibited the typical adaptations to resistance training compared to resistance training alone. Mind you, the RTET group significantly increased both 1RM and thigh circumference, just not as much as the RT group. The ET group failed to increase either 1RM or thigh circumference.

Today, a good 25 years later, we know much more about the subject. The interference effect has been investigated in a large number of studies. The original observations of Robert Hickson could be replicated several times. However, it should be noted that the interference effect has been observed in studies mainly in young trained men (less or not at all in older people and women) and is therefore not a generalizable result. In contrast, the addition of resistance training to an endurance training program does not result in a compromised adaptation to endurance training. This is an important finding, especially for endurance athletes. On the contrary, the addition of resistance training leads on average to an improvement in endurance capacity (see Sect. 15.4).

## 15.2 Why Muscle Protein Synthesis Is Not a Priority in the Presence of Energy Stress

Skeletal muscles require energy in the form of ATP for both force production and protein synthesis. If a muscle is now used for the purpose of force production, it makes sense from an anthropological point of view (flight, fight) if the available ATP is used for this purpose instead of using it for the synthesis of new proteins. For methodological reasons, there are (almost) no equivalent studies in humans (i.e. measurement of MPS during exercise). An exception is Dreyer et al. (2006), who were able to prove that MPS (mixed protein fraction) was reduced in young men during resistance training in the fasting state. This result was also confirmed by the same research group a few years later for the case in which resistance training was performed 1 h after ingestion of a drink containing amino acids and carbohydrates (Fujita et al. 2009). The molecular mechanisms of this acute inhibition have not yet been elucidated. It is often assumed that the accumulation of [AMP] and the resulting activation of AMP kinase (AMPK) triggers the inhibition. Indeed, AMPK inhibits the increase in MPS by dominantly inhibiting the mTORC1 *(mechanistic target of rapamycin [C1])* protein complex. Alternatively, there is the possibility that protein synthesis is negatively regulated by calcium-dependent kinases, which in turn are influenced by fluctuations in intracellular calcium concentration (amplitude and frequency). The latter is related to the pattern of muscle fiber activation (frequency of triggering action potentials on the cell membrane). Since the processes described occur within individual muscle fibers, they are localized. The interference effect therefore only applies to those muscles that are subjected to closely timed strength and endurance training.

The energy stress described here can of course not only occur during endurance training, but in all forms of training that involve a high energy consumption in the trained muscle. This also includes resistance training itself. The interference effect can therefore also occur if you repeat the same strength exercise far too many times and therefore train for too long. It sounds contradictory that resistance training can inhibit the typical adaptation processes to resistance training, but that's the way it is.

## 15.3 Misconception of Periodization

The concept of training periodization essentially involves the systematic, phasic or cyclic variation of the training program in terms of external force, power, work, etc. over a period of time. The concept is widely used and popular among both coaches and athletes, especially in sports with seasonally varying demands. The goal of training periodization is generally progressive or optimal (e.g., injury-free development) performance. In resistance training, for example, cycles of high training load are alternated with cycles of low training load because this is intended to prevent overtraining or plateau or decline in performance. But why does a plateau or even a decrease in performance occur in the first place?

As described (see Sects. 13.3 and 13.4), MPS and MPB are directly affected by mechanical and metabolic stress. During force production, the MPS is shut down because energy in the form of ATP is primarily used for force production rather than protein synthesis (see Sect. 15.2). After force production, the anabolic response of the muscle may be delayed depending on the intensity of training. Finally, microtrauma is accompanied by complex degeneration and regeneration processes that can take some time (see Sect. 7.5). Consequently, if you train too long, too often and/or too intensively, and if the intervals between two training sessions are too short or inappropriate for the same muscle, this can lead to the phenomenon of overtraining. If the training dosage is not correct, it is therefore to be expected that your muscle mass will increase more slowly than possible or, in the worst case, even decrease.

If you apply an inappropriate dosage in a high-intensity cycle that results in prolonged suppression of the MPS, the MPS will recover in the subsequent low-intensity cycle of a periodization program. It can then be expected that muscle fiber cross-sections will increase more rapidly during the low-intensity cycle and hypertrophy may continue to increase despite the lower demand.

This is also consistent with the following experimental observation. Young, untrained men completed 16 weeks of progressive (i.e., increasing training load) resistance training for the legs. Thereafter, the intensity (i.e., in this case, the training load) remained constant, but the training volume (i.e., number of exercises and/or sets) was reduced to varying degrees (to 1/3 or 1/9) in order to determine at what training dose the results obtained during the 16 weeks could be maintained (Fig. 15.1).

At the beginning of the 16-week training phase, the men performed 3 sets each of knee extensions, squats, and leg press of 8–12 repetitions at approximately 75–80% of 1RM on 3 days (Monday, Wednesday, Friday) per week (cadence and TUT, etc. are unknown). They then progressively increased the training load. After 16 weeks of training, they achieved 22 and 37% muscle fiber hypertrophy for type 1 and type 2 fibers, respectively (Bickel et al. 2011). The men were then divided into two groups. One completed training only once per week for the following 32 weeks (i.e. from week 16 to 48) with the

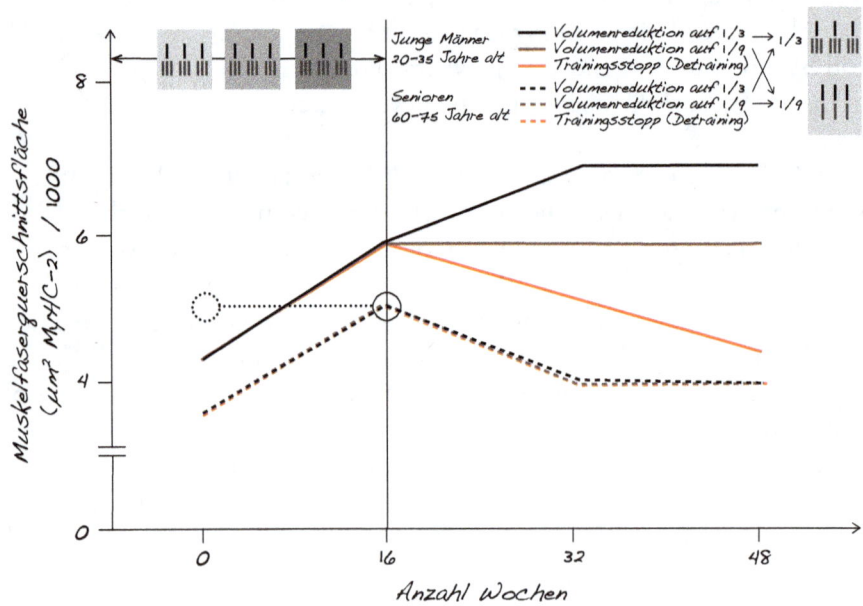

**Fig. 15.1** Time course of the development of pooled type 2 (MyHC-2A + MyHC-2X) muscle fiber cross-sectional areas during an initial 16-week resistance training phase followed by a 32-week phase of reduced training volume (1/3 or 1/9 of the original training volume or complete training stop) in adult young men and seniors. *MyHC* myosin heavy chains (see Sect. 5.3). (According to Bickel et al. 2011)

same number of exercises and sets (i.e. 1/3 of the volume) while the other reduced both the number of training days (1 instead of 3) and the number of sets (1 instead of 3) (i.e. 1/9 of the volume). Curious to see the results yet?

With 1/9 of the training effort (1 training per week of 3 exercises of 1 set per exercise at the same load as in the first 16 weeks), the cross-sections of both type 1 and type 2 fibers were maintained in the subsequent 32-week training phase. With 1/3 of the training effort (1 training per week of 3 exercises of 3 sets per exercise at the same load as in the first 16 weeks), the cross-sections of type-2 fibers continued to increase(!) in the subsequent 16 weeks and then stabilized at this level for the remaining 16 weeks (Fig. 15.1). From this scientific data we learn that, firstly, the concept of periodization is not the mechanism of adaptation and is therefore not causally related to the hypertrophy effect, and thus you do not necessarily *have to* periodize your training to gain massive amounts of muscle mass. Secondly, "more" is not automatically "better". The common perception that you generally need to train more the more muscular and stronger you become is wrong. Rather, the opposite is likely to be the case.

However, as you can see from Fig. 15.1, every reduction in training volume was associated with a decrease in muscle fiber cross-sectional areas in seniors. Only 16 weeks after the reduction in training volume (i.e. 32 weeks after the start of the study), the size of the fiber cross-sectional areas was almost back to the initial level. Seniors therefore seem to rely on a greater training volume and/or frequency to (maintain) the muscle hypertrophy achieved through resistance training. So, on the one hand, I recommend that you break away from the misconception that more training will generally and in all cases produce more or better results. At the same time, however, I also recommend that you break away from the misconception that you can "maintain" the results you have achieved so far in terms of muscle growth with less training in any case. Always train with the goal of triggering anabolic processes, because there are more than enough influencing factors that already work in the other direction. Finally, it should be noted that the size of the MyHC-2 fiber cross-sectional areas after 16 weeks of training was larger in the seniors than the MyHC-2 fiber cross-sectional areas in young men at the time the study started (time 0 in Fig. 15.1). Within 16 weeks, the seniors were thus able to "rejuvenate" their type 2 fiber cross-sectional areas by at least 30 years (see Sect. 19.7).

## 15.4 Does Resistance Training Make Sense for Endurance Athletes?

The endurance athlete has one main training goal. He or she wants to have the best possible performance during the sporting competition. In most endurance sports, the sporting task is to complete a given, long distance in the shortest possible time. The endurance athlete who has the greatest mechanical power or speed and can maintain it and/or delay fatigue better than his competitors has the best cards in his hand physically. Now, resistance training can affect this competitive power or speed in a number of ways. Before we go into these points, however, a distinction must be made. In endurance sports, where the athlete does not have to carry their own body mass, an increase in muscle mass can have a direct positive effect on competition performance. An example of this is a racing cyclist on a more or less flat circuit during a time trial. An increase in muscle mass in her legs can lead to an increase in peak power output and to an increase in average power output during the time trial. Based on cross-sectional studies, it has been postulated that there is a strong relationship between muscle mass in the legs and average time trial performance in elite female road cyclists (Mujika et al. 2016). However, a different situation arises when the female road cyclist is riding uphill or we consider the case of the long distance runner. In both cases, work must be done against gravity to get one's body mass up the hill or to maintain an upright body position while running. In these cases, a large increase in muscle mass can potentially have a negative impact on competitive performance. Therefore, we will now look at the situation where resistance training is performed in such a way that muscle mass does not increase or increases only slightly.

The competitive power of an endurance athlete is made up of two components. The first component is the mechanical power or velocity that he or she can theoretically produce indefinitely. This "base" is usually referred to as *critical power* or *critical velocity*. The second component corresponds to the limited energy store that the athlete must tap into as soon as he produces a power or velocity greater than the critical power or velocity. The greater this energy store, the more resistant the athlete is to fatigue during intermediate sprints, uphill climbs or headwinds. The energy store is therefore also of decisive importance during the final sprint. Resistance training leads to an increase in this energy store, even if the muscle mass remains the same.

Resistance training also leads to more efficient movements in endurance athletes. Many studies have shown that after a resistance training intervention, athletes need to consume less oxygen to achieve the same power or speed.

This suggests that movements became more economical and athletes required less energy to maintain the same power or speed. The background for the described increase in efficiency has not yet been conclusively clarified. However, some researchers assume that the stiffness of the muscle-tendon unit increases as a result of resistance training and that more energy can thus be stored and released during cyclic movements.

Finally, resistance training also has an indirect positive effect on endurance performance. Through full-body resistance training, the trunk muscles can be strengthened neuromuscularly, which can delay or even prevent incorrect postures when practicing the sport. In fact, these misalignments can lead to unwanted pain in delicate areas, forcing the athlete to quit even though they have not yet reached their endurance limit. All in all, properly executed resistance training makes a lot of sense for endurance athletes and should definitely be included in the training plan.

## 15.5 Why Resistance Training Hardly Makes Your Heart Fitter

Physical training is a fundamental component of the treatment and prevention of cardiovascular diseases. It leads to an improvement in the functional capacity of the body and to a reduced mortality rate in the affected patients via various mechanisms of action. The functional capacity of the body depends on many factors, including the cardiac output. Cardiac output is the number of litres of blood that the heart muscles can pump through the circulatory system per minute. It can be understood as a measure of the pumping function or pumping capacity of the heart and thus also indicates the "fitness" of the heart.

Cardiac output is calculated by multiplying the stroke volume (i.e. the volume of blood ejected into the circulation by the left ventricle via the aorta) by the heart rate (i.e. the number of heartbeats per minute, also called pulse rate). Consequently, a higher cardiac output can in principle be managed under stress if the stroke volume and heart rate are increased.

If, as a healthy person, you start your endurance training with a low cycling performance (or at a low "intensity level") or running speed and moderately increase the cycling performance or running speed every 3–4 minutes, you will notice (e.g. using a heart rate monitor) that your heart rate increases after each increase and settles at a new, higher value after 3–4 minutes. At the same time, the stroke volume also increases, so that the total cardiac output also increases with increasing cycling performance or running speed. What values are reached? In young untrained healthy male and female students, maximum heart rates of approx. 200 heartbeats per minute and maximum stroke volumes of approx. 100 (men) or 70 (women) millilitres per heartbeat have been determined. This results in a maximum cardiac output of approximately 20 (men) and 15 (women) L of blood per minute. For comparison, at rest, cardiac output was about 5 L per minute for men (heart rate of about 70 heartbeats per minute times stroke volume of about 70 ml per heartbeat) and 3.5–4 L per minute for women (heart rate of about 70 heartbeats per minute times stroke volume of about 55 ml per heartbeat). Young, untrained, healthy persons can thus increase the output of their heart by about four times during endurance exercise up to the tolerable limit!

The adaptability of the heart and circulatory system to physical training is both remarkable and fascinating. However, cardiac adaptations are exercise-specific, which means that different results are achieved depending on the type of exercise and the training methodology. For example, *high-intensity interval training* (HIIT or HIT for short) leads on average to an increase in maximum stroke volume and thus an increase in maximum cardiac output, whereas high-intensity resistance training typically does not. In other words, HIIT, unlike resistance training, increases the pumping capacity of the heart in healthy young individuals.

The reason for the different effects of HIIT and intensive resistance training lies in the different "coding" of the training stimulus, which forms the basis of the cardiac adaptation. During HIIT, depending on the level of power (e.g. power on the bike) or running speed, the stroke volume may be increased several times to the currently possible peak value and is also maintained at this value for several seconds or minutes. In principle, the higher the external mechanical power or speed produced, the higher the heartbeat and cardiac output generated, but the shorter the period of time during which you can maintain this power or speed. In contrast, during resistance training, the stroke volume and the cardiac output remain virtually unchanged or increase only slightly.

In both types of training, peripheral vascular resistance can increase during high-intensity exercise. Peripheral vascular resistance is essentially the resistance that the blood vessels outside the heart (arteries, veins, capillaries) offer to the flowing blood. The increase in peripheral vascular resistance causes a temporary, but sometimes marked, increase in mean arterial blood pressure. However, the increase in blood pressure during high-intensity resistance training on the leg press is many times greater than during HIIT on the bike.

In summary, during HIIT, the heart primarily has to pump a large amount of blood against a comparatively slightly increased peripheral vascular resistance. During high-intensity resistance training, on the other hand, the heart must eject blood against a large counterpressure at a roughly constant pumping rate. As a result, the regular inclusion of HIIT-like training sessions over a period of months leads to a balanced increase in heart mass and heart volume (so-called "eccentric" cardiac hypertrophy), whereas high-intensity resistance training primarily increases heart mass, but not (or only slightly) heart volume ("concentric" cardiac hypertrophy). Classically performed resistance training (one set or several sets, each with several repetitions in a row, with a slow or moderate rhythm of movement against high resistance) is therefore certainly not the method of choice if you want to increase cardiac output, a central component of your endurance performance. It won't help you if you take short breaks between strength exercises – heart rate is not a measure of training stimulus. If this were the case, watching a few exciting films would be enough to prepare for a marathon! However, both forms of training, HIIT and resistance training (especially isometric resistance training), have a positive effect on blood pressure values at rest and are equally recommended in this respect (for people with high blood pressure after medical clearance).

## 15.6 Summary

The combination of resistance and endurance training often not only makes sense from a health and sporting point of view, but it is even mandatory. Resistance training alone does not promote the functional capacity of your cardiovascular system. However, when resistance and endurance training are combined, an interference effect can occur in that endurance training can, under certain conditions, inhibit the typical adaptations to resistance training (increase in muscle mass and muscle force). This applies to those muscles that are used in a closely timed manner with resistance and endurance training, e.g. leg training in the fitness center followed immediately by jogging.

From a practical point of view, the possible interference effect can be significant or insignificant depending on the degree of inhibition and the objective of the trainees. For top athletes, milliseconds often determine victory or defeat in competition. The combination of resistance and endurance training should therefore be designed as optimally as possible so that the training adaptations can develop to the maximum. This can also be important for patients in rehabilitation or in preparation for surgery ("prehabilitation"). On the other hand, the possible interference effect is completely insignificant for people (including top athletes) who do neither the one nor the other form of training correctly, i.e. who do not train properly in terms of quality, intensity, frequency, duration, etc., or who do their training without effort.

To minimize possible interference effects, the following is recommended based on molecular biology research information:

Between a *high-intensity* endurance *training* session (*HIT, or HIIT*) and resistance training, there should be a break of at least 3 h for the muscles that were primarily used during endurance training. The reason for this is that the molecular signals triggered by resistance and endurance training, which form the basis for training adaptation, last for different lengths of time. In HIIT, the majority of them have subsided after 3 h, whereas the muscle-building signals last for at least 18 h after resistance training (see Chap. 13). To ensure that HIIT does not interfere or only slightly interferes with the muscle-building signal pathways of resistance training, the two training sessions should be performed at separate times, e.g. HIIT in the (early) morning and resistance training in the afternoon or evening.

- Between the two training sessions (HIIT or endurance training in the morning, resistance training in the afternoon or evening), the energy stores in the muscle should be replenished if possible.
- Immediately after resistance training and before bed rest, an optimal source of dietary protein should be supplied in the correct amount.
- If resistance training is carried out immediately after low-intensity endurance training for the muscles trained during this training (i.e. in the same training session), the adaptations to the endurance training are reinforced without the muscle-building processes of the resistance training being disturbed. In this case, resistance training even enhances the adaptation effect to endurance training. Moreover, in this case, the low-intensity endurance training does not interfere with the adaptation to the resistance training. Therefore, if you only do low-intensity endurance training, you can combine this with resistance training in the same training session, whereby you should perform the low-intensity endurance training before the resistance training.
- If you have organised your resistance training as part of a split programme, it is conceivable (there are no scientific facts on this yet) that you will complete both resistance training and HIIT in the same training session. The prerequisite for this is that the muscles trained in HIIT are not the same as those trained in the split program. For example, a possible combination would be chest/triceps in resistance training followed by HIIT on the bike. In this case, perform the resistance training before the HIIT.

- As mentioned, the term "endurance training" should be understood in the context of the interference effect in the sense of "energy stress". Energy stress can of course not only occur during endurance training, but in all forms of training that involve a high energy usage in the trained muscle. This also includes resistance training itself and means that the interference effect can also occur if you repeat the same strength exercise far too many times and thus train for too long.
- Finally, you can also use the possible interference effect specifically to reduce or avoid muscle hypertrophy. There are women and men who react to a resistance training program with an above-average muscle hypertrophy. However, depending on the individual ideal of beauty, this is not always desirable to such an extent, especially if the fat mass remains unchanged. In such cases, "more strength without muscles" is often desired. A possible strategy for this effect is the execution of a HIIT or a very long endurance training on the treadmill, bike, stepper or similar immediately after the resistance training for the legs.

To summarize:

- If you cannot perform the two forms of training in the same training session, do the HIIT first and the resistance training 3 h later at the earliest. A good practical implementation would be, for example, that you perform the resistance training on one day and the endurance training on the next day and then repeat this (several times) in the course of the week depending on the program or objective.
- If you are doing a low-intensity endurance workout, it is beneficial for increasing endurance and building muscle to do the resistance training in the same training session after the endurance workout.
- A hard leg workout in the weight room followed by HIIT (leg muscle) makes little sense if you want to maximize your muscle mass and strength. If you still don't want it any other way, in this case you should do the resistance training before the HIIT.
- In the weight room, train as hard as possible but as short as necessary. Too many exercise sets for the same muscle can weaken the muscle-building effect of resistance training under certain circumstances.
- Forget the interference effect if you already do not meet the basic requirement for any training adaptation, namely a qualitatively and quantitatively correct training, which is performed properly.
- Forget about the interference effect if you are primarily concerned with the health effects of training, because the general mortality rate decreases most

in percentage terms with increasing fitness when you move from unfit to fit (and not from fit to extremely fit). On average, you manage this transition, i.e. from unfit to fit, well even despite any interference effect!

# 16

# The Hunt for Hormonal Ghosts

## 16.1 Whole Body or Split Training?

Part of the daily routine in a gym, besides the workout, is the tiring debate of which training style is preferable: full-body or split training. As the name suggests, full-body training involves working out most muscle groups (legs, chest, back, arms, shoulders and core) together on one training day, one to three times a week (i.e. 48–72 hours apart for up to 7 days). In split training, the training of *the* different muscle groups is distributed over different days of the week. For example, the chest, back and arm muscles are trained on Monday and Thursday, while the leg, trunk and shoulder muscles are worked on Tuesday and Friday.

For reasons that are inexplicable to me, the split training mode is usually assigned to advanced users, while the full body training mode is assigned to novices. Yet, *a priori*, the training mode has nothing whatsoever to do with your personal training history. Which mode is chosen should primarily be based on your goals (see below). In any case, the primary selling point that gym operators or their instructors use to teach the full-body workout is based on the "propagation effect."

As I have explained to you, there are cellular propagation effects (see Sects. 9.15 and 9.16), but these are not what is meant here. The proponents of whole-body training claim that training large muscle groups such as the leg and gluteal muscles increases the release of anabolic hormones and that these would promote hypertrophy and strength gain of the entire body musculature and also of the smaller muscles. So in this idea, the propagation effect comes from the higher blood concentration of anabolic hormones. Is there really any truth to this? Do your arm, shoulder, back or chest muscles benefit in terms of muscle hypertrophy during a full body workout if anabolic hormones are released more when you train your legs as well? And what is meant by the term "anabolic hormones" anyway?

First to the last question. Hormones are biochemical messengers produced in hormone-specific glandular cells. In virtually all cases, they are secreted into the blood and can thus reach their target cells via the bloodstream, bind to them or diffuse into the cell and exert their functions there. When hormones reach their target cells via the bloodstream, they are said to be secreted in an endocrine mode. However, hormones can also be released by glandular cells into their immediate environment and act directly on neighboring cells without blood vessel passage, in which case a paracrine secretion mode is present. Skeletal muscle cells also act on their target cells via the secretion modes described above (see also Sect. 8.1). The muscle can therefore also be understood as a gland-like organ. Each hormone usually has multiple biochemical functions and is involved in several complex interactions and metabolic processes. In the context of our discussion (skeletal muscle), the term "anabolic" refers to the potential mass- and force-building functions of the hormone.

## 16.2 Why Testosterone Is Overrated as an Anabolic Hormone

If we look at the structure and composition of the male and female body, we notice, among other things, that the male body is on average more muscular than the female body (see Sect. 5.4). The development of this gender-specific difference takes place during puberty and is accompanied by a sharp increase in testosterone production in male adolescents. After completion of puberty until the age of about 40 (in males) or 45 (in females), the average testosterone concentration in the blood remains more or less constant. In healthy, non-smoking, American men from Framingham (Massachusetts), it averages about 724 ng dl$^{-1}$. However, the spread is very large, ranging from about 282–1322 ng dl$^{-1}$. In healthy, non-smoking women in the same American region, levels vary according to phase in the menstrual cycle. Follicular phase (approximately the first 10 days of the cycle): ca. 8–48 ng dl$^{-1}$ (median: 23.7 ng dl$^{-1}$), luteal phase (approximately the last 14 days of the cycle): ca. 11–63 ng dl$^{-1}$ (median: 28.5 ng dl$^{-1}$), ovulation (transition period between follicular and luteal phase): approx. 10–48 ng dl$^{-1}$ (median: 34.7 ng dl$^{-1}$).

The values are significantly higher in the luteal phase than in the follicular phase. However, this cycle-dependent fluctuation does not seem to be clinically relevant, since daily fluctuations are already greater in the same individual.

Testosterone thus seems to be somehow involved in the muscle formation and building process during the attainment of sexual maturity. The criminal error in thinking occurs when the correlation between increasing testosterone concentration in the blood of boys and increasing muscle mass mentioned at the beginning is firstly used to derive a general and therefore universally valid causal relationship and secondly the supposed causal relationship is applied to the adult organism. The concept that has been put together would therefore be that training-related fluctuations in the concentration of this anabolic hormone in adults *must* lead to quantitative changes in muscle mass and muscle force.

## 16.3 How Does Resistance Exercise Affect the Blood Concentration of Anabolic Hormones?

As mentioned above, all hormones have more than one function. For example, all anabolic hormones are involved in the energy balance of the body in some form. Testosterone and growth hormone play an important metabolic role in glycogen breakdown and fat mobilization. Insulin and IGF-1 (insulin-like growth factor 1) are mainly involved in glucose metabolism. When maintaining an external power or speed (intermittent or constant), substrate utilisation (fat and carbohydrate or fatty acids and glycogen or glucose) depends, among other things, on the level and duration of exercise (see Sect. 6.8). For example, the exercise-induced increase in the concentration of adrenaline and noradrenaline influences the release of free fatty acids into the blood, depending on the location or density of the corresponding receptors on the cell membrane of fat cells. Therefore, it is obvious to assume that during muscular stress, metabolically active hormones are released that promote (or inhibit) the mobilization of energy reserves in the body. In this sense, a physical strain would act as a stressor and trigger a stress-dependent hormone release.

In fact, it has been shown on several occasions that resistance exercise can lead to an acute release of anabolic hormones and an increase in their blood concentration. Incidentally, this applies not only to anabolic hormones, but also to catabolic hormones such as cortisol. The blood concentration of anabolic and catabolic hormones increases primarily immediately after the use of large muscle groups (e.g. leg and gluteal muscles). From a physiological point of view, this is also obvious, as voluminous muscles place high metabolic demands under stress. But how much do the concentrations actually increase and how quickly do they decrease again?

The testosterone concentration in the blood is subject to a diurnal cycle in men, i.e. it is highest in the morning, then decreases linearly by approx. 20–30% in the course of the day until the evening and builds up again at night. In the afternoon, at about 5 pm, the testosterone concentration of young men has already fallen by about 18–20%. If you then carry out intensive resistance exercise for the legs, the testosterone concentration rises rapidly and reaches a value at 7 pm that is very close to the morning resting value (peak value). By 8 pm, however, the value is back to what would be expected without training at that time. Typically, the training-induced release of testosterone therefore leads to a temporary, short (about half an hour) increase in the blood concentration of testosterone, but this is not or not significantly higher than the morning peak value.

This condition must be clearly distinguished from a supply of exogenous testosterone. It is well known that the administration of exogenous hormones (e.g. so-called anabolic steroids) for the purpose of performance enhancement in sports is prohibited (keyword doping), but nevertheless widespread. It is also assumed that the use of anabolic steroids is also very widespread in popular sports or in the context of fitness training and bodybuilding. The fact that the supply of exogenous testosterone interferes massively with the human hormone balance with varying degrees of sustainability and can lead to serious side effects is probably superfluous to mention at this point and shall not be discussed further. In any case, the administration of testosterone leads to both a markedly higher peak concentration of testosterone in the blood and a sustained high testosterone concentration compared to training-induced testosterone release.

In dose-response studies, it was shown in young untrained and non-training men that administration of 600 mg of testosterone enanthate (one possible route of administration), injected into the muscle as an intramuscular depot once a week for 16 weeks each, resulted in approximately a fourfold increase in basal testosterone concentration in the blood; at 300 mg, it was approximately a twofold increase. Muscle volume of the quadriceps muscle increased by approximately 9 (300-mg dose) to 14% (600-mg dose) over a total administration period of 20 weeks. The reason for the increase in muscle volume, as shown in several follow-up studies, is thought to be hypertrophy or increase in cross-sectional area of type 1 and type 2 fibres via promoting changes in MPS, MPB as well as satellite cell function.

In this context it should therefore be mentioned that in healthy men the administration (and later discontinuation) of prescription testosterone preparations can chronically alter protein metabolism, for example by delaying the *muscle full effect* after training and protein intake. Therefore, do not make the mistake of thinking that the above-average muscle mass of competitive bodybuilders is in any case causally related to higher protein consumption. This is because the possible doping alters the metabolic basis for protein build-up and breakdown.

From these considerations it is clear that the training-induced release of testosterone cannot be compared in any way with the administration of testosterone forms, either in terms of the magnitude of the change in concentration or its change over time (Fig. 16.1). The testosterone concentration increased approximately fourfold in young men by the supply (600 mg dose) is more like the difference in magnitude between the highest normal

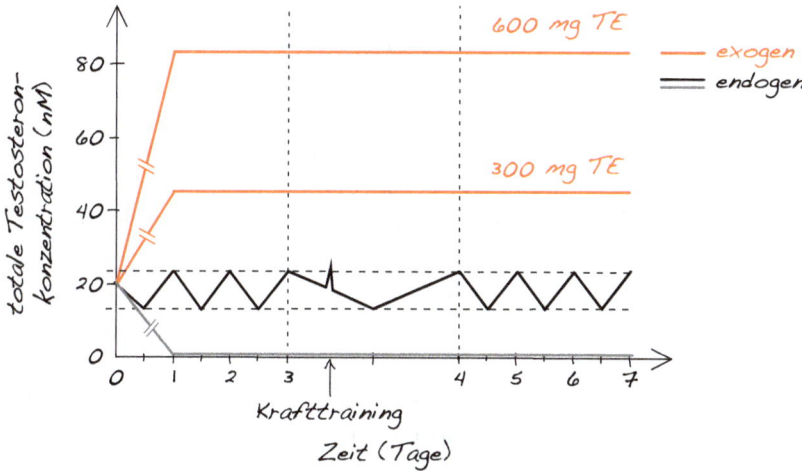

**Fig. 16.1** Natural daily variation of testosterone concentration in the blood of men. The natural concentration of endogenously produced testosterone is highest in the morning, decreases during the day and is then regenerated overnight (black curve). A single resistance exercise session results in a small and short-lived increase in testosterone concentration. In comparison, the change in testosterone concentration is shown with a regular application of different supraphysiological doses of exogenous testosterone (e.g. as testosterone anthate injected weekly into the muscles; red curves). When exogenous testosterone is administered, endogenous production of testosterone in the testes decreases due to negative feedback (grey curve). *TE* testosterone enanthate

testosterone concentration in a woman and the lowest normal concentration in a man (see above).

To test whether there is a causal relationship between the release of anabolic hormones during training and the hypertrophy response, a possible study design could be to have subjects train their upper arms for 15 weeks with the exercise "arm curls". Each arm is trained at approximately 48–72 h intervals, each on a separate day, and approximately 20 g of protein is administered immediately after the resistance exercise. One arm is always trained in isolation, the other always together with the leg muscles (immediately before or after leg training). I will abbreviate these two conditions accordingly below as A (arm) and AL (arm plus legs).

At the beginning of the training phase, the blood concentrations of anabolic hormones are measured before, during and after resistance exercise. At the same time, the acute response of the MPS to the two training stimuli (A vs. AL) is determined. Finally, after the 15-week training period, peak voluntary torque and muscle volume of the biceps brachii muscle will be measured using magnetic resonance imaging (MRI). Based on the theory of the propagation effect, the hypotheses would be as follows:

- Resistance exercise leads to a significant increase in blood concentrations of anabolic hormones only in AL.
- The increase in the concentration of anabolic hormones in AL is associated with a higher acute MPS, i.e. a higher acute anabolic muscle response.
- After several weeks of training, AL has resulted in greater muscle hypertrophy (a larger muscle volume) relative to A and can generate more torque.
- The greater muscle hypertrophy by AL relative to A is proportional to the greater acute release of anabolic hormones after exercise, or the greater increase in MPS with AL relative to A.

You probably already guessed it – there is no truth to the propagation effect. Apart from the first point, none of the hypotheses apply (West et al. 2009). The concentrations of anabolic (growth hormone, IGF-1 and testosterone) and catabolic (cortisol) hormones do increase rapidly and significantly exclusively with AL, but MPS does not increase more after AL than after A alone. Furthermore, the acute increase in hormone concentration (testosterone and growth hormone) during training is not proportional to muscle hypertrophy after the 15-week training period, meaning the subjects with the highest acute increase in blood anabolic testosterone or growth hormone concentration are not the ones with the most muscle hypertrophy. Whether you work your biceps alone (i.e., in a split workout) or with other muscle groups (e.g., in a full-body workout) does not matter for acute MPS or short- to medium-term hypertrophy and torque increase. As mentioned previously, local muscle intrinsic mechanisms such as processes associated with the cell membrane or tension sensing appear to be the primary driving forces behind muscle hypertrophy.

## 16.4 Summary

When you start resistance training, the amount of muscle growth it will produce cannot currently be predicted. For this reason, you should focus primarily on the quality of the training. Basically, muscle hypertrophy is an intrinsic process, meaning it starts and ends in the muscle that was trained. Whether you perform only the specific exercises A, B and C for a particular muscle, or complete these three specific exercises as part of a whole-body program, is basically irrelevant in terms of the muscle hypertrophy achieved for the muscle in question – as long as the muscle is subjected to the "same" mechanical and metabolic demands. The organizational form of your training is therefore basically of secondary importance for muscle growth.

However, if you want to do everything possible to exploit the hypertrophy potential of a muscle, it is advisable to perform functionally different exercises for that muscle (see Sects. 9.14 and 9.18). This is less feasible in a whole-body program, mainly because it is not possible to perform an infinite number of exercises in one workout with the same training quality and intensity. With a split program, the number of workouts per week increases, but the time required per workout decreases. The decision is yours.

# 17

# Men Are Not Martians and Women Are Not Venusians

## 17.1 What Does Planetary Science Have to Do with Gender-Specific Muscle Development?

As mentioned earlier, men have more muscle mass on average than women and various scientific efforts have been made to explain this difference in adults. Among other things, basal rates for MPS and MPB have been measured. Except for a single study that measured a higher (not lower!) basal MPS for females compared to males, all other studies failed to establish gender differences, either basally or after dietary protein intake and/or resistance exercise. However, two problems inherent in all studies were that they did not examine the maximal stimulatory effect after protein and/or carbohydrate intake, and they did not look at the entire phase of increased muscle anabolism after resistance exercise.

Recently, however, this gap in knowledge has been filled experimentally. For example, West et al. (2012) showed that the MPS of young men did not differ from that of women for the following circumstances: first in the morning at rest and in the fasting state, second in the morning at rest after ingestion of the maximum anabolic amount of whey protein (see Sect. 12.4), and third immediately and up to 28 h after resistance exercise (leg muscles) and ingestion of the maximum anabolic amount of whey protein. These data thus confirm the previous scientific consensus that the MPS of young men and young women do not differ, either basally in the fasting state or after maximal protein and training stimulation.

Interestingly, this study also measured the previously mentioned anabolic and catabolic hormones during training and afterwards. Of course, I don't want to withhold this data from you. While the concentration for the growth hormone, IGF-1 and cortisol was about the same for both sexes at rest and rose just as fast and high through training, the much lower basal testosterone concentration of the woman, in contrast to that of the man, remained unaffected by training. Therefore, in females, there was no exercise-induced increase in testosterone levels and yet the MPS increased at the same rate, starting from an equal MPS at rest. However, the exercise-induced release of growth hormone was virtually no different from that in men. These results clearly show that the training-induced increase in MPS is independent of the level of testosterone concentration after training and that stimulation of MPS is effective even at the relatively low blood concentration of testosterone in young women.

It therefore seems relatively certain that the rumour that MPS differs between women and men has been dealt the coup de grace with this study. At first glance, it may seem counterintuitive that adult males and females do not differ with respect to MPS. However, does this really surprise us? Based on the reasoning in the preceding sections and chapters, hardly. Muscle mass remains relatively constant in untrained adults, regardless of gender, after the completion of puberty until the fourth to fifth decade of life, and the relative gains in muscle mass and muscle force from resistance training do not differ between the sexes (Roth et al. 2001; Walts et al. 2008). In percentage terms from baseline, therefore, women gain on average about the same amount of muscle mass and force through resistance training as men. That women are "naturally" disadvantaged in this regard is a myth.

Even if differences in MPS and MPB were found between males and females at young and middle age, they would only imply differences in protein turnover (i.e. in the rate of renewal of existing muscle protein). Such differences cannot *a priori* explain why men have more muscle mass on average than women. To elucidate these mechanisms, more experiments are needed in childhood and adolescence, which is not justified and/or may be questionable from an ethical and medico-legal point of view. In any case, more studies are also needed in women and men, to explain the apparent differences between the sexes in the rapidity of muscle mass loss in old age, in physical inactivity and in muscle catabolic diseases.

In summary, returning to the question of what planetary science has to do with gender-specific muscle building, women and men are not from different planets and do not differ significantly in adulthood in terms of anabolic reactivity to resistance exercise as defined by the stimulation of the MPS, contrary to popular belief. The answer to the question of whether muscle protein metabolism differs between young men and women appears to be a definitive "no." Consequently, there is no basis for gender-specific training programs, and certainly no basis for the idea that muscle training is men's business. Rather, it is high time that men and women meet as equals in training practice as well. I therefore strongly advocate demystifying the stereotype that the "weaker sex" has to primarily engage in group classes (aerobics, yoga, etc.) and endurance training at the gym, and would generally encourage everyone, and especially women and older people, to build or maintain muscle mass and muscle force. However, despite all the sameness regarding muscle protein metabolism between young women and men, it is important to remember that the muscles of older men and women appear to respond differently to the aging process, lack of training, and loss of muscle due to disease. This possible gender-specific difference requires further scientific clarification.

## 17.2 How the Contraceptive Pill Can Affect Your Muscle Mass

In connection with the menstrual cycle of women, the question arises whether in women the anabolic reactivity of the muscles differs in the follicular and luteal phase of the menstrual cycle and whether the intake of an oral contraceptive (contraceptive pill or simply pill) influences the MPS. It was found that myofibrillar MPS in young women – measured at rest as well as 24 h after resistance exercise (2.5-fold increased relative to baseline at rest) – was the same in both phases (Miller et al. 2006). The same was true for collagen synthesis rates in muscle. The estradiol and progesterone concentrations in the blood were higher in the luteal phase than in the follicular phase, in accordance with the definition of the menstrual cycle.

About half of all young women in the so-called industrialized or service countries take a low-dose (<50 μg ethinyl estradiol) oral contraceptive (contraceptive pill) (Lidegaard et al. 2001; Thomson et al. 2007). Third-generation contraceptive pills also contain the progestins (synthetic progestins, see above) desogestrel or gestodene in addition to ethinyl estradiol (Thomson et al. 2007). Hansen et al. (2011) demonstrated that women taking a third-generation contraceptive pill (in this case Lindynette: 30 μg ethinyl estradiol and 0.0075 mg gestodene per day) had lower myofibrillar MPS (at rest as well as after weight training) than menstrual-cycle women or those taking a second-generation contraceptive pill (Cilest: 35 μg ethinyl estradiol and 0.25 mg norgestimate per day). No differences were observed with regard to MPB.

The same research group was also able to show in previous studies that the synthesis rate of tendon as well as muscle collagen at rest and after resistance exercise was lower in women taking an oral contraceptive (with ethinyl estradiol). These results may suggest that oral contraceptives, depending on their type, may have a negative effect on the adaptive capacity of muscles and tendons in women. This may be related to the fact that the incidence of sports injuries (number of new people injured) is higher in women than in men. More studies are clearly needed to investigate the relationship between endogenously produced and administered exogenous sex hormones and the adaptation of the musculoskeletal system in women, specifically also with regard to the different effects of various pill preparations.

## 17.3 XXY

In connection with the role of hormones in the onset and during puberty, reference should also be made to the 47, XXY or Klinefelter syndrome. The number 47 indicates that the body cells of males with this chromosomal abnormality carry 47 chromosomes instead of 46. This difference comes from the presence of twice the X chromosome (hence XXY instead of normally XY in males). Klinefelter syndrome is the most common chromosomal abnormality in males. It is associated with low testosterone levels at the onset of puberty due to testicular dysfunction.

The increased concentration of estradiol (one of the most important estrogens) is caused by the overexpression of the aromatase CYP19, which catalyzes the conversion of testosterone to estradiol. Incidentally, due to this metabolic pathway, the application of testosterone preparations in men can also lead to so-called gynecomastia, the enlargement of the mammary glands in men. The reduced testosterone production at the beginning of puberty and the resulting lack of effect of the hormone on the target organs leads to a delayed progression of puberty in men with Klinefelter's syndrome. Possible or typically observed consequences are a reduced formation of facial and body hair, muscle and bone mass and gynecomastia.

## 17.4 Summary

On average, healthy adult women have lower muscle mass than men of the same age. This gender-specific difference in muscle mass is formed during puberty and is indeed probably linked to the fact that during this early developmental phase testosterone levels rise to a markedly higher level in boys compared to girls in the long term. However, it would be a fallacy to believe that in adulthood the hormonal differences thus established have a decisive influence on training success in resistance training. In percentage terms, adult women gain about the same amount of muscle mass through several months of resistance training as men of the same age. In terms of the percentage change in muscle strength, women are even slightly ahead.

Generally, it was assumed until recently that pill use in women had no effect on lean mass. However, little to nothing is known about the direct effect of the pill on the processes of muscle building and breaking down, especially in combination with resistance training. Initial available data on this suggests that third generation pills can significantly inhibit muscle building. This is thought to be related to the type of progestin contained in the pill. However, nothing is yet known about the effects on muscle loss measured directly, nor about the isolated effects of estrogen and progestin. It is also largely unclear whether taking certain types of pills can dampen the boosting effect of resistance training on muscle growth. Despite the currently sparse data, it is worth checking this aspect in consultation with your doctor if no progress is being made in training despite correctly performed resistance training in combination with a sensible diet.

# 18

# Specificity of Adaptation to Training

## 18.1 Does Your Right Arm Benefit When You Exercise Your Left?

One reads in the literature of the cross-education effect, i.e. that when training one side of the body alone, the opposite side of the body also benefits from resistance training, primarily for neural reasons (increase in firing frequency; see Sect. 4.2). Results from meta-analyses show that the pooled effect of unilateral training on voluntary maximal effort of the contralateral (opposite) side is 7.8%. This corresponds to 35% of the effect on the ipsilateral (same) side. Pooling all available data led to the conclusion that unilateral resistance training can lead to modest increases in strength in the contralateral limb.

## 18.2 Initially with the Shotgun, Later with the Precision Rifle

The specificity of the training adaptation is also reflected in the acute stimulation of the MPS for the different protein fractions in the muscle. Wilkinson et al. (2008) trained the left or right thigh of young men during 10 weeks each with resistance exercise (5 sets of 8–10 repetitions at 80% of 1RM, tension duration and movement speed unknown) or endurance exercise (45 min of unilateral cycling at a power equivalent to performance at 75% of maximal oxygen uptake). Before and after the 10-week training period (i.e., in the untrained and trained condition), the researchers measured myofibrillar and mitochondrial MPS acutely (4 h) after the respective training with the same relative stress.

It was shown that acute resistance exercise in the untrained state led to a non-specific increase in MPS for both protein fractions. This means that resistance exercise can initially lead to the production of mitochondrial proteins depending on the training state or deconditioning status. This is likely why maximal oxygen uptake may initially increase in untrained individuals when they begin resistance training. However, the effects are small compared to those of endurance training.

As more and more training sessions were performed during the ten-week training phase, the stimulation of MPS also became more specific in that only myofibrillar (and not mitochondrial) MPS increased after an acute resistance exercise session. In contrast, the acute endurance training session stimulated exclusively mitochondrial protein synthesis both before and after the training phase. Accordingly, single-leg endurance training never (i.e., in either the untrained or trained state) acutely increased myofibrillar MPS. It is quite conceivable that muscle hypertrophy can occur in very untrained individuals at the beginning of endurance training with higher relative power, for example in the sense of HIIT (*high-intensity interval training*), parallel to the increase in peak power. But even here, the possible effects are rather small compared to resistance training.

## 18.3 Exerceuticals

However, the specificity of training adaptation and possible interference effects are not primarily related to external movement patterns or phenomena such as endurance training or resistance training, because how is a muscle supposed to know whether you are cycling, running or doing squats? In principle, it does not matter to the muscle what you need it for in terms of adaptation. What matters is the mechanical and metabolic imprint that the muscle experiences in the form of active and passive muscle fiber force, power, energy production and/or energy dissipation. All activated intra- and intercellular signaling is integrated at more or less localized sites and eventually leads to transcriptional and/or (post-) translational changes (see Sect. 8.2) that precede structural adaptations. Therefore, as described above, resistance exercise can also (temporarily) inhibit MPS if the energy stress (too many exercises and sets) is too great.

In other words, all training stimuli, whether labelled as endurance or resistance exercise, basically consist of exactly the same mechano-biological determinants (Toigo 2006a, b; Toigo and Boutellier 2006): for example, muscle fiber force change over time as a function of length change, force and length change frequency, muscle fiber energy production and dissipation. The resulting qualitative and quantitative mix of these determinants determines stimulus imprinting, integrated signal initiation and inhibition, and adaptation. I call these individual determinants exerceuticals in reference to the English term pharmaceuticals.

Following this line of reasoning, it becomes clear that classical movement patterns or even training modalities can be specifically modified to achieve specific, combined or simultaneous adaptations. In a series of experiments with young untrained women, resistance exercise trained men, and well-trained endurance athletes, we were able to demonstrate (Item et al. 2011, 2013; Mueller et al. 2014) that the superposition of classical squats (time under tension approx. 100 s, full ROM, slow movement execution until exhaustion) with Galileo vibration (i.e. side-alternating whole-body vibration) and sustained vascular occlusion (stopping blood flow to and from the legs) during squats and 3 min afterward resulted in simultaneous force and endurance adaptations (including muscle fiber hypertrophy, increases in lean mass, 1RM, peak torque and maximum power, capillarization, and endurance capacity). We call this type of conditioning vibroX (from *side-alternating vibration + resistance + sustained vascular occlusion exercise*).

## 18.4 Summary

If a previously untrained person starts resistance training, both myofibrillar and mitochondrial MPS increase during the first training sessions. In the untrained state, resistance exercise thus stimulates muscle development and mitochondrial biogenesis. However, this multilateral training effect fades with each subsequent training session and is no longer measurable after a few weeks. In other words, the training effect in terms of increasing protein synthesis rates becomes more specific over time. Thus, after only a few weeks of training, resistance exercise primarily stimulates myofibrillar MPS, but not mitochondrial MPS. This is one of the reasons why resistance training is generally not an effective method for increasing maximal oxygen uptake.

Resistance and endurance training represent the two endpoints on the continuum of training forms. In between there are many other forms of training. The muscle is not interested in the name of the training form it is currently performing. It simply decodes the mechano-biological determinants or exerceuticals acting on it, which can be thought of as a kind of barcode. Each training form ultimately consists of exactly the same mechano-biological determinants, only they are put together differently (quantitatively and qualitatively), i.e. they have a different barcode. How a muscle ultimately adapts to training depends on the exerceuticals acting on it.

# 19

# Why Muscle Training Is Not Optional

## 19.1 The Hidden Sides of the Skeletal Muscles

Maintaining the protein mass of essential tissues and organs such as the skin, brain, heart and liver is central to our survival. In the fasting state, these essential tissues and organs rely on a steady supply of amino acids from the blood. These amino acids serve as precursors for the synthesis of new proteins, which serves to compensate for the protein breakdown that occurs naturally in all tissues. Skeletal muscle represents the largest amino acid reservoir in the human body. In the fasting state, amino acids in muscle are mobilized by protein breakdown and supplied to the bloodstream to meet the amino acid needs of vital tissues and organs. In addition, these amino acids serve as precursors for hepatic gluconeogenesis (sugar formation in the liver). This is important for maintaining blood glucose concentrations, especially during periods of fasting. The protein mass of the essential tissues and organs as well as the blood glucose concentration in the fasting state can thus be kept relatively constant thanks to muscle protein. However, this is only true as long as there is sufficient muscle mass and/or the demand for amino acids does not increase too much.

In states of physical stress, triggered by sepsis (systemic inflammatory reaction of the organism to an infection, e.g. by bacteria and viruses), advanced cancer, AIDS, burns, traumatic injuries, etc., the requirement for amino acids from muscle protein breakdown is markedly higher than in the fasting state. In severe burn injuries, for example, the daily protein requirement may increase from about 1 to over 4 g per kilogram of body mass. In such cases, MPB is strongly stimulated and can hardly be stopped even with intravenous administration of amino acids. It is therefore not surprising that people with limited muscle protein stores react worse to such stress conditions than those with good muscle protein stores. For example, individuals with a high degree of burns are less likely to survive if they have a small muscle mass than if they have a large muscle mass (burns are classified into four degrees depending on the layers of skin involved and the extent). Less well known is that muscle protein metabolism can contribute significantly to daily energy expenditure and therefore play an important role in the prevention of fat-related overweight and obesity in the long term. The reason for this is that both MPS and MPB are energy-consuming processes that occur continuously as described. The exact energetics to muscle protein turnover in living humans is still unknown, however, based on the MPS, a conservative estimate of this can be made: The average MPS (i.e., daily food-dependent fluctuations are accounted for) is approximately 0.075% per hour. Thus, approximately 1.8% of the existing protein mass is resynthesized per day. Absolute protein synthesis can consequently be calculated from pure muscle mass. Assuming a young man has a muscle mass of 50 kg, the daily protein synthesis to maintain this mass is about 0.9 kg. In contrast, for a senior woman with 13 kg of muscle mass, the daily muscle protein synthesis may be 0.23 kg. Since the incorporation of 1 mol of amino acids requires approximately 4 mol of ATP of energy, and 1 mol of ATP contains approximately 20 kcal (83.7 kJ) of energy, the MPS-related energy expenditure in the young man's example is approximately 485 kcal (2.03 MJ) per day, whereas for the senior woman it is approximately 120 kcal (502.4 kJ) per day. The hypothetical difference of 27 kg muscle mass therefore translates into a corresponding energetic difference of about 365 kcal (1.53 MJ) per day. If we consider extremes, for example a very well trained bodybuilder with a frail senior, the differences are of course even greater.

Very conservatively estimated, the energy expenditure for the MPS increases or decreases by approximately 10 kcal (42 kJ) per day for each additional or lost kilogram of muscle mass. Now, if the young man loses 10 kg of muscle mass over time due to inadequate and/or ineffective protein intake combined with lack of training, but continues to consume unchanged amounts of energy, this would theoretically result in a daily energy surplus of 100 kcal (420 kJ) over the long term. One kilogram of body fat contains about 7700 kcal (32.24 MJ) of energy (i.e. 7.7 kcal per gram of fat tissue). Thus, the excess of about 100 kcal per day would lead to a daily increase of about 13 g of fat. With the same general conditions, this means an annual fat increase of approx. 4.7 kg.

The energetic effects of maintaining muscle mass on the energy balance of the entire body are therefore not negligible. This is especially true in light of the fact that the energy expenditure for MPB was not considered in the above calculation and the actual energy expenditure was underestimated rather than overestimated. Therefore, the energy expenditure of an appropriately large muscle mass can contribute to the prevention of fat-related overweight or obesity (adiposity).

Disturbances in muscle metabolism due to disuse or reduced use can also have other effects on chronic metabolic diseases. It is known, for example, that muscular underuse leads to a reduced sensitivity of the muscle to insulin. The consequences of this are systemic hyperinsulinemia (increased blood insulin concentration) and hyperglycemia (increased blood glucose concentration) and the gradual development of type 2 diabetes (adult-onset diabetes) including associated cardiovascular disease.

Finally, our bone strength adapts to the applied muscle forces, influenced by modulators (Toigo 2013, see Sects. 19.2 and 19.3). The development of muscle strength and mass in youth and the maintenance of these two parameters in old age are therefore important for bone health and for the prevention of osteoporosis (bone loss) and bone fractures.

This list of interactions between skeletal muscle and other organ systems is by no means complete. For example, skeletal muscle also "communicates" with the brain, liver, pancreas, and adipose tissue, among others. The means of communication include, as described, mechanical forces (in the case of muscle-bone interaction) and chemical factors called myokines (in reference to Gr. *myos* for muscle and the term cytokine). These myokines include all cytokines and other peptides that are produced in muscle fibers and spread locally or throughout the body via autocrine, paracrine, or endocrine release mechanisms.

As the largest organ in the human body, skeletal muscle must be understood not only as part of our system for locomotion, but also as a secretory organ, i.e. a gland, at the same time. In recent years, several hundred peptides have been identified that are secreted by muscle cells during activity and exert their effects in other target organs. The finding that skeletal muscle sends different signals to other organs of the body depending on the stress it is subjected to thus provides the conceptual basis or a new paradigm to study and understand the undisputed positive health effects of exercise on human health.

## 19.2 The Muscle-Bone Unit

During childhood and adolescence, bones and joint surfaces adapt to everyday mechanical loads as they grow. The goal of this adaptation process is to improve bone strength while minimizing the risk of fracture and the amount of "material" (i.e. bone mass) required for this purpose. The underlying mechanisms also occur in adulthood, although once the growth plates have closed, there is no further longitudinal growth of the bones. In healthy individuals, bone mass and geometry are regulated by the opposing mechanisms of bone synthesis (bone deposition) and bone breakdown (bone resorption). Thus, the relationship between bone synthesis rate and bone breakdown rate determines whether bone mass is increased or decreased at each defined time interval. However, changes in bone are not limited to changes in size (i.e. length and/or diameter), but also include changes in bone geometry, i.e. the spatial arrangement of bone mass. In principle, the regulation of bone mass is therefore similar to the regulation of muscle mass via the actuators of the MPS and MPB.

There are several theories that have been used to try to explain how and when bones adapt depending on the mechanical situation. One of the best known theories in this context is the "mechanostat theory" (Frost 1987). Central to this theory is the concept that mechanical forces and bones constitute a feedback loop with negative feedback. In this control loop, a so-called "mechanostat" records the bone deformation and analyses it in terms of a comparison between the actual value and the setpoint value. The "mechanostat" responds to deviations of the actual value from the setpoint by adapting the manipulated variable to bring the actual value into line with the setpoint. The regulator or "mechanostat" is the network of mature bone cells (osteocytes) in the bone. The actuators that adjust the actual value to the target value are represented by osteoblasts (specialized bone cells that build up bone) and osteoclasts (antagonists of osteoblasts). Bone deformation thus represents the controlled variable in this control loop, which is kept constant, whereby hormones and cytokines, among other things, can modulate the sensitivity of the regulator or mechanostat. Bone mass and geometry (as surrogates for bone strength) are thus adapted to the acting mechanical forces in such a way that the regular introduction of the same forces causes the same bone deformation in each case. Since bone deformation can be characterized by a variety of properties (e.g., deformation speed, frequency, and type of bone deformation) that can influence the functional adaptation of the bone, nowadays one speaks of habitual deformation stimulus in order not to have to commit to single properties. In mechanostat theory, however, no assumption is made about the origin of the mechanical forces that lead to bone deformation. In agreement with Thompson's (1917) notion that bone mass is dependent on the development of muscle mass and based on the data of Zanchetta et al. (1995), Schiessl et al. (1998) postulated that due to anatomical leverage ratios, the largest forces repeatedly acting on bone under physiological conditions do not originate from gravity but from muscles ("muscle-bone hypothesis"). As a consequence, muscles (resp. the muscle force) and bones (resp. the bone strength) form a functional unit, the so-called muscle-bone unit (Anliker and Toigo 2012; Schoenau et al. 1996; Toigo 2013).

In a large-scale cross-sectional study, we were able to demonstrate the strong positive correlation between maximum (muscle) force and bone strength in humans *in vivo for* the first time (Anliker et al. 2011). 323 female and male participants aged between 8 and 82 years performed multiple single-leg hops to determine the maximum voluntary ground reaction force (see Sect. 2.3) and, in addition, bone variables of the lower leg were determined using peripheral quantitative computed tomography. An important result was that the measured maximum voluntary force could explain 84% of the variability in the measured bone strength. Further studies from our laboratory demonstrated this strong relationship between maximum voluntary force and lower leg bone mass/geometry in school children, young soccer players, previously anorectic women, and women with varying body fat percentages.

In addition to this strong mechanical influence on bone, however, it is becoming increasingly apparent that non-mechanical factors can also influence bone positively or negatively. Recent research suggests that muscles and bones communicate with each other and with other organs via chemical signals. The totality of soluble factors secreted by muscle and bone is called the muscle or bone secretome. The secretome is dependent on all combined systemic and local influences (e.g., exercise, diet, hormones) on the tissues at any given time. Consequently, not only does mechanical information in the form of force flow between muscle and bone, but chemical information is also exchanged in both directions. These non-mechanical factors can have an effect independent of the mechanical stimulus.

Relatively little is known about the relative influence of mechanical and non-mechanical factors on bone remodeling. In healthy post-menopausal women, it has been estimated that mechanical and non-mechanical factors each contribute approximately 50% to bone remodeling in the lower tibia (Christen et al. 2014). In-house study data also suggest that high fat mass, together with low-threshold chronic inflammation, may negatively affect bone mass and strength in pre-menopausal women. However, significantly more study data are needed in this area to provide a more comprehensive picture of the influence of non-mechanical factors on the muscle-bone unit.

## 19.3 The Bone-Building Potential of Training and Exercise Purely from the Perspective of the Bone Deformation Achieved: Practical Tips

As mentioned, the greatest force repeatedly applied to bone comes from actively produced muscle force. Thus, the greatest voluntary bone deformations during everyday activities, sports or training also come from muscle force. If we now look exclusively at the mechanical component of bone adaptation, we can compare the "anabolic potential" of different movement or loading patterns. Generally, because of the term "strength training", it is assumed that this is the best form of training to strengthen the bones. If this were true, "strength training" should result in the greatest bone deformities compared to other forms of training or sports. But is this really true?

To study the potential bone-strengthening effect of a form of exercise, one first needs a reference point. Strictly related to the tibia, this reference point corresponds to the bone deformation that occurs during walking (5 km/h). The reason for this is that in post-menopausal women, normal walking normally results in no or minimal increase in bone strength (Cavanaugh and Cann 1988; Nelson et al. 1991). Thus, for forms of exercise that are similar to or lower in degree and rate of bone deformity than walking, the likelihood that they can further stimulate bone to strengthen is a priori small in adults. Such forms of training, as shown in scientific studies, include, for example, cycling, training on a cross-trainer and resistance exercise on a leg press machine (Milgrom et al. 2000a). Running fast outdoors (17 km/h) and simple jumping exercises (e.g. single-leg hops and zigzag jumps on a hard surface) were different: Compared to walking, these forms of exercise or stress resulted in significantly higher bone deformation than walking (Burr et al. 1996). Incidentally, at least as high bone deformation values as during fast running and hopping were shown during basketball rebounding (Milgrom et al. 2000b).

From the point of view of the habitual bone deformation stimulus at the lower leg, only very fast running or sprinting, maximum single-leg jumps in various directions and sports such as basketball appear to have the potential to be effective strengthening exercises for the tibia. Always assuming, of course, that the bone strength of the person exercising can be increased at all and that the non-mechanical molecular and cellular environment allows this.

It is interesting to note that it is not so much the jumps that are responsible for the greatest tibial deformations. Rather, it is the landings on the forefoot (without heel contact), especially if they are coupled with a renewed upward momentum. Why do the greatest bone deformities occur during landing? Because only maximal muscle force leads to the greatest bone deformation, and muscles can only develop their maximum force under pliometric conditions (Anliker and Toigo 2012). This is exactly the case during the landing or braking phase.

Here are a few simple tips on how you can try to stimulate the bones in everyday life with simple means:

- Complete as many steps as possible every day.
- Take the stairs whenever available.
- When climbing the stairs, make sure to take two steps at a time if possible. When doing so, shift your full bodyweight onto your toes and raise your heels.
- When descending, also consciously place your body on the forefoot from time to time. While doing so, keep your knee and hip extended so that you have to slow down the downward movement of your body with the calf muscles alone. Do not allow the heel to bounce.
- Occasionally change the orientation of your upper body when going up and down the stairs: for example, stand sideways to the stairs and take the steps sideways.
- Buy a skipping rope and perform the jumps barefoot on the forefoot with the knees and hips extended, without the heels touching the solid ground.
- Do a few sprints outdoors from time to time. *High-intensity interval running* does the trick, too.
- In general, please note that strong (gym) shoe cushioning as well as treadmills or soft or flexible surfaces reduce the degree of bone deformation and are therefore not to be preferred from the bone's point of view.
- A little variety in life can't hurt: Leap Frog, Hopscotch and many other bouncy games can be played with your children, nephews and grandchildren.

Last but not least: For strengthening the forearm bones, (negative) pull-ups are more effective than dumbbell exercises or machine exercises for the upper arm or forearm from the point of view of the bone deformation stimulus achieved in the process (Földhazy et al. 2005). Another good exercise is to slow down the upper body falling to the ground, e.g. from a kneeling position on the ground. Very advanced users can also let themselves fall forward standing with an extended body, braking the falling body to a standstill with their arms before it touches the ground. Conclusion: Negative training (i.e. training with pliometric muscle force generation) with maximum effort is positive for your bones in terms of the deformation stimulus!

In addition to these forms of activity, it is also urgently recommended to exercise the muscular and circulatory system as diversely as possible due to the still mostly unknown non-mechanical influences. This includes all evidence-based training measures that bring positive health effects.

## 19.4 Training During Pregnancy

In connection with the pleiotropic effects of training and the health effects for the mother as well as the child, it is important to point out the important role of training during pregnancy. In the past, it was feared that exercising during pregnancy would have a negative effect on the fetus. However, these fears have not been borne out or proven with scientific studies, on the contrary. There is a large body of data that clearly indicates that exercise during pregnancy has a positive effect on several health parameters of both mother and child. A summary of the scientific data from epidemiological studies in the USA, Canada and Scandinavia clearly shows that exercising during pregnancy prevents gestational diabetes, hypertension and excessive body mass gain. In addition, exercise positively affects the timing of birth, the body mass and composition of the child, and learning development during childhood (Mudd et al. 2013). Therefore, the prevention of chronic diseases and possibly the basis for the child's later health begins in the womb. The concept of myokines therefore provides a logical basis to better understand the transmission of training effects from mother to child.

## 19.5 "From the Age of 25, Muscle Force and Mass Go Downhill": If You Believe So!

According to estimates by the World Health Organization (WHO), demographic trends will cause the proportion of people over 60 to multiply from around 600 million to around 2 billion worldwide between the years 2000 and 2050. One result of this development is that the age group of the over-80s is growing fastest in the industrialized and service countries. This poses a major challenge to the health care system because aging is associated with an increased prevalence of several pathological conditions such as vascular disease, type 2 diabetes and osteoporosis. Age-associated loss of muscle mass, called sarcopenia (Janssen and Ross 2005), may both increase the risk of these conditions and be predictive of performance decline and loss of mobility.

For example, the decrease in the cross-section and number of type 2A muscle fibers is related to the decrease in the speed of force or torque development (RFD, see Sect. 22.5), external mechanical power or peak torque (see Sects. 1.9 and 1.11). Furthermore, with age there is increased infiltration of fat into the muscle tissue and changes affecting the connective tissue (tendons, fascia, etc.). These changes can adversely affect lateral and longitudinal force transmission (see also Sects. 4.5 and 9.15), even without altering fiber cross-sections and/or fiber type distribution. Another reason for the observed decrease in performance is probably the loss of coordination, mind you understood as neuromuscular coding of movement. Regardless of the cause, the decrease in RFD may negatively affect motor function and be associated with increased incidence of falls (Janssen et al. 2004).

Age-associated sarcopenia begins on average between the ages of 40 and 50 (but note: the decline in maximal external mechanical power begins in young adulthood despite training) and progresses at approximately 6% per decade (Janssen 2010). Although sarcopenia is a general phenomenon, the extent to which individuals are affected may vary with respect to the timing of onset, magnitude and rapidity of decline as well as the previous peak muscle mass. The extent and speed of muscle mass loss do not therefore necessarily have to lead to threatening health impairments in every case. However, particularly in older people, phases of muscular underuse or immobilisation (e.g. as a result of illness/hospitalization) lead to an exacerbated reduction in muscle mass (Suetta et al. 2009). Accordingly, even a seemingly trivial reduction in the number of steps per day can already accelerate muscle mass loss in older people. In 70-year-old healthy men, a reduction in the number of steps per day to approx. 1500 (reduction of approx. 75%) within 2 weeks led to a reduced MPS, a measurable decrease in fat-free mass, a decrease in insulin sensitivity and an increase in inflammation markers (Breen et al. 2013).

## 19.6 Anabolic Resistance

Anabolic resistance generally refers to a relative insensitivity to anabolic stimuli such as dietary protein (or essential amino acids) and/or strength training. Although various causes can lead to temporary or sustained anabolic resistance, the term has been associated primarily with the aging process. The reason for this is that in several studies by the same research groups it has been observed that older people – compared with young people – respond to the same anabolic stimuli (strength training and/or essential amino acid intake) with a smaller increase in MPS (Fig. 19.1) and that this relative resistance can be (partly) overcome by higher protein intake (see Sects. 12.4 and 14.1). Thus, the term "anabolic resistance in old age" was born. Several factors have

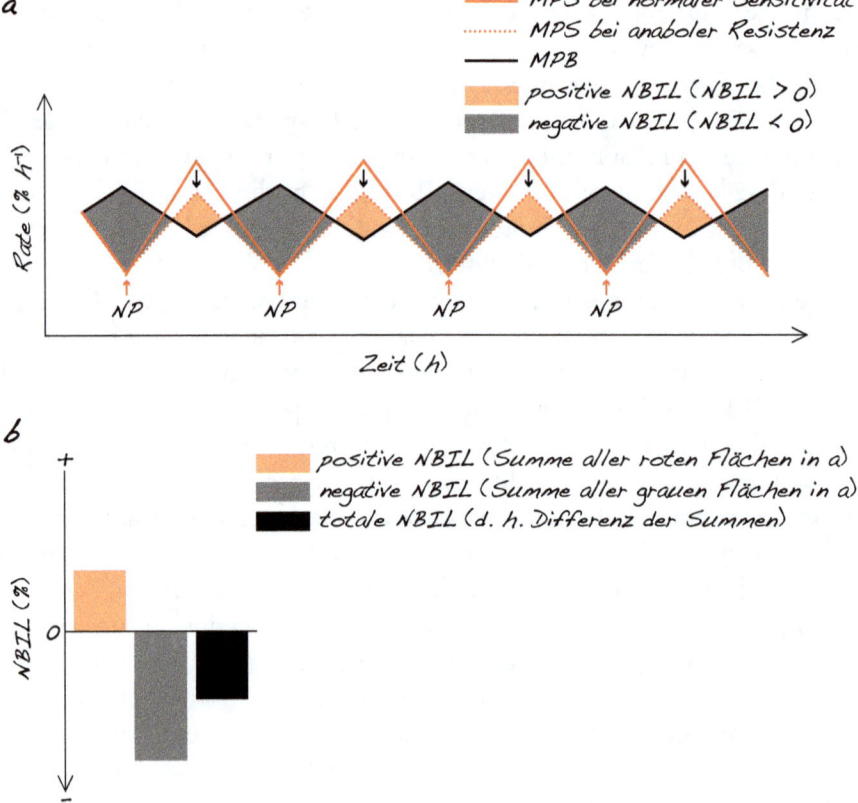

**Fig. 19.1** Anabolic resistance. (**a**) For a defined amount of dietary protein (DP), the increase in MPS can be smaller in the case of anabolic resistance (for the same amount of protein ingested). (**b**) The result is that the net muscle protein balance (NBIL) can become negative when viewed over weeks, months and years (NBIL <0). This can lead to loss of muscle mass. Note that muscle mass loss over time comes from a decreased muscle anabolic response to dietary protein, not from an increase in the rate of breakdown or an overall decrease in MPS. The relatively decreased anabolic reactivity may also manifest with other anabolic stimuli such as strength training. MPS, muscle protein build-up rate; MPB, muscle protein breakdown rate; NBIL, net muscle protein balance; *DP* dietary protein

been suggested as possible reasons for a possible relative anabolic resistance in old age, e.g. impaired digestion and absorption of dietary protein, increased retention of amino acids in the splanchnic region (in the viscera), a decrease in amino acid availability after a meal, decreased muscle blood flow (possibly due to insulin resistance, see below), a decrease in amino acid transport and/or uptake by muscle fibers, and finally, profound or subthreshold inflammatory processes. As far as the last point is concerned, it has been possible to measure increased levels of corresponding inflammatory markers in the blood as well as in the muscles of elderly people. However, since muscular or physical inactivity (i.e. lack of exercise) is considered to be *the* very cause of chronic inflammatory processes in the body, it is reasonable to conclude that the decrease in muscle activity associated with age, rather than age *per se*, is responsible for the possible anabolic resistance. Indeed, recent study results suggest that anabolic resistance to strength training and/or essential amino acids does not exist in healthy, physically active older people (Moro et al. 2018, see Sects. 12.3, 13.1 and 14.1).

Presumably the phenomenon of anabolic resistance is similar to that of insulin resistance: in both cases the underuse of skeletal muscle leads to relative insensitivity – in the case of insulin resistance to insulin (the muscle fibers consequently take up less glucose from the blood), in the case of anabolic resistance to amino acids and/or strength training stimuli. In general, a lot of exercise in everyday life should therefore be beneficial, as should frequent, regular endurance training and/or other sports (in older people there is usually no interference effect, see Sect. 15.1). Polysportive training can therefore have a very positive effect on the combined anabolic effect of strength training and dietary protein by increasing the sensitivity of the muscle to these anabolic stimuli. This is a point that young muscle trainers should certainly take to heart.

Another possible cause of sarcopenia is decreased activation of satellite cells in response to exercise or general muscle stress. This particularly affects the satellite cells located around the type 2A muscle fibers. Remember that satellite cells are muscle-specific stem cells (see Sect. 8.3)? In response to muscular stress or training, satellite cells can proliferate, differentiate and fuse to repair segmental muscle fiber injuries.

It stands to reason, therefore, that a decrease in the number of satellite cells equates to a decrease in regenerative capacity (or, more generally, adaptive potential). Consequently, reduced satellite cell numbers may lead to impaired skeletal muscle function in old age, which in turn may explain the more frequent muscle injuries and longer recovery time in seniors compared to younger people. The local molecular and cellular environment in which satellite cells reside is often cited as the reason for this impaired satellite cell anabolic reactivity.

It is assumed that this environment in old age can impair the function of satellite cells due to the described fat and connective tissue infiltration, reduced capillarisation, profound inflammatory processes as well as marked hormonal changes. *Notabene it* could be shown that satellite cells, when isolated from muscles of older untrained people and grown in cell culture, can perform the same number of cell divisions until their division capacity is exhausted as isolated satellite cells from muscles of young people (Mouly et al. 2005). It therefore appears that the proliferative capacity of satellite cells need not be impaired *per se* in old age, but is more indicative of a less anabolic environment.

## 19.7 The Anti-aging Effect of Resistance Training

With increasing age, anabolic reactivity can therefore decrease or anabolic resistance increase. As described, there are various explanations for this, but the common denominator is probably the (too) low level of muscular ATP production (i.e. muscular activity), whether during everyday activities or training. This is by no means to say that the muscles of older people are poorly adapted to training in absolute terms – quite the opposite! I don't know of any other measure that could hold a candle to resistance training in terms of anti-aging effect.

How far back do you think you can turn the wheel of time when you start resistance training? Functionally speaking, by how many years will you become younger? At least 30 years! There are two types of scientific support for this, from so-called cross-sectional and longitudinal studies.

In cross-sectional studies, for example, different age groups are compared with each other with regard to one or more characteristics. However, the people in the different age groups are not the same, which means for the above example that the young people are different from the older people.

In a cross-sectional study, for example, male high-performance sprinters between the ages of 20 and 80 were compared with each other. By the way, athletes aged 35 and older who participate in high-performance sports are called master athletes. People like to use master athletes as a scientific model to isolate the effects of aging *per se* from the decline in muscular activity that usually occurs with age. However, one of several problems is that master athletes are already individuals (genetically) selected for specific mechanical and physiological characteristics. It is therefore unclear whether and to what extent the results are transferable to all other individuals.

Another problem is that training for typical sports can also decrease drastically with age. In the example of the sprinters mentioned above, the 18- to 33-year-old sprinters trained for about 11.5 h per week, while the 70- to 84-year-old sprinters were still active for about 5.9 h per week (about 6 *vs.* 4 training sessions). It is striking that the training effort (not to be confused with the effective training time) for strength training decreased markedly: from 5.2 to 0.9 h per week. In view of the fact that these people hardly trained according to the aspects outlined in this book, it is clear that the term "master athlete" is relative or by no means expresses the "ideal state". It would most likely be more informative to examine people who, from the outside, have integrated muscle training seemingly unspectacularly as a natural and fixed part of their lives and proceed according to the concepts and recipes in this book.

In any case, even the top sprinters do not seem to be immune to the general adaptations mentioned at the beginning: Decrease in the cross-sectional area of type 2A and type 2X muscle fibers and muscle cross-sectional areas of vastus lateralis muscle, rate of force development, and peak isometric force (Korhonen et al. 2006). The distribution of muscle fiber types in terms of the number of muscle fibers per type remained unchanged. Therefore, due to the changes in fiber cross-sectional areas, there was a different distribution of muscle fiber types in terms of area: from an average of approximately 41% type 1 fibers between 22 and 35 years of age to approximately 47% at 70 to 84 years of age. *Notably*, the cross-sectional areas for type 1 fibers did not change, so that the shift in the area distribution of muscle fiber types was due to the decrease in the cross-sectional areas of type 2 fibers.

This, in turn, could explain some of the observed slowing of strength development and, along with the decrease in muscle cross-sectional area, the decrease in peak isometric strength. Unfortunately, since it is not known how the strength training of these subjects was specifically designed, it remains unclear, despite the master status, whether the decreases were age-related or perhaps, in part, training-related.

But the more important aspect follows now. The values of 70-year-old sprinters were compared with those of 40-year-old untrained men. The result of the comparison was that 70-year-old sprinters did not differ from untrained men 30(!) years younger in terms of muscle fiber cross-sectional area, peak isometric force, and rate of force or torque development (RFD). Studies retrospectively (looking back) relating individuals' years of training patterns to muscle condition in old age yielded similar results: muscle fiber cross-sectional areas of all MyHC fiber types in the M. vastus lateralis were larger in individuals who had been resistance training for years (more than 50 years of sports experience in sprint training, shot put, high jump and long jump with regular resistance training 2–3 days per week) than for individuals who had been inactive for years (more than 50 years of no regular training) or endurance trained (more than 50 years of long distance or orienteering running or cycling three to five times per week) (Aagaard et al. 2007). Endurance training therefore does not appear to be the method of choice for radial hypertrophy from this perspective either, which is not surprising given the concepts outlined in Sects. 15.1 and 15.2.

Longitudinal studies, unlike cross-sectional studies, examine the development within the same individuals of a group over time. The time span studied can vary enormously, from a few days to several decades. However, the latter is very rare for feasibility reasons. Especially as far as training is concerned, there are no controlled prospective long-term studies (e.g. from puberty to old age). However, there are many training studies that demonstrate the effectiveness of strength training. For example, Kosek et al. (2006) and Bickel et al. (2011) demonstrated that 65-year-old previously untrained men and women were able to increase the fiber cross-sectional area of type 2 vastus lateralis fibers to the level of 30-year-old untrained individuals within 4 months(!) (see Sect. 15.3 and Fig. 15.1). The strength training consisted of three exercises (knee extensions, leg press and squats). For these three exercises, 3 sets of 8–12 repetitions each were performed on 3 days per week (e.g. Monday, Wednesday and Friday) (90 s rest between sets). Unfortunately, again there is no better description of the training stimulus, and the diet (specifically protein intake) was not controlled or optimized. During the same period, total body lean mass significantly increased by about 1 kg, while fat mass decreased by about 1.5 kg. There were also marked increases in 1RM of up to 49% (Kosek et al. 2006), which clearly also indicates significant neuronal adaptations.

Therefore, don't let anyone tell you that you are on the decline automatically because of your age. Conversely, I would advise you not to use the same fallacy as an excuse for not training. It is true that as an older person, relative to younger people, you probably exhibit less anabolic reactivity and your structural adaptations to training are less accentuated. Nevertheless, older muscles show remarkable adaptability to training, which should definitely be exploited. This should be especially true if training and (protein) nutrition are properly designed and executed. Go for it and draw from the fountain of youth of muscle training!

## 19.8 Summary

Muscles not only have an influence on the external appearance and locomotion, but also perform very many vital functions. Firstly, muscles represent the largest amino acid reservoir in the human body. The body draws from this reservoir in many vital situations. In fasting states, and much more so in states of physical stress (e.g. inflammatory responses, cancer, burns), the body relies on muscle as a protein store to meet increased protein or energy demands. Second, the maintenance and remodeling of muscle mass involves energy expenditure. Consequently, as muscle mass increases or decreases, the daily energy expenditure changes. Third, with exercise, you provide vital information not only to your muscles, but to virtually all organ systems in your body. The muscles release chemical factors during activity, which are sent to other organs via the bloodstream. This is, among other things, the causal explanation for why muscle training is healthy and why inactivity can cause illness in the long term.

The bone is adapted according to the "minimax" principle. The bone should be as light as possible, but as strong as possible in order to withstand the habitual stress. In order to fulfil this task, the bone mass and architecture are continuously adapted to the stress by comparing the occurring bone deformations with the target value and activating build-up or breakdown processes. The greatest forces repeatedly acting on the bones come from the voluntary muscle force. If you want to strengthen your bones in a targeted manner, you have to load the bones beyond the habitual stress. From the point of view of bone deformation in the lower leg, only very fast running or sprinting, maximum one-legged jumps in various directions and sports such as basketball seem to have the potential to be effective strengthening exercises for the lower leg bone. However, it is important to remember that any form of physical activity results in the release of chemical factors from the muscle, which can have a positive effect on bone health.

Seniors respond to the same anabolic stimulus with a smaller increase in MPS on average compared to younger people. This effect is referred to as "anabolic resistance". With a constant MPB, the phases with negative NBIL therefore outweigh the phases with positive NBIL over a longer period of time, which leads to muscle loss. The reason for anabolic resistance is usually low-grade or subliminal inflammatory processes in the body. Since physical inactivity is usually considered to be the cause of these inflammatory processes, it can be suspected that decreasing physical activity in old age is an important cause of the decreased anabolic response and not the aging process *per se*. Physical activity therefore appears to be the best option for reducing this diminished anabolic response. In addition, strength training can lead to substantial increases in muscle mass and strength even in older individuals. Within a few months, previously untrained seniors can increase the cross-sectional area of their muscle fibers to the level of untrained young individuals. The positive effects of resistance training should therefore be exploited at any age.

# 20

# At the End of the Day, What Makes You Aesthetic?

## 20.1 The Difference Between Muscle Mass and Body Mass

When you stand on the scale at home, the scale displays a mass in kilograms – your body mass. The body mass is in turn the sum of the masses of the individual body components. Chemically, your body mass is therefore the sum of fat, protein, carbohydrates, water and minerals. Anatomically, however, your body mass is the sum of fat tissue, muscle tissue, internal organs, bones, and remaining components. Training and nutrition can influence the mass of these body components, and the effects can vary depending on the stimulus applied to the different components.

Your scale cannot tell you what has happened inside your body. If it suddenly shows more body mass, you cannot automatically assume that this is more muscle mass. You may have simply taken in more energy than you needed as a side effect of your daily workout routine. This would lead to an increase in fat mass and therefore also in body mass.

Normally, both a large body mass and a high body mass index (BMI, body mass in kilograms divided by body length in meters squared) are representative of a person's fat rather than muscle mass. However, people with above-average muscle (e.g., bodybuilders) may well be classified as overweight (BMI $\geq 25$ and $<30$ kg m$^{-2}$) or even obese (BMI $\geq 30$ kg m$^{-2}$) according to BMI. However, unlike untrained individuals, such cases are not fat- but muscle-related obesity. Therefore, in highly muscular individuals, BMI is not suitable for determining any fat-related obesity that may be present.

Conversely, a BMI in the normal weight range (BMI ≥18.5 and <25 kg m$^{-2}$) or even underweight (BMI <18.5 kg m$^{-2}$) does not automatically mean that your fat mass is normal or low. It could also be that you simply have (too) low muscle mass.

Unlike some sports (e.g. marathon running, mountain biking, etc.) where body mass can be a factor influencing or limiting performance and/or competitions are based on weight classes (e.g. boxing, wrestling, etc.), body composition is more important than body mass when it comes to your physical appearance. Therefore, it is hardly worthwhile to desperately try to achieve a certain body mass. Instead, focus on your body composition, because you can significantly change your appearance through fat loss and muscle gain without changing your body mass. The same applies to measuring circumferences, for example of the upper arm. Even in the simplest case, for which we assume only three major components (muscle, fat and bone volume), you can only infer a change in muscle volume from a change in circumference if the other two variables are constant, i.e. do not change in the same period of time. As mentioned earlier, bone mass is relatively constant in active adults (see Sect. 19.2), but fat mass is not. It is therefore not much use comparing circumferences (even less so between people) unless you know the composition. What is important for appearance is not so much the circumference but that the muscle volume (or muscle mass or muscle cross-sectional area) is relatively large and the fat volume (or fat mass or fat cross-sectional area) is relatively small (Fig. 20.1).

## 20.2 If Measuring, Then Correctly

When you measure something, you should do so using a method that meets scientific standards. This is the case when the measuring device is precise and accurate, where precision includes only the measurement precision of the device, or the measuring device error that occurs when measuring repeatedly under identical conditions. Accuracy refers to the degree of agreement between the value obtained and the correct or true value of the quantity being measured, and the portion of the measurement error that is not caused by the measuring device error. The true value is usually not known. Precision and accuracy of a measured value or a measurement method are usually specified under the term "test-retest reliability". The parameter for test-retest reliability is a percentage value that corresponds to the typical total measurement error. Included in this percentage value is the device measurement error and errors

# 20 At the End of the Day, What Makes You Aesthetic?

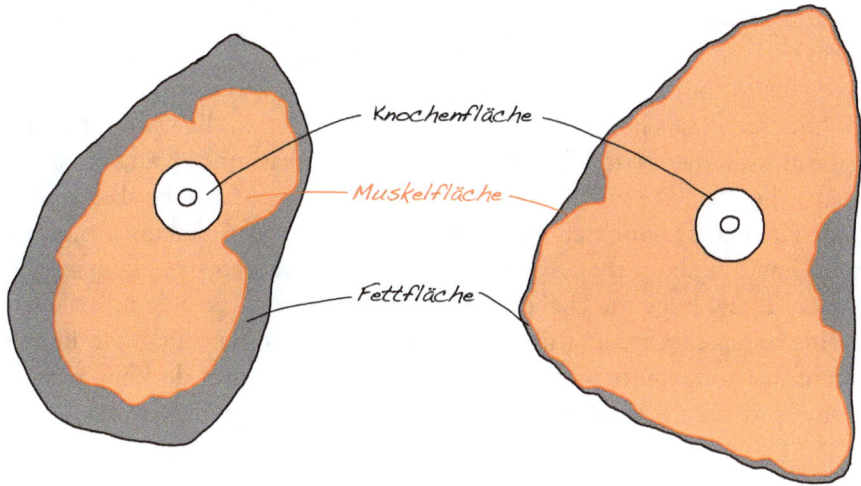

**Fig. 20.1** Cross-section through an untrained (left) and a trained (right) upper arm. (The anterior and posterior muscles of the upper arm are shown as one area). In this example, the areas are symbolic of the masses. In the trained upper arm, the ratio of muscle to fat mass is much greater than in the untrained upper arm. In order to make the muscles more prominent, the percentage of fat must be reduced by increasing the muscle mass combined with a reduction in the fat mass. Depending on the measurement method, the percentage fat refers to the mass, area or volume of the body or body segment under consideration

introduced by the person operating the instrument (e.g., due to different handling or positioning of device components, etc.) or by the participants themselves (one time you appear fasted, another time after eating, one time before exercising, another time after exercising, etc.). I know this all sounds very theoretical and you may be wondering what relevance this has for you personally?

Assume the case that you measure the fat mass of your body in the gym. Then you start your training program and after half a year you would like to check whether and how much the training has paid off, i.e. you would like to know how your body composition has developed in that time. In order to be able to answer this question, you or the person carrying out the measurements must know the test-retest reliability for all the measured values obtained. Specifically, you need to know the *least significant change* (LSC). The LSC value indicates how large the measured change (increase or decrease) must be at least in order to be able to speak of a real change. It corresponds to 1.5 to 2 times the typical percentage measurement error (see above).

Here is a practical example. In the initial test, a fat mass of 20 kg was determined. Let us assume that the LSC for the fat mass in kilograms is 10 % for the measurement method used. In this case, the fat mass at the control or repeat measurement must differ from the initial value by at least 2 kg in order to be able to speak of an actual change. It is pointless to discuss changes of a few hundred grams in this case, because such fluctuations lie within the range of the measurement error. The more accurate the measuring apparatus and the smaller the LSC, the smaller the changes must be in order to be able to make valid statements about training success. Therefore, before taking a measurement, find out about the LSC associated with the various measurement variables and how large the changes should be in order to be able to make any reliable statements at all. This will give you, among other things, an impression of the competence of the specialist and also a basis for deciding whether the measurement is at all meaningful in the proposed time interval.

## 20.3 Fat Loss

If your body's energy metabolism is higher than the energy you supply it with through food, you have a so-called negative energy balance, or in other words an energy deficit. If this state of negative energy balance persists over a longer period of time, you lose body mass. This body mass is lost because the body utilizes itself to cover the energy deficit. It does this by partially dissolving its endogenous energy reserves. The body's own energy stores are the glycogen stores in the muscles and liver, the fatty tissue, but also the muscles. The goal of a consciously induced negative energy balance is, of course, in most cases the reduction of fat mass. Basically, a negative energy balance can be achieved in three ways: (1) increasing the energy turnover through more physical activity, (2) reducing the energy taken in with food, (3) a combination of the two points mentioned. If we now look at the effect of the three types on body composition after an intervention, different results emerge.

The way in which the negative energy balance is achieved has no influence on fat mass. Untrained overweight women and men in young and middle adulthood lose fat mass in all three variants with a given energy deficit. However, the situation is different when muscle mass is maintained. If the energy deficit is created purely by dieting, there is a good chance that fat-free mass will also be lost. Since muscle mass is a large component of fat-free mass, dieting will result in muscle mass loss unless resistance training is performed at the same time. Consequently, if a negative energy balance is the long-term goal, it should always be accompanied by resistance training. In addition, recommendations for protein intake to reduce lean mass loss range from 1.6

to 2.7 g/kg/d. The magnitude of the energy deficit, as well as the type and intensity of training also have an influence on the change in muscle mass.

## 20.4 Why You Do Not Continue to Lose Weight Despite Even More Exercise

The total amount of energy that a person needs per day in order to cope with or maintain all their life processes is called the total daily energy expenditure (TDEE), which is measured in kilojoules[1] per day. The TDEE reflects the sum of all metabolic activities in the body that originate from the various organ systems such as the immune system, the reproductive system, the digestive system, the musculoskeletal system, etc. These metabolic activities serve, among other things, to manage or maintain the body's life processes. These metabolic activities serve, among other things, to maintain the body's functions in physiological balance, to maintain structures, to renew or remodel them, to enable growth and breakdown processes, and to regulate body temperature. But they also serve to move our bodies – or objects in general – to slow them down and keep them still against gravity.

It is this energy turnover that comes from the musculoskeletal system that can vary greatly from day to day. There are days when you probably hardly move at all, whether because of a night of drinking, rainy weather or other reasons or excuses. In this case, the energy expenditure of the musculoskeletal system contributes very little to TDEE. On other days, however, you move more than average, e.g. because you do all the housework, gardening and shopping and also go to the gym. On days with a lot and/or strenuous physical work, the energy expenditure of the musculoskeletal system can easily exceed the combined energy expenditure of all other organ systems and then determines the majority of the TDEE.

In summary, TDEE can be broadly classified as two sources of metabolic activity and associated energy turnover:

(a) Musculoskeletal metabolic activity or musculoskeletal energy expenditure (MSE)
(b) Non-MSE, i.e. all other metabolic activities in the body.

---

[1] The abbreviation for kilojoules is kJ. One kJ is equal to 1000 J, where 1 J is approximately equal to 0.24 calories (cal). Thus, 10,000 kJ or 10 megajoules (MJ) equals about 2400 kilocalories (kcal). Note that the indication in cal or kcal is obsolete and will gradually disappear.

The myriad positive health effects associated with the MSE are scientifically undisputed. However, it is virtually unknown how an increase in MSE will affect TDEE in the long run depending on the size of the increase. "Whaaaaaaat?"…you are probably thinking to yourself now. "Well, that's obvious! The greater the MSE, or in other words, the more exercise and training in everyday life, the greater the TDEE." In fact, this view, that with each increase in MSE, TDEE also increases linearly (i.e., proportionally to MSE), is consistent with the still-prevailing scientific and medical opinion, including that of the World Health Organization (WHO).

This understanding has shaped institutional health promotion to recommend increasing TDEE via increasing MSE as part of the measures to control or prevent fat-related obesity. The underlying idea here is to raise TDEE via an increase in MSE such that it becomes greater than total daily dietary energy intake. If this is the case, one speaks of a "negative energy balance". However, since energy can neither be destroyed nor produced, this situation theoretically means that the body must use its own energy stores to cover the energy deficit. The hope, of course, is always that this will primarily involve the fat stores, to put it bluntly.

Of course, many supposed training and nutrition experts have also internalized this concept and therefore tell their readers and customers who want to lose weight that they will lose more fat or should lose more fat, the more, longer and/or harder they train with a constant, possibly reduced energy intake.

However, contrary to these assumptions, an increasing number of scientific studies on the long-term effect of training on metabolic rates suggest that the relationship between MSE and TDEE is far more complex than previously thought: Instead of increasing TDEE linearly with increasing MSE, our metabolism seems to adapt in such a way that above a certain MSE the increase in TDEE is dampened, contrary to expectations, i.e. it does not continue to increase linearly (Pontzer 2015). In other words, there probably exists an individually different saturation point in TDEE, above which any further increase in MSE does not result in a further increase in TDEE. Up to this saturation point, however, TDEE increases linearly with increasing MSE.

If after a certain point, the saturation point, the TDEE does not increase further despite increasing MSE, this can only mean that the non-MSE decreases from then on. This would mean that in the case of (too) high MSE, the body would restrict the other metabolic processes, e.g. production of thyroid hormones, sex hormones, etc. This in turn can have long-term negative effects on non-MSE, general drive (fatigue, exhaustion), reproductive ability, susceptibility to infection (immune system), susceptibility to injury, etc. The reduction in non-MSE is the evolutionary price we pay, so to speak, for limiting TDEE. Increasing the MSE beyond the saturation point of the TDEE can, in this sense, have a similar negative effect on the non-MSE as an excessive reduction in food or energy intake (i.e., a diet severely reduced in energy relative to your energy requirements). It is worth noting here, however, that the dampening effect on non-MSE is not necessarily all negative. On the contrary, reducing non-MSE is also likely to reduce inflammatory processes in the body. The anti-inflammatory effect of exercise, for example in cardiovascular and rheumatic diseases, is well documented in the scientific literature.

From an evolutionary biological point of view, the strategy of limiting TDEE upwards seems to be advantageous for natural selection, for every conceivable ecological scenario. For example, for many organisms, periods of starvation or food acquisition are necessarily associated with an increase in MSE, i.e., movement. Without movement, there can be no food or energy intake for these organisms. This was probably also the case for our ancestors from the time of hunter-gatherers. If, in such a situation, TDEE were to increase linearly and without limit with increasing MSE, TDEE would be maximized precisely during the temporal period when physical energy requirements or the risk of famine are greatest. The chance of survival would decrease. Conversely, as MSE increases, limiting TDEE at the expense of non-MSE would limit energy requirements and thus reduce mortality risk. However, there are also organisms in which MSE is greatest when food stores are accumulated during periods of high food availability. Such a scenario, i.e., high food availability and intake with limited increase in TDEE due to physical work, would maximize physical energy reserves (i.e., fat, carbohydrate, and protein). I am afraid that this is the situation of people who are very physically active or do a lot of exercise or physical work, but at the same time also consume excessive amounts of energy through food.

Although we are only at the beginning of this important question scientifically, there are good data that indicate that in humans the TDEE is a regulated quantity. Should this fact be definitively confirmed by many further studies, it would have an enormous practical relevance for society, not only for doctors and nutritionists, but also for the general fitness sector and (elite) sports. Indeed, it is likely that especially elite athletes with very high MSE (in training and competition) have a much higher saturation point in TDEE, probably primarily genetic and/or due to decades of training. This would make you more tolerant of MSE than the average person, which is a selection advantage for elite sports. Accordingly, such athletes are successful primarily not necessarily because they train so often, long, and hard, but because they can handle those training and competition workloads without, or at least with less, sacrifice to the non-MSE. In other words, elite athletes can probably handle such high energy workloads, while others would have long since landed in an area that is still generally referred to as "overtraining".

In summary, therefore, my advice is this:

- If you haven't started yet, start now and increase your MSE by moving around in your daily life, playing sports and working out, because it's healthy. Most of you are probably still far from the energetic saturation point (see above).
- Exercise and do sports primarily to get fit or to stay fit and not to supposedly do penance for your "eating sins". This may also be fun, but it does not necessarily have to be.
- Train with brains. Among other things, be aware of what exactly you want to train and how you can achieve this goal most efficiently and effectively. Do not waste unnecessary training time, i.e. time that does not bring you any physical or mental added value despite the training.
- Use forms of training that increase your non-MSE in the short and long term, i.e. that you also convert more energy at rest. Resistance training, more specifically muscle growth training, is good for this.
- Don't make the mistake of thinking that "more" always equals "better". If you are not getting closer to your aesthetic goals despite continuous increases in training volume or MSE, you should not continue to blindly follow this path and increase MSE even more just because it "theoretically" should work after all. The same goes for exaggerated reductions in energy intake.
- Accept the fact that the likelihood of you ever having a real six pack is relatively small, and the likelihood of then being able to maintain that six pack throughout the year and over decades is even much smaller.
- Eat sensibly, i.e. do not consume more energy than is possible for you to implement. How much that is, can be very different for each individual.
- Don't copy the enormous training workloads and consequently the extremely high average MSE of elite athletes, because these athletes are probably at the top not because of, but despite these training volumes. This means that one of the important prerequisites for certain sports (e.g. triathlon) may be precisely the "tolerance" for an above-average MSE.

Be critical or sceptical of so-called "metabolic analyses" that are nowadays advertised on the public fitness market. There are no official, scientifically validated rules on how to interpret the test results and, above all, which behavioural changes in terms of training and nutrition etc. can be derived from them. Misinterpretations do more harm than good. Apart from this, the scientific validity and repeatability of such analysis results can be fundamentally questioned.

## 20.5  About Problem Zones and Cellulite

When asked about their goals or wishes, fitness trainers often receive the same answer from women: the tightening of problem areas (abdomen, legs, buttocks) or body toning in general. How do trainers respond? Ideally, they explain to those interested in training which factors influence the outer appearance, which of these factors can be changed by training and diet and how, and what can be measured and how. In the worse case, the trainer reflexively (i.e., unthinkingly or ignorantly) recommends doing specific abdominal, leg, and butt exercises for the purpose of fixing the problem areas. You will then be frustrated to find, weeks or months later, that the firmness of your abdomen has not changed and that the shape of your buttocks and thighs may even have developed in the opposite direction to that desired. This may be the case, for example, if your muscles hypertrophy more than average, but the fat mass remains unchanged. In such a scenario, the bulges or volume of the body region (e.g. thighs/buttocks) increase.

**Local Fat Burning: Does Abdominal Exercise Make Belly Fat Disappear?**
A wishful thought of many is that the completion of specific exercises for abdomen, legs or buttocks makes the fat mass in these areas disappear. There are no limits to the imagination when it comes to the choice of words for such a phenomenon – there is talk of "melting away" or even "drying away", ideas that are of course also nourished by countless TV commercials about curious training equipment. The idea is that through specific exercise *per se* and through multiple repetition of the same movement, the effect of selective fat burning is initiated. I fear that it will remain wishful thinking.

Nevertheless, you know, perhaps also from observations of your own body, that certain fat deposits are more stubborn than others. In order to understand whether local fat burning (*spot reduction*) is theoretically possible at all, we need to take a brief look at the mechanisms of lipolysis (fat breakdown) in the human body. Human fat cells, so-called adipocytes, contain fat droplets in which triacylglycerols (three fatty acids esterified with glycerol) are found. Whether such triacylglycerols are mobilized from the fat droplets and enter the bloodstream as cleaved fatty acids and glycerol depends on the balance between pro- and anti-lipolytic influences on the fat cell.

These influences in turn depend on the signalling of various receptors in the cell membrane of the fat cells. For example, if insulin binds to the insulin receptors of the fat cell, this has an antilipolytic effect, i.e. inhibits lipolysis. Conversely, the binding of catecholamines (e.g. adrenaline and noradrenaline, which are released during exercise, among other things) to $β_{1/2/3}$-adrenergic receptors has a prolipolytic effect. In contrast, the binding of catecholamines to α-adrenergic receptors has an antilipolytic effect. It is known that depending on body region and sex, fat cells have a different mix of pro- and antilipolytic receptors on their surface. Whether fatty acids and glycerol can be mobilized from fat cells thus depends on the one hand on the receptivity of the fat cell to prolipolytic signals and on the other hand on the molecular and cellular "niche", i.e. on the pro- and antilipolytic agents (hormones, cytokines, etc.) in the immediate environment of the fat cell.

Men have more $α_2$-adrenergic receptors in the cells of abdominal fat compared to women. This could be part of the reason why men have a greater tendency to accumulate fat in the abdominal region relative to women. Similarly, in women, the preferential accumulation of fat in the gluteofemoral region (upper thigh area and buttocks or hips) could be under the influence of a locally stronger antilipolytic receptor function. Sex hormones are also thought to influence the distribution and formation of fat deposits. Thus, gluteofemoral storage of fat is associated with increased production of estrogens in girls or testosterone in boys during puberty. Some testosterone is aromatized to estradiol (see also Sect. 17.3) and may therefore play an important role in the formation of gluteofemoral fat deposits. In general, however, nothing to little is known about local and sex-specific differences in $β_{1/2/3}$ – and α-adrenergic receptor function and their regulation. In any case, training of local muscle groups does not seem to have a significant effect on them.

**Strength Training Against Cellulite?**
Cellulite ("orange peel skin") is a cosmetically disturbing dimpling of the skin and not a pathological skin change. Cellulite almost exclusively affects women. Between 85 and 98% of all women over the age of 20 show signs of it, although the frequency of occurrence can vary by ethnic group. However, cellulite can also occur in men, but usually as a concomitant of certain medical conditions such as hypogonadism (abnormally low testosterone levels).

A distinction is made between four degrees of severity of cellulite:

- Grade 0 is characterized by a smooth skin surface when lying and standing. If you pinch the skin, wrinkles and furrows appear, but the typical mattress phenomenon is not visible.

- Grade 1 is determined by a smooth skin surface when lying and standing. When pinching, the typical mattress phenomenon appears.
- Grade 2 is characterized by a smooth skin surface when lying down; when standing, the mattress phenomenon appears spontaneously.
- Grade 3 is manifested by the mattress phenomenon spontaneously while lying as well as standing.

Cellulite is thought to be caused by four main factors:

- sex-specific differences in the structure and composition of the skin and subcutaneous fatty tissue: in those affected, the connective tissue at the boundary between the dermis and subcutis (border lamella) appears to be weaker. As a result, the subcutaneous fatty tissue has an increased tendency to bulge outwards – i.e. into the dermis. The clinical correlate is the formation of the typical cellulite symptoms: dents and dimples. In addition, the subcutaneous adipose tissue of affected individuals shows fewer connective tissue septa and consequently larger fat lobules.
- vascular changes
- chronic inflammatory processes
- genetic predisposition

Treatment attempts range from topically applied skin creams to invasive methods such as laser assisted lipolysis or liposuction. However, given the complex and multifactorial etiology (history of development), it is not surprising that a single treatment attempt is not very effective. In the context of this book, the question is what is known regarding the effect of exercise and diet on cellulite.

The answer is: not very much. This much is clear though: with a higher degree of severity of cellulite, a mere decrease of body mass, BMI and thigh circumference does not lead to a significant improvement of the skin appearance. A study of 51 participants with visible cellulite examined the effect of a weight loss program on severity (Smalls et al. 2006). The measures ranged from bariatric surgery (e.g. insertion of a gastric band) to drug treatment and fat-reducing diets.

Improvement of the cellulite appearance was observed in most of the participants, although it also worsened in some. Improvements occurred in those cases where the loss of body mass was significant, the percentage of fat in the legs decreased, and BMI and severity of cellulite were high at baseline. Cellulite worsened in cases where BMI was lower at baseline, body mass reduction was lower, and most importantly, the percentage of fat in the legs did not change; however, there was a decrease in skin tone.

A (diet-related) loss of body mass *per se* therefore only leads to a reduction of cellulite if the percentage of fat in the affected region is reduced. This occurs when the fat mass decreases more than the muscle mass or the fat mass decreases while the muscle mass remains unchanged. However, this can still have no effect on cellulite if the skin has less tension due to the previous expansion.

Although there are still no studies on the specific effect of various training interventions on cellulite, the following can be assumed based on the observations made above: If the amount of fat in the body is reduced through training and diet such that the regions in question are also affected, *and if* muscle mass is increased in the target region at the same time, the percentage of fat in the cellulite region and thus the anti-cellulite effect should be greatest. At the same time, the reduced volume decrease (due to the muscle mass increase) may reduce or even prevent the formation of skin wrinkles. The hypothetical result of simultaneous fat reduction and muscle mass increase is the relative skin tightening.

## 20.6 Is There an Optimal Time of Day for Muscle Training?

One question often asked by exercisers is whether there is an optimal time of day for resistance exercise. Admittedly, for most people this question does not arise at *all*, as they struggle with the problem of integrating training into their daily routine. Furthermore, it is often unclear what is actually meant by "optimal", because the emotionally optimal time (e.g. the most motivation or similar) does not necessarily have to correspond to the training time that leads to optimal adaptation (if the latter time exists).

Nevertheless, the question is generally very interesting, because it is potentially, in the long term, relevant for the health of the whole organism. The observation underlying the question is that virtually all organisms (from bacteria to plants to animals) have physiological, biochemical, and behavioral rhythms. In mammals, sleep-wake rhythms, heart rate, blood pressure, body temperature, kidney activity, liver metabolism, and secretion of many hormones are controlled by an endogenous timing system. This endogenous timing system is called the circadian clock (from Latin *circa* for around something/about and *dies* for day). Circadian rhythms comprise biological cycles with a periodic duration of approximately 24 h. Their function is to prepare the body for daily environmental changes. In the liver, for example, most genes (see Sect. 8.2) with a rhythmic expression pattern encode enzymes and regulatory proteins involved in food processing and energy metabolism. The expression of these proteins therefore fluctuates according to or anticipates the pattern of food intake.

The central circadian pacemaker is located in the suprachiasmatic nucleus (SCN) of the hypothalamus, a section of the diencephalon. As the central clock, the SCN functions independently of external influences. If the SCN is missing, arrhythmic behaviour patterns occur. In hamsters, for example, it has been shown that removal of the SCN led to a loss of the usual day- and night-dependent drinking and movement behavior. Transplantation of a healthy SCN (either from a hamster or a mouse) restored the rhythms according to the rhythms of the donor, i.e. the drinking and locomotor rhythms of a hamster with implanted SCN from a donor mouse corresponded to those of a mouse.

However, it was later discovered that peripheral tissues (as mentioned above, for example the liver, kidney, etc., but also skeletal muscle) have their own circadian rhythms independent of systemic influences. The actual basis for the central and peripheral circadian rhythms are considered to be mechanisms around the molecular clock, i.e. molecular signalling, which takes place primarily in the nucleus of most (if not all) cell types in our body. At the level of the individual cell, including the muscle fiber, the presence of a molecular clock is considered a necessary mechanism for tuning cellular activity to daily environmental changes. From an evolutionary perspective, the ability to synchronize the molecular clock, and thus intracellular physiology, with the clocks of other tissues and the external day-night cycle is therefore an important prerequisite for adaptation to changing environmental influences.

It is considered certain that the mechanism of the molecular clock is inherent to each individual body cell and can run autonomously. The trick, however, is that the timing of the molecular clock can be influenced by environmental stimuli. This can happen to the extent that the rhythm of the molecular clock is adjusted or reset. Such stimuli are called Zeitgeber (German for timer). The timing of the central clock in the SCN is primarily determined by light stimuli. Thus, light from natural and artificial (televisions, lamps, computers, mobile phones, etc.) sources influences the central circadian clock.

However, the circadian rhythm in peripheral tissues (for example in skeletal muscle) can be uncoupled from the central circadian rhythm, i.e. gene expression in the center and periphery oscillates out of phase. Such a dyssynchrony can occur, for example, during shift work or represents the chronobiological basis for the so-called jet lag. Long-term dyssynchrony between the central and peripheral circadian clocks can lead to health problems. While light is the primary zeitgeber for the central circadian clock, other zeitgebers can affect the peripheral clock independently of the central clock. These stimuli include the timing of food intake and/or exercise (or muscular activity).

This fact could be proven in experiments with mice. Mice are nocturnal animals that consume most of their food at night. If the mice are forced to consume all their food exclusively during the day (by providing food only then), the circadian rhythm in the peripheral cells is completely changed, but phase shifts in the central circadian rhythm in the SCN do not occur. Regarding the role of training as a zeitgeber, a human study on the vastus lateralis muscle demonstrated that a single resistance exercise session (10 sets of 8 repetitions of unilateral knee extension at 80 % of 1RM with 3 min rest between sets, no more precise training session data available) alters the expression of genes controlled by the molecular clock, 6 and 18 h after training. This suggests that training or muscle activity acts as a zeitgeber. Characteristically, mice in which essential genes controlled by the molecular clock have been knocked out are weaker, have fewer mitochondria, and have reduced mitochondrial function.

Taken together, these results show that food intake and muscle use can act as dominant zeitgebers in peripheral tissues and that circadian rhythms in peripheral tissues may be decoupled from central timing in the SCN by these light-independent influences. Specifically, the circadian rhythm in skeletal muscle can be reset independently of the central clock by changing the timing of exercise and/or the timing of food intake. These findings therefore shed new light on the impact of exercise on human health: muscle training provides timing information to both skeletal muscle cells and other peripheral tissues through the mechanisms described.

It is questionable whether and to what extent the findings from the experiments in mice can be extrapolated to humans. In principle, however, the animal experiments suggest that one or more training times may exist that can be regarded as optimal in terms of synchronization between the central and peripheral clocks and the strengthening of circadian rhythms. The actual question, therefore, is not so much whether there is an optimal time in the course of the day when training is most effective, but which training and nutritional times are optimal for you to synchronize your internal clocks and stabilize/strengthen circadian rhythms. Thus, it is likely that your chronobiological status will provide another basis for the unfolding of training adaptations. Until the optimal timing is known, training regularly based on the timing seems like a reasonable alternative. Likewise, listening to your rough chronotype seems reasonable. "Owls" tend to be active late into the night and sleep correspondingly longer in the morning, or should, but can't due to societal constraints (e.g. work). "Larks" tend to go to bed early and get up very early in the morning.

## 20.7 The Path from Training Stimulus to Muscle Adaptation

As discussed elsewhere (see Sect. 18.3), all training stimuli, whether labelled as endurance training, resistance training, CrossFit or vibration training, consist fundamentally of the same mechano-biological determinants (Toigo 2006a, b; Toigo and Boutellier 2006), which include changes in muscle fiber force over time as a function of length change, force and length change frequency, and muscle fiber energy production and dissipation. I call these mechano-biological stimuli exerceuticals (in reference to the specific action of *pharmaceuticals*). The imprint of the training stimulus is determined by the qualitative and quantitative mix of these exerceuticals. When you train in a certain way, the specific mix of stimuli meets your individual response matrix (Toigo 2006a). The response matrix includes all factors that interact with the training stimuli or that can influence the translation of these stimuli into a molecular and cellular response. These factors include, for example, (epi-) genetics, age, sex, nutrition, immune status, chronobiology, disease states, etc. The training stimuli are translated into a molecular and cellular response based on the interaction with the response matrix, which then (when repeatedly applied) lead to local and systemic adaptations. These adaptations are in turn the basis for the functional (increased muscle force, speed, endurance, etc.) and health effects of training.

## 20.8 Summary

The body mass, which can be determined with a commercial scale, says nothing about the composition of the body. For health and appearance, the proportions of muscle and fat mass are crucial. This is equally decisive if you want to document your training progress. For this purpose, there are various measurement methods with which the individual components can be measured or estimated. In order for you to be sure that a change has occurred, the change must be greater than the LSC for the measured variable. The more precisely the device measures or the measurement is carried out, the smaller changes may be interpreted as "true" changes.

You can achieve a low fat mass primarily by adjusting your eating habits and food quality. Through training, you can also influence the substrate utilisation, i.e. from which energy store (carbohydrates, fat, protein) the body converts the energy. Everyone should do resistance and endurance training because this is central to health. On average, resistance training increases muscle mass. This also increases the energy metabolism. However, for this to have a caloric effect, substantial changes are required. Endurance training, depending on the intensity and duration of the training, is associated with an energy metabolism, but this is rather small in absolute terms. Therefore endurance training is more suitable to stabilize the shape. In both resistance and endurance training, the interesting effect in terms of fat loss is that substrate metabolism can be altered in the hours/days after training so that fat oxidation takes up a higher proportion in relative terms.

The wishful thinking of many is that doing specific exercises for the abdomen, legs or buttocks will make the fat deposits in these areas disappear. I have to disillusion you – it will remain wishful thinking. However, you may know from your own experience that certain fat deposits are more stubborn than others. Why? Our fat cells are exposed to both fat loss stimulating and fat loss inhibiting signals. However, these signals can only have a corresponding effect if they bind to the appropriate receptors that are located on the surface of the fat cells, according to the lock-and-key principle: a certain key (e.g. the signal substance that promotes fat loss) only fits a certain lock (the specific receptor for this signal substance). Thus, whether fat cells release fat for burning depends on the number and type of both signals (keys) and receptors (locks). The distribution of receptors that promote and inhibit fat loss can vary by sex and body part. For example, fat cells in the abdominal region in men have more fat loss inhibitory receptors relative to other fat deposits. In women, this affects fat cells in the hip, buttock and thigh regions. Little to nothing is known about how these differences occur and how receptor distribution is regulated. Until now, if you want to lose fat, you should focus on regularly triggering fat loss-promoting signals in your body and avoiding fat loss-inhibiting signals through a combination of exercise and nutrition (not just nutrition). Eventually, even the most stubborn areas will shrink…hopefully. Constant dripping wears away the stone!

# 21

# Nature's Whim: The Extent of Adaptation to Training Is Individual

## 21.1 Interindividual Variability of Adaptation to Training: The New Mantra?

Due to the complexity of the response matrix, it is clear that a relatively large interindividual variability in training adaptation can occur. This means that even if two people train in exactly the same way, the outcome may be significantly different. For example, from studies of identical twins, it is estimated that the heritability of adaptation of maximal oxygen uptake to 20 weeks of standardized endurance training is 47 % (when corrected for age, sex, baseline values for maximal oxygen uptake, body mass and composition) (Bouchard et al. 1999). The influence of the genetic component in the adaptation of muscle size and muscle force is probably even greater. Studies put the heritability of hypertrophy and muscle force increase at approximately 70 % (environmental influences and technical errors are therefore 30 %) (Pérusse et al. 1987). We must therefore move away from the concept of the mean. It is true that resistance training on average leads to a larger muscle cross-sectional area and a higher performance, but this is by no means true to the same extent for all people.

In terms of sample size, there are two major studies that have examined interindividual variability in adaptation to resistance training. The first is a multicentre (multiple national and international sites) study (Hubal et al. 2005). In the aforementioned study, the effect of three months of upper arm muscle resistance training on biceps muscle cross-sectional area (quantified by magnetic resonance imaging), 1RM, and peak torque was investigated. The study included a total of 585 participants aged between 18 and 40 years. 243 were women and 342 were men. Training was performed using the non-dominant arm only (i.e. not the arm used spontaneously for throwing) and included three different biceps exercises (preacher curl, concentration curl, standing biceps curl) and two different triceps exercises (triceps press and triceps kickback).

The objective of the study was only the biceps adaptation. The triceps muscle was only trained in order to prevent imbalances. All training sessions were supervised and lasted approx. 45–60 min. The actual progressive training program then consisted of the following phases: Weeks 1–4: 3 sets of 12 repetitions per exercise with the 12RM load (a load that can be moved 12 times over the ROM at maximal effort); Weeks 5–9: 3 sets of 8 repetitions per exercise with the 8RM load; Weeks 10–12: 3 sets of 6 repetitions per exercise with the 6RM load. Unfortunately, more detailed training information is not available here either. The cross-sectional area of the biceps increased by an average of 20.4 % (standard error of the mean [SEM] 0.6) in the men. However, the values obtained ranged from -2.5 to +55.5 %. A virtually identical result was observed in females. The cross-sectional area increased by a mean of 17.9 % SEM 0.5; range of values -2.3 to +59.3 %).

Peak torque also increased on average: by +15.8 % for males (SEM 1.1; range -24.3 to +148.5 %) and by +22.0 % for females (SEM 1.1; range -31.5 to +93.4 %). Finally, similar improvements were also seen for the 1RM: Men +39.8 % (SEM 1.4; range of values 0 to +150.0 %), Women +64.1 % (SEM 2.0; range of values 0 to +250.0 %) (Hubal et al. 2005). The extent of interindividual variability (see value ranges) was impressive. There were participants in both sexes who lost muscle cross-sectional area and muscle force with this specific training program! In terms of cross-sectional area, there were a few individuals in both sexes who were classified as *low responders*, and about 2 % of women and about 3 % of men who were classified as *high responders*. These individuals responded extremely weakly *(low responders)* or strongly *(high responders)* to this specific training protocol.

In the second study, the effect of interindividual variability on the adaptation of muscle size and muscle force of the thigh muscles was investigated. For this purpose, a research group analyzed all data from resistance training studies conducted in their own laboratory from 1996 to 2011 (monocentric study) (Ahtiainen et al. 2016). Changes in thigh cross-sectional area or thigh lean mass were collected using ultrasound, magnetic resonance imaging, or dual-energy X-ray absorptiometry. The resistance training studies lasted between 20 and 24 weeks. The training was monitored by professionals. The studies featured different training protocols, but all were aimed at producing muscle hypertrophy. Data from 287 study participants between the ages of 19 and 79 were ultimately included in the analysis. Muscle size increased by a mean of 4.2 % (standard deviation [SD] 6.3) in women and 5.1 % (SD 5.9) in men. The small difference between men and women was not statistically significant. The 1RM increased by a mean of 24.2 % (SD 13.8) in women, which was significantly higher than the increase in men (+19.4 %, SD 9.5). This study also examined the effect of age on changes in muscle size and 1RM. For this purpose, participants were divided into three age groups (<45 years, 45–60 years, >60 years). Muscle size and 1RM increased similarly across all age groups percentage wise and there were no significant differences in increases between age groups. Younger and older participants were thus able to benefit from resistance training to the same extent percentage wise.

If we now look at the value ranges of the changes achieved in muscle size and 1RM, the large intraindividual differences again become apparent: For muscle size, the percentage changes ranged from −11 to +30 % and for 1RM from −8 to +60 %. Regarding muscle size, 14.6 % of all participants recorded no increase or even a decrease during the training phase. In contrast, approximately 3 % of the participants recorded no increase or even a decrease in 1RM. For the value ranges of both variables, there were no differences between sexes or between age groups. Interestingly, there was only a very weak relationship between change in muscle size and change in 1RM. Thus, it was shown that a study participant with a negative change in muscle size could certainly achieve an improvement in 1RM at the same time. The changes in the two variables therefore do not necessarily go hand in hand.

It follows that it is not correct to speak of a "low response" *in general* on the basis of a "low response" in a measurement variable. This is even more true because the studies did not simultaneously investigate whether the *low responders* could be successful with a different training program and/or a different training dosage, frequency, and/or duration. In any case, the values for most of the measured variables are widely scattered around the mean, and one can observe both *low responders* and *high responders* for each measured variable. For some measurement variables, the proportion of *low responders* is as high as 15 % of the population, and in extreme cases, such as insulin sensitivity after 20 weeks of endurance training, more than 20 %! A challenge for the future is therefore to understand the basis for this interindividual variability so that targeted (target group-specific) and effective training measures can be formulated.

## 21.2 Twice as Much Muscle Mass: Without Training!

The ability of humans to physiologically adapt to training varies, depending on the training stimulus or, more precisely, the exerceuticals applied and the interaction with the response matrix. In addition to the influence of dietary protein, age, etc., it is considered undisputed that some of the variability is familial. The familial contribution in turn comes from variations in the DNA sequence of genes (see Sect. 8.2) that we inherit from our parents. With regard to muscle hypertrophy and muscle force increase, a few single genetic polymorphisms (i.e. gene variants) are known to date, but these can only explain a small part of the variability in adaptation to resistance training. However, as described in this section, there are genetic polymorphisms that lead to an extremely muscular and strong phenotype even in the absence of training.

These include, for example, mutations in myostatin *(MSTN)*. Myostatin belongs to the TGF-β *(transforming growth factor-β)* molecular family and plays a critical role in the regulation of skeletal muscle mass. Mice in which the *MSTN gene has* been knocked out by genetic mutation have twice as much muscle mass (evenly distributed over the entire body) compared to a normal (wild-type) mouse. The doubling of muscle mass is the result of hyperplasia and hypertrophy of muscle fibers. Even just inhibiting the activity of the myostatin protein, for example by binding to an inhibitor, can lead to an increase in muscle mass in mice. Myostatin thus has at least two functions. One is the regulation of the number of muscle fibers that form during development, and the other is the postnatal (after birth) regulation of muscle growth. Inactivation of myostatin results in marked muscle enlargement in mice, cattle, sheep, dogs, and humans, so the function of myostatin appears to be conserved across species.

In humans there is a scientifically well-described case of a boy who was born at the Charité in Berlin. This boy stood out for his unusually pronounced musculature. Using ultrasonography, the muscle cross-sectional area of the quadriceps muscle was determined 6 days after birth and compared with reference values of other boys. The result was impressive: the boy had a muscle cross-sectional area of 6.7 $cm^2$, which was more than twice as large as that of normal boys (3.1 $cm^2$). In other words, the muscle cross-sectional area of the quadriceps muscle was 7.2(!) standard deviations higher than the corresponding mean value from measurements of ten control boys. Conversely, the subcutaneous fat layer thickness was 2.9 standard deviations smaller than the mean. At the age of 4.5 years, the boy was able to hold two 3-kg dumbbells horizontally with extended arms.

In this boy, a loss-of-function mutation in the *MSTN gene* was detected. This is a mutation that leads to the production of a non-functional myostatin protein. So this boy's cells were not producing functional myostatin. Bookmarked, this boy was twice as muscular as others, but without training! In people with exceptionally or extremely high muscle mass, it is therefore difficult to say whether they look the way they do *because of* training or *in spite of* it. In any case, it is *a priori* not useful to try to copy the training methods of genetically selected people, because they are hardly causally related to the phenotype.

There are natural inhibitors that influence the function of myostatin or proteins of the TGF-β superfamily in the body. These include, for example, follistatin, FLRG and Gasp-1. If one now takes genetically manipulated mice in which the myostatin gene has been knocked out and overexpresses follistatin (excess production of follistatin), there is a quadrupling of muscle mass instead of the usual doubling. This suggests that myostatin is not the only member of the TGF-β superfamily that affects the amount of muscle mass. It also suggests that there are other gene mutations that may have a milder but still relevant effect on the quantity of muscle mass. Naturally, the pharmaceutical industry has also become aware of such molecules and is researching at full speed to develop appropriate active substances that are intended to counteract muscle atrophy. It is a matter of time before the first myostatin signal inhibitors are introduced, irrespective of whether their application and cross-system efficacy make any sense at all from a physiological and regulatory point of view.

In addition to gene mutations, epigenetic influences can also affect response strength and thus adaptability to training. Epigenetic modifications are changes in gene expression that are *not* due to a change in DNA sequence. Epigenetic modifications include, but are not limited to, changes in DNA accessibility and readability (e.g., through chemical modification of DNA and/or histones) and post-transcriptional changes. Epigenetic influences may thus also contribute to the observed interindividual variability in adaptation to training.

## 21.3 What Can Be Expected in Terms of Average Muscle Growth?

Back to the averages. What is the average magnitude of hypertrophy that can be expected from resistance training (understood as a general term)? This question was investigated in a recent meta-analysis (Wernbom et al. 2007). In general, the scientific longitudinal studies lasted between 30 and 180 days. The quadriceps studies in particular lasted between 14 and 180 days (on average 79 days). The average increase in muscle cross-sectional area for these studies was 8.5 % (range 1.1–17.3 %). For miometric-pliometric resistance training (classic form of training), the rate of increase in cross-sectional area averaged 0.13 % per day and was approximately the same for men and women.

Elbow flexor training studies lasted between 30 and 180 days (on average 91 days), with an average increase in muscle cross-sectional area of 15.8 %. For miometric-pliometric resistance training, the rate of increase in cross-sectional area averaged 0.20 % per day. These numbers may be true on average, but you must remember two things. First, for the individual, meaning you, the results may be completely different (see above). Secondly, the numbers do not allow you to extrapolate what the absolute potential is for increasing muscle mass and muscle force, either on average or for the individual.

When an untrained person starts training, the result is essentially unpredictable. For averages, therefore, ask about the sample size (i.e., number of measured values or study participants) and the statistical distribution underlying those averages. Although you still won't be able to predict how strong your training adaptation will actually be, you will at least have a reasonable idea of the possible and most likely outcomes and be better able to rank your progress.

The concept of interindividual variability is certainly a valuable tool to study molecular and cellular adaptation to training. However, studies on this subject have at least one problem: they more or less deliberately ignore the fact that exerceuticals can vary from individual to individual for apparently the same training. Just because two individuals produce the same external torque, mechanical work or power, in relative terms, does not mean that the muscular (internal) torque or other internal mechanical variables are the same for the muscle or muscle fibers studied (see Sect. 1.10). Thus, as long as it is not clear to which internal stimuli the examined muscle fibers were actually exposed, the proportion of the supposed interindividual variability of exerceuticals and response matrix cannot really be separated. We are therefore still far from a scientific basis for tailored and comprehensive training recommendations for the general population. Instead of unreflectively parroting the mantra of interindividual variability, we should examine the entire axis between external training stimulus, internally acting exerceuticals, their interaction with the response matrix, and finally experimental or methodological variability. Only then will we be able to assign the possible variability of a training adaptation between individuals to the corresponding variability determinants. Nevertheless, the available data impressively show that the influence of (epi-)genetics on the magnitude of training adaptations is likely to be many times larger than the potential effect differences between single-set training and multi-set training that are up for (sham) debate (see Sect. 13.6).

## 21.4 Why We Sometimes Confuse Cause and Effect in Training Too

On our way through life we stumble over fallacies again and again, and systematically. Rolf Dobelli, a Swiss author and entrepreneur, has unmasked 52 treacherous cognitive errors in a book (Dobelli 2011). One of them, which is important in the context of training and nutrition, is the imitation illusion (called *swimmer's body illusion in* the book): You stand in front of the mirror in the morning and examine yourself from head to toe. You don't like what you see (anymore), and you decide you want to change the shape of your body. You know, the usual requests: more muscle (but yes, not too much) and less fat. How do you proceed? Logically, the first thing you think about is who is closest to your ideal: marathon runners, perhaps? Too skinny and lopsided for you. Bodybuilder? Too broad and bulky. Swimmers? Yes, in them you see elegant, well-built bodies. Now the next logical step is to copy the training program of a top swimmer, preferably an Olympic champion, and train accordingly. But is that really goal-oriented?

In all likelihood, after a few months of hard training, you'll find that your dream body has remained wishful thinking (or maybe you'll get lucky and find your "biological niche"). You would not be the only one who has fallen for the illusion that imitation can bring about the desired appearance. Without this illusion of imitation, much of advertising would probably not work. As an example, we might mention the many models who advertise cosmetics, or female bodybuilders who stand in for nutritional supplements, training equipment or similar.

The cognitive error is that top swimmers don't have the characteristic physique primarily because they swim a lot, but because physique is, among other things, a selection criterion for being a top swimmer. The same is true for all other biological specializations. Likewise, cosmetics do not make women or men models. Models just happen to fit the current ideal of beauty, or they fit the beauty template of the exponents of the fashion industry (fashion designers, photographers, etc.). Here, too, "beauty" (however defined) is a selection criterion, because without it these people could not advertise cosmetics. In imitation, then, there is a danger that we confuse a selection criterion with the result of a particular activity. In other words, we confuse cause and effect. Copying behavior is firmly anchored into our genes because, from an evolutionary biology perspective, it can be beneficial for survival. Suppose you are sitting in a movie theater. Suddenly you smell and see smoke. I hardly suppose that you then start looking for the source of the smoke to make sure that there is indeed a fire burning – of course not. You run after or ahead of the others, heading for the emergency exit. You can worry about the cause of the smoke when you are safe. The problem is that a nonsensical idea, wrong behavior, etc., doesn't become more right by many people believing it to be right. If thousands claim nonsense, that doesn't make it truth. Just because many claim that multi-set training (or in the opposite case, single-set training), barbell training (or machine training), or whole-body training (or split training) is more effective does not automatically mean that the claim is true.

Advertising systematically exploits our weakness of imitation, for example, through so-called testimonials – people like you and me, who make advocacy statements. Just look for a homepage on which a weight-loss product is advertised. You will come across countless affirmative comments: Stefan: "I took product XY and lost 10 kg of fat mass and gained 5 kg of muscle mass in 2 weeks as a result!" Julia: "Congratulations on your bombastic success! For me it also worked brilliantly -10 kg body mass in 3 weeks – and all without training!" After a dozen such affirmations, most people believe that there must be something to it.

Well, it is one thing to copy behaviors of your own volition. That is human. More serious is the fact when we let ourselves be blinded by one aspect and conclude from this to the whole picture. From particularly striking characteristics, for example muscle mass, we automatically infer unknown qualities such as professional competence. The striking characteristics do not necessarily have to be of a physical nature only. Expert status can also be signalled in other ways: in the case of doctors by their white coats, in the case of researchers by the number of publications, in the case of bank managers by their suit and tie, and so on. There are also other signals such as invitations on radio and television, books, presence in social media (Facebook, Twitter, etc.). In a similar way to how we perceive the products of a manufacturer with a good reputation as being of higher quality, we assume that the statements and writings of such experts are worth something or have substance in terms of content.

## 21.5 Summary

Similar to height, muscle mass and muscle force are physical characteristics that can vary greatly between individuals. One reason for these differences is that the magnitude of the expression of these characteristics is partly family-related. Scientific data show that muscle mass is about 70% inherited and about 30% influenced by environmental factors. Similarly, the increase in muscle mass that can be achieved with exercise is largely hereditary. While most women and men achieve a moderate increase, there are a few individuals who have exceptionally large increases and others who have no increase in muscle mass. Accordingly, in order to achieve exceptionally large muscle mass and/or muscle force, suitable (epi-)genetic conditions are required, both for high initial values and for trainability. Hard training in combination with adequate nutrition supports you in the development of your individual potential.

# 22

# Neural Aspects of Resistance Training

## 22.1 Force Versus Exercise Competence

When a previously untrained person starts resistance training, amazing things happen in the first training phase. Almost every exercise session, the exercise load can be increased. Studies with untrained men confirm this observation. After just three to four exercise sessions, the exercise load can be increased by up to 25% on equipment that is simple from a motor point of view, such as the knee extension machine. At this point, no increase in muscle cross-sectional area is detectable or measurable. In the subsequent exercise sessions, the increase in exercise load is still greater than would be expected on the basis of the increase in muscle cross-sectional area. Consequently, factors that are not directly related to the mass, geometry and/or composition of the muscle also contribute to the increase in exercise load.

The first factor involves inhibition of the coactivation of muscles that can counteract the desired external force application. Evidence for this mechanism comes from studies of antagonist muscle activity in the presence of agonist activity. For example, in one study, ten young untrained men trained their knee extensor (agonist) muscles for 8 weeks. The exercise consisted of 30 maximal intentional isometric force productions for 3–4 s with more than 30 s rest between each repetition, which was performed three times per week. Peak voluntary isometric force was measured at the beginning of the study and after 1, 2, 4 and 8 weeks. Muscular activity of the knee flexor (antagonist) muscles was also obtained during this measurement. Before the training phase, the antagonist musculature had an activity of 14.7% of its peak value at maximum intentional effort of the agonist musculature. After only three exercise sessions, coactivation decreased to 11.5%. At the same time, the measured force during knee extension increased significantly. In the aforementioned study, the increase in measured knee extension force within the first exercise sessions was largely explained by the inhibition of antagonist coactivation (Carolan and Cafarelli 1992).

The second factor concerns frequency coding (see Sects. 4.2 and 9.4 and Box 9.1). By increasing the maximal firing frequency due to training, the "force" (better: the external load) can be increased even without increasing muscle mass. As a reminder, during maximal intentional force production, all motor units available for this motor task are generally recruited and the motoneurons fire at the current highest possible frequency. During the course of a training phase, this peak firing frequency of the motor units increases. After a resistance training phase, the motor units reach a higher firing frequency during maximal intentional force application for the same motor task, resulting in an increase in externally measured force or load.

The third factor is the so-called intermuscular coordination of agonists. On the one hand, this refers to the additional involvement of agonists, which may not yet be activated in the untrained state. Primarily, however, one means the coordination of the initial activation, the duration and the applied force of all muscles/muscle groups involved in the motor task. The more coordinated the actions of the muscles involved, the stronger the effect on the externally measured mechanical quantities such as force, torque, power or impulse.

In contrast to these three factors, both "intramuscular coordination" (see Box 9.1) and the synchronization of motor units (i.e., the simultaneous "firing" of action potentials for several motor units) are not scientifically plausible explanations. In a recent, scientifically rigorous study, my research colleagues even concluded that synchronization is an epiphenomenon, i.e., that the synchronization of motor units is not part of a physiological design but should be seen as a random product of numerous neuronal interactions (Kline and De Luca 2016).

In summary, in adult individuals, a major reason for increases in exercise and/or competition loads is motor, or neural, learning. This effect and the associated potential for increase is proportional to the complexity of the motor task, i.e., the "difficulty" of the exercise. Thus, multi-joint exercises such as the squat or similar, which are often presented as a measure of "force", can be improved over a period of years, presumably farafter the actual hypertrophy potential of the corresponding muscles has been exhausted. Consequently, the observed increases in exercise and competition loads are primarily due to improvements in exercise-specific motor skill and ability as a result of the three factors mentioned above. So if someone tries to convince you that he or she has multiplied his or her "(maximum)force" within a certain period of time through training, you know better now: what is actually meant is "motor skill competence", no more and no less. The learned motoric exercise competence is exercise-specific, i.e. it cannot be easily transferred to other exercises. If you train or practice the squat endlessly in an exercise-specific manner, the best case scenario is that you improve your performance on this exercise or variations of it. A direct transfer of the relative improvement to other exercises such as the seated knee extension or similar is not *a priori* given (see also Sect. 22.4).

## 22.2 Is a Bigger Muscle Also a Stronger Muscle?

The use of tissue dimensions as a surrogate for maximal intrinsic muscle force is limited mainly because of four reasons. First, the force generated by a non-fatigued muscle depends on the activity of the motor units. This activity is a function of the number of motor units recruited and the firing rate (see Sect. 4.2). Of these two force-coding mechanisms, only the first is affected by muscle fiber size. Indeed, for a given recruitment and unchanged firing rate, the force response will be higher if the number of parallel actin-myosin cross-bridges (i.e., the number of parallel sarcomeres or fiber cross-sectional area) is increased. As discussed, in large muscles, all motor units are recruited at approximately 85–95 % of peak force. If you measure your peak voluntary force (equivalent to 100 %) before and after several weeks of resistance training and find that it has increased, the reason for this, as explained in Sect. 22.1, is either an increase in firing rate and/or an improved distribution of activity between agonist and antagonist and/or improved intermuscular coordination (which includes an increase in intermuscular muscle fiber cross-sectional area).

Second, muscle force is also dependent on the relative area occupied by the activated muscle fibertypes relative to the total cross-sectional area (see Box. 5.2). As discussed, human muscle fibers produce 1.4- to 2.1-fold more tension (force per cross-sectional area) during active lengthening than during active shortening, depending on fiber type, with maximal isometric tension up to two times higher in fast fibers than in slow fibers (Fig. 5.2). The optimal shortening velocity and power characteristics also behave similarly, which are significantly higher in type-2 fibers than in type-1 fibers (note: the mechanical and kinetic properties of actin-myosin interaction during pliometric force production are virtually the same for type-1 and type-2 fibers). Thus, for any given physiological muscle cross-sectional area during mio- or isometric muscle action at a given recruitment and firing rate, the force is higher when the area fraction occupied by type-2 fibers is higher. It follows that the force, for the same total physiological muscle cross-sectional area, may vary depending on the area distribution of muscle fiber types. In isolated muscle, therefore, it is to be expected that for two individuals who have the same physiological cross-sectional area for a given muscle, the isometric peak force will be higher in the subject who has a greater area of type-2 fibers.

Third, it can be assumed that the correlation between muscle mass or (physiological) muscle cross-sectional area and task-specific peak force is greatest when the hypertrophied muscle fibersare actually used in the motor test task (see sport-specific training, Box. 9.5). If this is not the case, you will have larger muscles, but the measured task-specific peak force may not change much, if at all. It can therefore also be statedthat the correlation between muscle mass and peak force also depends on the choice of force test.

Fourth, in adults, the size of a joint could limit the maximum force that can be applied to the bones, regardless of the current muscle size (Toigo 2013). From a cross-sectional study of 323 individuals, it is known that both maximum force (multiple one-legged hopping on the forefoot, see Sect. 2.3) and tibial bone strength increase during body growth and peak around age 20 (Anliker et al. 2011). In the population studied, these values then remained constant or decreased slightly over the rest of the lifespan. These results are consistent with previous observations that muscle and bone mass increase proportionally during childhood and that much of the bone mass is accumulated during puberty. This implies that bone mass is essentially adapted to the mechanical forces typically applied during and at the end of puberty. It is suggested that not only the bone mass but also the joint surfaces must be adapted to these peak loads and that after the end of length growth (closing of the growth plates) there is no significant physiological increase in the same joint surfaces and maximum voluntary force (discussed in Toigo 2013).

Consistently, the few available studies indicate that during puberty the articular surface, not the cartilage thickness, increases and that after a six-week unilateral immobilization phase of the knee there are no lateral differences, neither in the tibial cartilage thickness nor in the articular surface. Since the physical material properties (*stress* and *strain*) of articular cartilage are given or there is no scientific evidence that these material properties change in healthy individuals (in contrast to pathological conditions such as osteomalacia), the maximum force that can be applied without damage depends on the articular surface. During childhood and puberty, the joint surface adapts in direct proportion to the muscle forces acting on it. Conversely, after the completion of length growth, the muscle force that can be applied would have to be limited as a function of the joint area reached in order to prevent cartilage and bone damage. However, there is currently no direct scientific evidence for or against such a mechanism (Toigo 2013).

For a non-deconditioned, healthy adult individual, it is therefore not to be expected that maximum voluntary transmittable muscle forceand consequently bone strength can be significantly increased physiologically (i.e. through training). Conversely, relative (i.e., relative to young adulthood) deconditioning, for example, as a result of being sedentary or bedridden, leads to a decrease in maximal voluntary muscle force and, in the worst case, a decrease in the force transmitted to the bone, which in turn leads to a decrease in bone strength (Toigo 2013). From these considerations, we learn that muscle hypertrophied by training in adults does not automatically lead to more external force, because the force transmitted to bone via the articular surfaces is likely controlled. What is generally considered an "increase in force" in adults is often no more than an increase in specific exercise competence through motor learning (see Sect. 22.1).

## 22.3 Are 100 Newtons Equal to 100 Newtons?

Regarding physics, the question must be answered with yes, regarding our central nervous system obviously with no. Imagine the following experiment (based on Rudroff et al. 2011). You are sitting comfortably on a chair, your right upper arm is at the side of your upper body, your right elbow joint is supported on a pad with your shoulder lowered, and your right forearm is parallel to the floor (i.e., there is a 90° angle between your forearm and upper arm). You wear an orthosis on the right forearm, through which the external force is applied. In the first case, I attach a tear-proof, non-elastic cord at the level of the wrist, which is connected in a line to a force sensor. This force sensor is in turn linearly anchored to the ground via a tear-resistant, non-elastic cord. As soon as you try to bend your arm, the sensor measures the isometric tensile force of the muscle-tendon unit. First, however, your peak voluntary force is recorded. To do this, you build up the peak force within about 3 s and with maximum effort over 3 s; it corresponds to the highest force value recorded by the sensor. Now, at given times in a rested state, you are asked to develop 20, 30, 45 and 60 % of the previously measured peak force and to maintain this for as long as possible (you receive feedback via representation of the force). This motor task is therefore a so-called *force task*.

For the second task (which also takes place in a rested state), I mount objects unknown to you on the orthosis whose weight force also corresponds to 20, 30, 45 and 60 % of the previously measured peak force. In this case, however, you should concentrate on the angular position between the lower and upper arm. This should remain at 90° for as long as possible. This is therefore a *position task*. In both cases your elbow flexors produce exactly the same external force, but in the first case you concentrate on keeping the force value constant, while in the second case the focus is on the angular position in the elbow joint. Crux: Is the *time to task failure* the same or different for the two cases? Most of us would probably assume that it is the same in both cases, since the muscle force is also the same. However, this is by no means the case for all force levels. For force levels of 20 % and 30 % of peak force, it takes only half as much time for the force to decay in the position target task as in the force target task. This means that despite producing the same force in the position task relative to the force task, you will fatigue much faster at low force values (Rudroff et al. 2011). However, the higher the force produced, the smaller the difference. At 45 % of peak force, the difference in time to performance decline is already only 25 % and at 60 % of peak force there appears to be no difference for this motor task (Rudroff et al. 2011).

The mechanistic reason for this observation is still unclear. It is thought that the central nervous system, as a function of motor intention, decides at the onset of the movement whether it is a force or position target and employs a different muscle activation strategy depending on this. Specifically, it is believed that during a movement task with a positional goal, the γ-motoneurons in the spinal cord that innervate the muscle spindles are more activated. This increases the reflex sensitivity of the muscle spindles, meaning that the muscle spindles are more sensitive to changes in length in the muscle and thus to changes in angular position. Increased afferent feedback through the muscle spindles allows positional deviations to be corrected better or faster, but this is at the expense of fatigability. Apparently, at relatively high forces (60 % of peak force in the above example), the central nervous system no longer distinguishes between positional and force targets. Incidentally, it is worth noting that the percentage drop in force for each level of force tested was the same for both force and position targets.

## 22.4 Core Training

Since the late nineties, the term *core training* has been used repeatedly in the prevention and/or treatment of back problems. The idea of core training is based on the scientific knowledge that the time sequence of activation of the various trunk muscles is altered in patients with chronic back ailments compared to non-symptomatic people. However, this finding is much older. As early as the late sixties, it was demonstrated that coordination between muscles can be impaired in the case of injury and pain. These ailments are now to be remedied with trunk stabilization training. By this training, trainers and therapists mean the ability and skill to maintain a specific trunk position, hip position, balance and movement control during body movements or in isometric positions. Exercises prescribed by trainers and therapists theoretically aim to improve stabilization skills. Two key assumptions underlie the choice of exercises. First, that a deep "core" musculature exists in the trunk that functions independently of the superficial trunk muscles, and second, that a "dysfunction" of this deep "core" musculature is responsible for decreased trunk stability. The aim of trunk stabilization training is therefore to activate these deep muscles specifically and independently of the superficial trunk muscles in order to correct their dysfunction. This is roughly the mantra of trunk stabilization training. However, well-known knowledge and scientific studies question the basis of trunk stabilization training (Lederman 2010).

First, the division of the trunk musculature into a deep, stabilising "core" musculature and a superficial musculature that is responsible for movements does not correspond to the functional anatomy of the trunk musculature (Lederman 2010). Indeed, in contradiction to this arbitrary classification, it turns out that in the stabilization of the trunk, all muscles that can contribute to the fulfillment of function in the specific situation are active, regardless of the "label" we give to the muscles. It is therefore not plausible that individual muscles should *a priori* be more important than others for trunk stability.

Second, although the argument that trunk muscles are activated with a time delay in individuals with back pain has been scientifically demonstrated, it has not yet been shown that this time delay is causally related to back pain. Moreover, it is equally unclear whether trunk stabilization exercises can reverse this time delay.

Third, there is no direct evidence that trunk muscle "force", however measured, has a causal influence on back pain. This becomes apparent when looking at muscle force levels during everyday activities. When walking or standing, only a maximum of 5 % of the peak force of the trunk muscles used is needed to stabilise the trunk. Even when we carry a load of over 30 kg while standing, no more than 5 % of the peak force of the muscles used is required (Lederman 2010). A loss of muscle force in the trunk muscles as an explanation for back pain therefore seems very unlikely (the only exception being if the current peak force were to drop to a value below 5 % of the initial peak force). This argument therefore also counters the marketing message that isolated resistance training of the back muscles is inherently more effective or efficient than other forms of training, or even the sole remedy for back pain. This latter point was explored in a large-scale study several years ago. To investigate the effect of active therapy on chronic low back pain, 132 affected study participants completed three months of training. The participants were divided into three experimental groups with different training programs: (a) physiotherapy, (b) machine-based resistance exercise with fixed pelvis, or (c) aerobics/stretching. Several functional tests were performed before and after the training phase (Mannion et al. 2001a) and questionnaires on psychological well-being, self-rated impairment level and socio-demographic characteristics were completed (Mannion et al. 2001b). In addition, muscle biopsies of the back muscles (M. Iliocostalis/M. Longissimus) were collected from a subgroup of 45 participants (Käser et al. 2001). The results on the three different study areas were as follows. Maximal voluntary isometric torque (i.e., figuratively speaking, "peak force") increased during the training phase in each measured direction of trunk motion. The group with the machine training was able to achieve a slightly greater improvement in this regard compared to the other two training groups. In isometric and dynamic fatigue tests, all participants performed better after the training phase, with no differences between the training groups. Muscle fiber cross-sectional areas of all muscle fiber types were not increased by the training interventions. In addition, there was also no change in the areal distribution of muscle fiber types. Consequently, the improvements in the functional tests could not be explained by changes in muscle fiber properties. For this reason, in the final step, the research group investigated which factors most influenced self-rated impairment, independent of the training program. Prior to the training phase, the most significant influencing factors were as follows (in order of decreasing importance): Pain, psychological distress, anxiety-driven avoidance behaviors, muscle activation levels, lumbar range of motion, and gender. The change in self-rated impairment during the training phase could only be explained by changes in pain, psychological distress, and fear-driven avoidance behaviors. Consequently, the improvement in discomfort was primarily based on the modification of the determining psychological factors and not on the improvement of the functional variables. Since physical activity *per se* led to an improvement in these psychological factors, this resulted in a decrease in ailments. This does not mean that resistance training is ineffective in all cases. Thus, the authors of a meta-analysis published in 2015 conclude that resistance training of the entire body (i.e. not only of the back muscles) as well as stabilization/coordination training can have a small but significant effect on the reduction of chronic, non-specific low back pain (Searle et al. 2015; see, however, the text below regarding stabilization training).

Fourth, trunk stabilization exercises are often intended to deliberately tense only individual muscles. So far, it has not been scientifically proven that people can specifically activate individual trunk muscles independently of the other trunk muscles.Imagine, for example, that you are in a plank position. Their job is to keep the trunk in its natural physiological position as much as possible and to prevent the trunk from lowering. The lowering of the trunk is prevented by the interaction of all abdominal muscle parts (e.g. central and lateral abdominal muscles). Feel free to try to willfully disable either muscle or muscle group in this position… You will not succeed. In an exercise task, all muscles covering this function are active at all times. This also makes sense throughout, as it distributes the load over several muscles or muscle groups and can thus delay the fatigue of individual muscles or muscle groups.

Fifth, the point of specificity of training adaptation discussed earlier comes into play. The adaptations of the nervous system to training are primarily movement specific. If trunk stabilization exercises are performed lying down, your specific exercise competence will increase over time (see Sect. 22.1). Whether a transfer to trunk stabilization in standing and sitting will be successful remains an open question. Moreover, trunk stabilization exercises are often not performed in the same context as everyday movements, which means that a transfer of training effects in favour of everyday activities such as standing for long periods of time or similar is questionable.

These five points provide a possible explanation for the lack of scientific evidence for clinically relevant relief or prevention of chronic non-specific low back pain through trunk stabilization training. Trunk stabilization training, according to the current state of scientific evidence, is unlikely to have a meaningful effect on reducing the aforementioned back ailments and, from a clinical perspective, is no more effective than other forms of training or manual therapy (Saragiotto et al. 2016). Trunk stabilization training is also no better than any other form of training when it comes to preventing injuries in everyday life or sports. This is not surprising, because the training effects achieved for the trained muscles are firstly small and secondly specific to the trained exercises.

Considered as a whole, the data on the relative effect of the various forms of training is unclear. In the case of non-specific, chronic back ailments, it is therefore recommended first and foremost to move the trunk in as varied a manner as possible. "Varied" here refers to the applied force, the mode of muscle action (miometric, isometric, pliometric), the training methods (e.g., isolated back muscle training only or whole-body training, machines or free exercises, etc.), range and direction of motion, number of repetitions, rate of force development, etc. To find out over time what works best for you personally, it is recommended that you only change one training variable at a time, while keeping all other factors constant. This way you can better localize the hopefully positive training effect and thus also reproduce it in the long term.

## 22.5 Rate of Force Development

As you learned in Sect. 1.12, the term "fast force" is not only misleading, it is simply wrong. It implies that there is a "fast" force and that it is a separate entity. In fact, however, it is not the force that is fast, but your neuromuscular system that can develop the force at different rates. What is meant is the *rate of force development* (RFD) or the *impulse*. To illustrate this concept, please imagine the following experimental set-up. You are sitting strapped to a dynamometer. The device looks similar to a knee extension machine, except that it can be used to measure force, among other things. The left leg is relaxed and fixed in a comfortable position. The measuring arm for the following experiment is positioned on the right shin. After a brief warm-up, the measuring arm is moved to a predetermined measuring position (e.g. the knee angle should correspond to 110°; 180° would correspond to full knee extension). The force sensor is located in the measuring arm. You are now given the task of exerting as fast and as hard as possible against the measuring arm after a start signal. However, the measuring arm remains fixed during the entire measurement and you consequently push isometrically against it. We now look at how the force develops during the first 200 ms of the measurement. At the very beginning, the force increases slowly and then goes into a steep rise. The increase in force then flattens out and after a certain time reaches the peak value for this exercise task (from 200 ms). The RFD can now be determined for different time intervals. Usually the intervals between 0–50 ms, 0–100 ms and 0–200 ms are used. The RFD simply corresponds to the linear slope, which can be determined with the help of the difference quotient from two different points lying on the straight line (Fig. 22.1a). For example, for $RFD_{100\ ms}$ these two points are the measured force at time 0 ms and the measured force at time 100 ms. Now, if the force is 0 N at time 0 ms and just under 500 N at time 100 ms, the $RFD_{100\ ms}$ is 5 N/ms [(500 N-0 N)/(100 ms-0 ms)]. The $impulse_{0-100\ ms}$ then corresponds to the determined integral (shown as an area) under the graph of the force function in the integration range from 0 to 100 ms (Fig. 22.1a). Which factors now have an influence on the rate of force development and how can these factors be influenced by training?

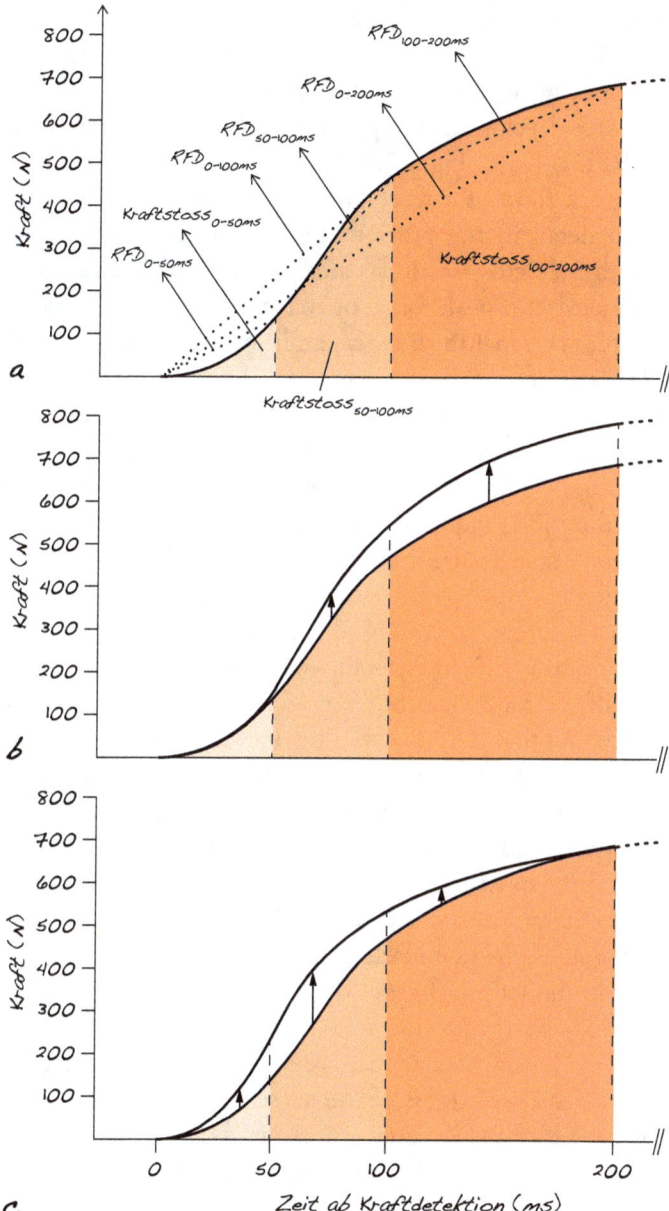

**Fig. 22.1** Measured force as a function of time. (**a**) Determination of the *rate of force development* (RFD), or impulse, in a defined time interval for a specific, isolated movement task such as knee extension on a dynamometer. (**b**) Possible influence of peak force increase on RFD in the late phase of force increase. (**c**) Possible influence of the timing of motor unit activity on the early phase of the force increase

1. The magnitude of peak force has a positive influence on the rate of force development. If peak voluntary force is increased by resistance training with or without muscle hypertrophy, this can have a positive influence on the rate of force development, especially in the late phase of the increase in force (i.e. $RFD_{100-200\ ms}$, Fig. 22.1b). The various possible reasons for the increase in peak force as a result of resistance training have already been described in detail in the previous sections and chapters. Note that an increase in muscle cross-sectional area in adulthood does not necessarily lead to an increase in peak force, or that the increase in peak force is not necessarily proportional to the increase in muscle cross-sectional area (see Fig. 3.3 [Pennation angle] and Sect. 22.2). For example, a simultaneous increase in the pennation angle can reduce or eliminate the potential force-increasing effect of the increase in cross-sectional area.
2. In addition to the magnitude of the peak force, the second critical factor is the time duration required to achieve a given force percentage. Improvements in this quantity have a positive effect on the rate of force development in the first phase (i.e., $RFD_{0-100\ ms}$, Fig. 22.1c). The underlying mechanism is that the timing of the activity of the motoneurons shifts forward. For example, Van Cutsem et al. (1998) showed that after several weeks of ballistic training, not only does the firing frequency of the motor unit increase, but that the activity of the motoneurons is shifted forward in time: the motoneurons fire earlier and faster, making the shape of the force curve steeper, especially in the first 50–75 ms. Changes in the areal distribution of type-1 and type-2 muscle fibers may also affect the RFD in the early phase. If the muscle fiber cross-sectional areas of type-2 fibers increase more compared to type-1 fibers, this will lead to an increase in the rate of force development as the muscle becomes intrinsically faster. Thus, polymorphisms in the actinin-3 gene *(ACTN3)*, which contribute to intraindividual variability in the proportion of type-2X fibers, may also affect RFD.
3. In addition to neuromuscular adaptations, resistance training can also lead to an increase in the stiffness of the muscle-tendon unit. This adaptation has a positive effect on force transmission and thus, theoretically, on the rate of force development. However, human science data supporting this adaptation mechanism is still lacking.
4. Finally, there are genetic factors that influence lateral force transmission between muscle fibers (see Sect. 9.15) and can therefore contribute to variation in specific force, i.e. force per square centimetre of muscle cross-sectional area, between individuals. In other words, two individuals with the same muscle cross-sectional area may generate different amounts of specific force due to polymorphisms in, for example, the *PTK2 gene*. This,

in turn, may affect the amount of peak voluntary force generated and thus the RFD in the late phase of the force increase.

## 22.6 Summary

What is colloquially referred to as "strength" has little to do with the physical concept of force and even less to do with actual muscle force. Rather, it refers to the physiological, mechanical and psychological competence to move and/or hold a load in an exercise-specific manner. This competence is based on a mutually beneficial collaboration of muscle-tendon-bone unit and nervous system. Put simply, by "strength" most people mean the exercise-specific ability and skill to move a (heavy) load from A to B or to hold it in position.

There are three main reasons how, in the absence of muscle hypertrophy, this exercise competence can be increased. First, the activity of the antagonist is reduced by the repeated execution of a movement of the agonist during the execution of the corresponding exercise (reduced coactivation). Second, resistance training results in an exercise-induced increase in the firing frequency of the motor units utilized (Frequencing). Finally, repeated exercise execution leads to an increase in intermuscular coordination, i.e. the timing of the activation of the different muscles or muscle groups involved in the motor task.

If muscle mass increases in adults during a time period (training phase), it is often assumed that the externally measured force or load will also increase proportionally. However, this is often not necessarily the case. First, motor unit activity is a function of the number of motor units used and their firing frequency. However, the latter is not affected by muscle fiber size. Second, muscleforce depends on the relative proportion occupied by different muscle fiber types. Third, the relationship between muscle mass and muscle force exists primarily when the hypertrophied muscle fibers are used in the test task. Fourth, in adults, the maximum force that can be transmittedto the bones could be dependent on joint area rather than muscle size. Finally, in pennated muscles, the concomitant increase in pennation angle may reduce the positive effect of muscle cross-sectional area increase on force.

The scientific evidence on trunk stabilization training is nowhere near as good as its widespread use in sports and fitness settings would suggest. For example, there is no scientific evidence that deep "core" muscles function independently of other trunk muscles and that individuals can effectively learn to activate any "core" muscle independently of other muscles. Similarly, what is learned for a specific exercise can hardly be applied to all movement patterns consciously or unconsciously. Nor has it been scientifically proven to date that reduced core muscle force makes individuals more prone to back pain. Finally, it has not been scientifically proven that the common trunk stabilization training *a priori* positively differs from any other form of trunk training regarding treatment and/or prevention of back pain. However, the same also applies to isolated resistance training of the back muscles on machines. Due to the unclear scientific data, it therefore appears to make sense to move and train the trunk (or spine) as diversely as possible in the case of non-specific, chronic back ailments.

Forget terms like "quickness" or "explosive power". They are scientifically wrong and lead to unclear thinking. Instead, it is better to use "rate of force development" or "impulse" and consider which phase of force development you are referring to when using the term (cf. Fig. 22.1a). The rate of force development is determined by the peak voluntary force and the time to reach a certain percentage of that peak force. The former factor has a preferential effect on the late (Fig. 22.1b), the latter on the early (Fig. 22.1c) phase of force increase. Both factors are in turn influenced by neuromuscular and musculoskeletal factors.

In adulthood you can normally train the peak voluntary force and the time to reach a certain percentage of this peak force, but hardly the maximum force that can be introduced into the bones via the joint surfaces. All methods that lead to an increase in peak force and the time it takes to reach a certain percentage of this peak force are suitable for training the rate of force development. The latter factor in particular includes exercise execution with the motto of completing the movement task "as fastand hard as possible". However, whether a movement is externally visible during the execution of the exercise plays a secondary role here, meaning that you can also train the rate of force development very well with isometric muscle actions.

# 23

# Anabolic Enhancers

## 23.1 Vitamin D

More than 400 years before Christ, the Greek historian Herodotus of Halicarnassus is said to have recommended sunbathing as a therapy against physical ailments. Based on this recommendation, athletes of the ancient Olympic Games are said to have taken sunbaths before and after their training sessions in order to increase the training effect. Whether true or not, the sun has apparently been attributed a healing effect for a long time.

It is now known that the ultraviolet radiation of relatively short wavelengths (UVB) of the sun is the most important source for the formation of vitamin D in the body. Vitamin D has a variety of functions in the body. The best described is the function in bone metabolism. For example, studies have discovered a link between vitamin D deficiency and osteoporosis, as well as an increased risk of bone fractures. There are also indications that vitamin D deficiency may increase the risk of other diseases. However, the data are inconclusive and both direct evidence and mechanistic studies of the effect function of vitamin D are lacking. The discovery that vitamin D receptors are also located in skeletal muscle (and other tissues) leads to the assumption that the effect of the active form of vitamin D, i.e. $1\alpha,25$-dihydroxy-vitamin $D_3$ ($1\alpha,25(OH)_2\ D_3$), takes place in the corresponding tissues via the triggered receptor signals.

Since the vitamin D synthesis capacity of the skin, the vitamin D concentration in the blood and also the maximal muscle performance decrease with increasing age in the population average, it is not surprising that a connection between vitamin D and muscle function is also suspected. This relationship has been experimentally confirmed in cross-sectional studies of elderly subjects. In addition, several studies have shown that an insufficient concentration of vitamin D (more precisely: total 25-hydroxyvitamin D [25(OH)D]) in blood serum is associated with age-related muscle mass loss (sarcopenia). Conversely, supplementation of vitamin $D_3$ (cholecalciferol) was shown to be associated with increased muscle performance in vitamin D deficient individuals. There is also evidence that supplementation of vitamin $D_3$ may lead to an increase in muscle fiber cross-sectional areas. However, the evidence is unclear and it appears that older individuals with vitamin D deficiency may benefit from vitamin $D_3$ supplementation, but not individuals in young adulthood. Thus, the inconsistent study results may also be due to differences in the dosing regimen. While the daily oral intake of a moderate dose (800–1000 *International Units,* IU) tends to have a positive effect, the effect seems to be absent with single megadoses of e.g. 150,000 IU every 3 months. For comparison: For the prevention of vitamin D deficiency, a daily intake (taken orally) of 400 IU (infants in the first year of life), 600 IU (children in the second and third year of life and persons between 3 and 60 years of age, including pregnant and breastfeeding women) and 800 IU (persons over 60 years of age) is recommended in Switzerland for all persons with minimal sun exposure. However, these recommendations are unlikely to be adequate for athletes with substantially increased energy and nutrient requirements. For adults, the maximum recommended tolerable level of vitamin $D_3$ per day is 4000 IU. This corresponds to the safe upper intake (daily dose).

It has been postulated that older individuals respond to the same anabolic stimuli with a smaller increase in muscle protein synthesis (MPS) compared to younger individuals – a phenomenon called "anabolic resistance of aging" (see Sect. 19.6). The possible anabolic resistance in the elderly is thought to be, at least partly, due to low-grade or subthreshold inflammatory processes. Since vitamin D can lead to a reduction in inflammatory processes, the question arises as to whether supplementation in addition to resistance training can increase the effect of resistance training. However, the studies conducted to date on this subject have not been able to prove the existence of such a mechanism in older individuals. Resistance training alone led to an improvement in muscle force and function in all studies. However, the additional intake of vitamin D supplements was not able to further increase these improvements. These results could also be interpreted to mean that the possible existence of "anabolic resistance" is not a phenomenon associated *a priori* with age, but is rather related to the person's level of activity and health.

As mentioned, the UVB radiation of the sun is the most important source for the formation of vitamin D in the body. Across Europe, however, there is insufficient UVB radiation between November and March. In the north, UVB radiation is even very low between September and April. During this time, the skin can produce very little vitamin D, resulting in seasonally fluctuating vitamin D concentrations in the blood, with significantly lower levels during the winter compared to the summer months. This also raises the question of whether adaptations to resistance training are lower in winter due to lower vitamin D levels, and whether this can be counteracted by vitamin $D_3$ supplementation. This very question was recently investigated in a study (Agergaard et al. 2015). Healthy young and older men performed 12 weeks of progressive resistance training during the winter months. Four weeks prior to the training intervention, half of the participants started supplementation with vitamin $D_3$, while the other half were given a placebo. Both groups took the supplements daily until the end of the training phase. With supplementation of approximately 50 μg vitamin $D_3$ (approximately 2000 IU) plus 800 mg calcium per day during the aforementioned 16 weeks (the last 12 weeks of which were in combination with resistance training), blood concentrations of vitamin D increased and were significantly higher at the end of the training phase compared to the training group with placebo supplementation. Nevertheless, no additional effect on muscle mass and muscle force increase in the thigh muscles was found (Agergaard et al. 2015). In other words, men with theoretically "optimal" vitamin D levels (approx. 90–100 nmol/L) did not achieve better results than those with lower levels lying on the border between normal and undersupplied (approx. 50 nmol/L). Unfortunately, no corresponding results are yet available for women.

In summary, it can be stated that primarily older and/or weak individuals with an existing vitamin D deficiency benefit from vitamin $D_3$ supplementation with regard to muscle size and force development. The reason for this may be the reduction of inflammatory processes that inhibit muscle growth. What does this mean for you? Focus primarily on properly executed resistance training in combination with a adequate protein intake, because as it seems from the available data, optimal vitamin D concentrations in the blood serum ([25(OH)D]) do not bring you additional positive effects compared to just normal values with regard to muscle mass and muscle force increase during resistance training in the winter months. Since natural dietary sources of vitamin D (especially in fatty fish such as wild salmon) are limited and vitamin D is essential for many body functions as described, it is nevertheless recommended to use a vitamin $D_3$ preparation from the pharmacy to prevent vitamin D deficiency. In addition, take every opportunity during the winter months to soak up the sun sensibly and proportionately (i.e. without harming your skin), because light is also important for us humans for other reasons.

This is particularly true for highly trained athletes, as several studies have shown that the prevalence of vitamin D deficiency is high in this population. Backx et al. (2016) showed that almost 70 % of the total 128 male ($n = 54$) and female ($n = 48$) athletes studied had deficient (50–75 nmol/l) or clearly insufficient (<50 nmol/l) 25(OH)D concentration in blood serum. However, by taking 2200 IU vitamin $D_3$ daily, the affected male and female athletes were able to restore sufficient serum 25(OH)D concentrations within 3 months. After 12 months of supplementation with 2200 IU vitamin $D_3$, 80 % of all male and female athletes had a sufficiently high serum 25(OH)D concentration (Backx et al. 2016).

## 23.2 β-Hydroxy-β-Methylbutyrate (HMB): Top or Flop?

For many years, anabolically active nutrients have been sought for skeletal muscle. Early stable isotope tracer studies revealed that essential amino acids (EAA) were the primary drivers behind the nutritionally-stimulated increase in MPS. These studies were further refined in subsequent years, leading to the finding that MPS can be robustly stimulated by the EAA phenylalanine, valine, and leucine alone. Meanwhile, a plethora of studies in cell culture, animal models, and humans confirmed the result that leucine is one of the most potent EAAs in terms of enhancing MPS. As a branched-chain amino acid (BCAA), leucine acts both as a trigger for the initiation of MPS and as a substrate for newly produced muscle proteins.

As a BCAA, leucine can be converted to β-hydroxy-β-methylbutyrate (HMB) in muscle (as well as in the liver and kidney). This suggests that HMB may have a direct anabolic effect in muscle cells. For example, it has been shown that supplementation with 3 g HMB per day during a three-week resistance training program in healthy, untrained, young men tended to increase lean mass and exercise loads moved relative to a placebo, which was explained by an anticatabolic effect (Nissen et al. 1996). Rodent and cell culture studies also showed that HMB increases MPS via a mechanism similar to leucine, inhibits the decrease in MPS that usually occurs in catabolic states, and can reduce muscle catabolism by reducing muscle protein breakdown (MPB). The anti-catabolic effect of HMB is also supported by the results of several human studies whose experimental model was muscle catabolism:

AIDS, cancer and COPD (chronic obstructive pulmonary disease). In summary, the data suggest that HMB may positively influence muscular protein metabolism by increasing MPS and/or inhibiting MPB.

Only recently, however, this has been experimentally proven. Wilkinson et al. (2013) demonstrated that the oral administration of 3.42 g HMB (more precisely HMB solution, see below) was slightly less effective in stimulating MPS compared to 3.42 g leucine. Further, HMB resulted in a 57 % decrease in MPB. The decrease in MPB observed after protein or EAA ingestion is usually attributed to the nitrogen-sparing effect of insulin (see Sect. 12.8). However, unlike leucine, EAA or protein, HMB is not insulinotropic, i.e. it does not stimulate insulin secretion. Similar to leucine, HMB thus increased MPS and decreased MPB, but unlike leucine did not lead to an increase in blood insulin concentration (Wilkinson et al. 2013). These results are therefore in line with the study results on the anticatabolic effects of HMB in the preclinical studies mentioned at the beginning.

Recently, a meta-analysis was published that summarized the scientific data on HMB intake with concurrent (resistance) training (Sanchez-Martinez et al. 2017). The analysis included 6 studies with a total of 193 study participants. The participants were mainly young trained men or even competitive athletes. The study duration was on average 6.8 weeks and participants received 3 g of HMB per day, with the exception of one study where participants received 6 g of HMB per day. All studies had a control group in which participants received a placebo supplement. Despite a slightly greater mean increase in lean mass and a slightly greater reduction in fat mass in the HMB group, there were no significant differences in these two variables between the HMB and placebo groups. In addition, there were no differences between the two groups in the improvement of 1RM on the bench press and leg press. Based on current scientific data, HMB supplementation does not appear to have any additional benefit on increasing lean mass or 1RM in trained individuals. However, the failure to detect a difference between groups in this analysis could be due to the short study durations and small effect.

It is noteworthy to mention that there are several forms of HMB that could differ in bioavailability. The typical HMB supplement consists of the monohydrate of a calcium HMB salt $[Ca(HMB)_2 \cdot H_2O]$. The peak concentration of HMB in blood plasma is reached after approximately 60 to 120 min after oral intake, depending on the dosage (for 1 g CaHMB after 120 min). Ingestion of CaHMB should therefore occur 60–120 min before resistance training (termination). Free HMB (free acid in a pH-buffered solution or as a gel) was tested for the first time in 2011. It was found that for 1 g, the peak concentration in blood plasma was already reached after 30 min and this was about twice as high for free HMB as for the same amount of CaHMB. found, in a later study, no difference in peak HMB concentration in blood plasma was found between the two forms (Wilkinson et al. 2017). Furthermore, the two forms resulted in a comparable increase in MPS and inhibition of MPB. Whether there are differences in the bioavailability of free HMB and CaHMB and whether these differences have an effect on muscle protein metabolism currently remains unclear. The commonly recommended amount of HMB is 38 mg per kilogram of body mass per day, or approximately 3 g of HMB for an 80 kg person. However, similar to protein, this dosage would need to be based on lean or muscle mass rather than body mass. Anyway, chronic administration of 3 g of HMB per day is considered safe for both young and older adults, provided the product used is pure and of high quality.

## 23.3 Fish Oil as an Anabolic Enhancer

Long-chain omega-3 polyunsaturated fatty acids (n-3 LCPUFA) – such as eicosapentaenoic acid (EPA), docosahexaenoic acid (DHA) and docosapentaenoic acid (DPA) – are essential nutrients with great potential benefits for our health. In general, the compounds play important roles in brain growth and development, blood pressure regulation, kidney function, blood clotting, and inflammatory and immunological responses. Specifically, EPA and DHA have anti-inflammatory properties and reduce cardiovascular risk. n-3 LCPUFA are found in foods such as fish and fish oil, milk and seaweed, and of course there are supplements available.

Recently, there has also been increasing scientific evidence that n-3 LCPUFA have an anabolic effect on skeletal muscle. For example, in animal models studying muscle wasting (burning, cancer, etc.), low-dose supplementation with n-3 LCPUFA (i.e. 1–2 % of total daily energy intake), alone or in combination with amino acids, was shown to help maintain whole-body protein synthesis, net protein balance (NBIL), and muscle mass. A study of individuals over 65 years of age also demonstrated that after eight weeks of supplementation with 3.36 g n-3 LCPUFA (1.86 g EPA and 1.5 g DHA) per day, the increase in MPS in response to a defined insulin and amino acid concentration in the blood was greater compared to placebo, i.e the anabolic reactivity increased (Smith et al. 2010). However, basal MPS remained unchanged. Finally, Ryan et al. (2009) showed that supplemental intake of n-3-LCPUFA was able to attenuate the loss of lean mass in cancer patients undergoing surgery (esophageal cancer). Concurrent ingestion of n-3-LCPUFA during a resistance training intervention resulted in a greater increase in isometric peak torque in older women compared to training without supplementation (Da Boit et al. 2017). Furthermore, an additional positive effect on muscle quality, calculated as torque per square centimeter of muscle cross-sectional area, could be detected. These effects could not be detected in older men. Furthermore, supplementation with n-3-LCPUFA did not lead to an additional increase in isokinetically measured peak torque in either women or men.

The exact mechanisms of action for the muscle anabolic effects of n-3-LCPUFA remain unclear. However, it can be speculated that they are related to the anti-inflammatory properties, as burn injuries, cancer, and aging are all conditions associated with an increased inflammatory status in the body. Chronic inflammatory processes are in turn linked to loss of muscle mass. However, the fact that the same supplementation pattern (3.36 g n-3 LCPUFA per day, of which 1.86 g EPA and 1.5 g DHA) also leads to anabolic effects in young, healthy individuals aged 25–45 years advocates more of a direct effect of n-3 LCPUFA on skeletal muscle. According to the European Food Safety Authority (EFSA 2012), the daily additional intake of up to 5 g (EPA and DHA combined) of long-chain omega-3 fatty acids is safe. Again, however, it is important to use pure and high quality products. The IFOS (The International Fish Oil Standards Program) can be helpful in finding a suitable product (IFOS 2013). This is an independent testing and certification program for omega-3 fish oil and products.

## 23.4 Creatine Supplementation: Why? What for?

As described in Sect. 6.4, the creatine kinase-phosphocreatine (CK-PCr) system, i.e. the phosphagenic system, has at least three functions (Wallimann et al. 2011):

- If a cell converts a lot of energy in a short time, ATP is kept constant at the expense of the larger PCr store. The ATP concentration can thus be buffered.
- It serves as an energy transport system (shuttle) between the sites of ATP synthesis (e.g. mitochondria) and ATP consumption (e.g. myofibrillar ATPase).
- It serves as a regulator of metabolism (e.g., Cr stimulates mitochondrial respiration).

As a reminder, the enzyme creatine kinase (CK) catalyzes both the regeneration of ADP to ATP (creating Cr from PCr) and the conversion of Cr to energy-rich PCr. The presence of Cr therefore plays a central role for the amount of PCr present and thus for the charge state of the muscle fiber. In energetically charged cells, the ratio between PCr and Cr is approx. 2/3 to 1/3. The daily Cr consumption of the body for a 70 kg untrained person is estimated at approx. 2–4 g (excretion as creatinine via the urine). Less than half of this (approx. 1–2 g per day) is produced by the organism itself. The remainder must be supplied via diet, with Cr occurring primarily in fresh, raw fish and meat (Cr is heat-labile) and to a lesser extent in milk (Wallimann 2008).

However, the Cr requirement can vary greatly. With large muscle mass (95 % of the Cr in the body is stored in the muscles) and muscular effort, the requirement can rise to over 5 g per day. If dietary Cr intake is less than the requirement, for example in athletes, vegetarians/vegans, and elderly, there may be a relative Cr deficiency in the cells (Wallimann 2008). Cr deficiency can also occur when the body's own biosynthesis is compromised (e.g. in the case of genetic defects). Oral supplementation of Cr can increase total Cr content (Cr + PCr) in muscle by an average of 5–20 %, depending on individual conditions. The immediate effect of this energy storage increase is delayed muscle fatigue – high external (or internal) mechanical power output can be generated for longer before performance degradation occurs. This means that in resistance training you can move/hold a given load for longer, or move/hold a slightly higher load for the same exercise duration. This can be beneficial for muscle mass and muscle force increase (see Sect. 13.7). In certain cases, however, the effect of Cr may be absent in athletes, and this has been linked to a concomitant intake of caffeine. However, a causal relationship is rather doubtful (Wallimann 2008).

As a dietary supplement, Cr is typically taken in the form of Cr monohydrate. The vast majority of all studies have been conducted with this molecule, or the majority of scientific evidence is based on Cr monohydrate. Cr is a legal (i.e., not on the doping list) ergogenic substance and is considered safe in the long term if no more than daily consumption (3–5 g) is taken per day (Wallimann et al. 2011). However, the latter is only valid if the product is absolutely chemically pure. Only consume a product containing Cr if the manufacturer of Cr can guarantee certified production with scientifically documented purity of the product.

Certain dosing regimens provide for a loading phase of 5–7 days (followed by a maintenance phase of indeterminate duration), during which 20 g per day (four times 5 g throughout the day) are taken. While this dosage is considered safe for the 5–7 day period, it is not recommended for prolonged use. During the loading phase, there may be an increase in body mass of approximately 1–2 kg. This increase is associated with the supplied Cr reaching the lumen of the muscle fiber via osmotically active sodium- and chloride-dependent creatine transporters (in the sarcolemma). This means that the sodium chloride transported into the cell lumen together with Cr can lead to an increase in the intracellular water content in the muscle fibers. However, the increase in body mass that occurs acutely due to water retention is only temporary, as the salt and water content in the muscle fibers is regulated. Nowadays it is assumed that, depending on body mass, no more than 5–10 g of creatine per day are necessary, even in the loading phase.

As an alternative to a loading phase, simply supplementing with approx. 0.05 g Cr per kilogram of body mass (approx. 3–5 g per day; corresponds to the maintenance dose after the loading phase) is an option from the beginning. It is recommended to consume the Cr product together with sufficient liquid (1 g creatine per 100 ml water) and carbohydrates. The latter favour the absorption into the muscle cells. The replenishment of Cr stores is faster if the intake takes place within approx. 1.5 h after training. Once the Cr stores are filled, no further increase in effects is to be expected. Taking breaks can be useful depending on the situation, but are not mandatory in every case. Especially for vegetarians/vegans, people suffering from stress and elderly people a regular intake can be justified. It is often forgotten that the effects of Cr are pleiotropic, i.e. they affect many organ systems and cells simultaneously. Thus, the CK-PCr system plays an important role not only in the energy metabolism of fibers of the skeletal and cardiac muscles, but also in the brain, in nerves and sensory cells as well as in sperms (Wallimann et al. 2011).

## 23.5 Summary

Every day, products are touted to support muscle growth and consequently act as anabolic enhancers. This chapter has described four substances that can have a positive effect on muscle mass and hypertrophy, at least in specific populations.

Regarding vitamin D, older individuals, highly trained athletes and female athletes with an existing vitamin D deficiency primarily benefit from supplementation with vitamin $D_3$ with regard to muscle mass and muscle force increase. In young individuals with "optimal" or slightly reduced vitamin D levels, supplementation has no additional benefit. Due to the diverse and essential effects of vitamin D in the body, however, you should make sure that you take enough vitamin $D_3$, especially during the months when there is little sunshine. If in doubt, it is advisable to have the concentration of 25(OH)D in the blood serum measured by your family doctor or directly in a certified laboratory. If the serum concentration is too low, an attempt can be made to raise the blood concentration with a daily supplementation of 2200 IU vitamin $D_3$ for 3 months (i.e. follow-up after 3 months). This dose corresponds to the described dose that led to a restoration of [25(OH)D] in highly trained athletes within 3 months (Backx et al. 2016) and is well below the recommended maximum tolerable amount of vitamin $D_3$ per day for adults.

HMB is a metabolic product of leucine and could therefore itself exert a direct anabolic effect. The isolated intake of HMB leads to a stimulation of the MPS and a simultaneous inhibition of the MPB. Unlike EAA or protein, these processes occur insulin-independently. At the current time, however, the scientific data does not indicate any additional benefit of HMB supplementation compared to resistance training alone without supplementation.

Omega-3 polyunsaturated fatty acids can have an anabolic effect on skeletal muscle. Especially in older individuals, it can be assumed that the anabolic effect is related to the anti-inflammatory properties. However, since a positive effect has also been shown in younger individuals, omega-3 polyunsaturated fatty acids could also have a direct influence on skeletal muscle.

Intramuscular PCr stores can be increased by taking Cr monohydrate. In resistance training practice, this allows a given load to be moved/hold longer or a slightly higher load to be moved/hold for the same exercise duration. This can have a positive effect on muscle mass and muscle force increase. However, the effect of Cr is not limited to skeletal muscle, but affects many organ systems simultaneously. These systems include the heart muscle, brain, nerves, sensory cells and sperms.

# 24

# Go for It!

One conclusion to be drawn from the considerations in Sect. 21.3 is that wherever something desirable to you is advertised, whether it is muscles of steel, a bikini figure, beauty, higher income or professional success, you should look and listen carefully. Question who is speaking to you and with what motive this is being done. Be skeptical and don't believe everything. Challenge training and nutrition experts whenever you meet them, for example by asking questions about terminology and training principles, as trivial as that may sound. Avoid asking 'why' questions, as these imply that the statement itself is true. Rather, ask how and on what data the statements are based. Don't be blinded by striking characteristics and arbitrary examples ("I can lift 300 kg and therefore I know how all other people on this planet can do the same", "I have already trained many people with success like this" etc.).

By reading and engaging with this book, you will have acquired many scientific concepts and recipes that will give you the content tools to navigate in the sea of training and nutrition opinions on your own. So, the best conditions to start training today (if you haven't done anything yet) or to take another look at your training plan.

Go for it! Your age or sex doesn't matter – it's never too late to start muscle training. The sooner you start the better, and make a lifelong commitment to it. Use your newfound muscle mass and muscle force to be more physically active in life in general. Take the stairs instead of the elevator. Walk a lot every day. Get in touch with nature and do more poly-sports, i.e. play and endurance sports as well as resistance training and go dancing from time to time (this trains your sensorimotor system and thus also your brain). Muscle activity animates many different organ systems in the body and thus conveys positive health aspects, because human nature is inextricably linked to movement.

And keep yourself up to date, because science doesn't stand still (and certainly spins in circles sometimes). Gaining scientific knowledge is a dynamic process and requires the ongoing integration of high-quality study results from a wide range of disciplines. Have the courage to put your newly acquired knowledge into practice and experiment with it. I sincerely wish you much success – let's go!

# References

Aagaard P, Magnusson PS, Larsson B, Kjaer M, Krustrup P (2007) Mechanical muscle function, morphology, and fiber type in lifelong trained elderly. Med Sci Sports Exerc 39:1989–1996

Agergaard J, Trostrup J, Uth J, Iversen JV, Boesen A, Andersen JL, Schjerling P, Langberg H (2015) Does vitamin-D intake during resistance training improve the skeletal muscle hypertrophic and strenght response in young and elderly men? – a randomized controlled trial. Nutr Metab 12:32

Altenburg TM, de Ruiter CJ, Verdijk PW, van Mechelen W, de Haan A (2009) Vastus lateralis surface and single motor unit electromyography during shortening, lengthening and isometric contractions corrected for mode-dependent differences in force-generating capacity. Acta Physiol 196:315–328

Andersen JL, Aagaard P (2000) Myosin heavy chain IIx overshoot in human skeletal muscle. Muscle Nerve 23:1095–1104

Anliker E, Toigo M (2012) Functional assessment of the muscle-bone unit in the lower leg. J Musculoskelet Neuronal Interact 12:46–55

Anliker E, Rawer R, Boutellier U, Toigo M (2011) Maximum ground reaction force in relation to tibial bone mass in children and adults. Med Sci Sports Exerc 43:2102–2109

Areta JL, Burke LM, Ross ML, Camera DM, West DW, Broad EM, Jeacocke NA, Moore DR, Stellingwerff T, Phillips SM, Hawley JA, Coffey VG (2013) Timing and distribution of protein ingestion during prolonged recovery from resistance exercise alters myofibrillar protein synthesis. J Physiol (London) 591:2319–2331

Backx EM, Tieland M, Maase K, Kies AK, Mensink M, van Loon LJ, de Groot LC (2016) The impact of 1-year vitamin D supplementation on vitamin D status in athletes: a dose-response study. Eur J Clin Nutr 70:1009–1014

Bamman MM, Hunter GR, Newton LE, Roney RK, Khaled MA (1993) Changes in body composition, diet, and strength of bodybuilders during the 12 weeks prior to competition. J Sports Med Phys Fitness 33:383–391

Bandegan A, Courtney-Martin G, Rafii M, Pencharz PB, Lemon PWR (2017) Indicator amino acid–derived estimate of dietary protein requirement for male bodybuilders on a nontraining day is several-fold greater than the current recommended dietary allowance. J Nutr 147:850–857

Bawa P (2002) Neural control of motor output: can training change it? Exerc Sport Sci Rev 30:59–63

Bergström J (1962) Muscle electrolytes in man. Scand J Clin Lab Med 14:511–514

Bickel CS, Cross JM, Bamman MM (2011) Exercise dosing to retain resistance training adaptations in young and older adults. Med Sci Sports Exerc 43:1177–1187

Biering-Sørensen B, Bruun Kristensen I, Kjaer M, Biering-Sørensen F (2009) Muscle after spinal cord injury. Muscle Nerve 40:499–519

Blazevich AJ, Cannavan D, Coleman DR, Horne S (2007) Influence of concentric and eccentric resistance training on architectural adaptation in human quadriceps muscles. J Appl Physiol 103:1565–1575

Boakes JL, Foran J, Ward SR, Lieber RL (2007) Muscle adaptation by serial sarcomere addition 1 year after femoral lengthening. Clin Orthop Relat Res 456:250–253

Bohé J, Low JF, Wolfe RR, Rennie MJ (2001) Latency and duration of stimulation of human protein synthesis during continuous infusion of amino acids. J Physiol (London) 532:575–579

Boirie Y, Dangin M, Gachon P, Vasson MP, Maubois JL, Beaufrère B (1997) Slow and fast dietary proteins differently modulate postprandial protein accretion. Proc Natl Acad Sci USA 94:14930–14935

Bouchard C, An P, Rice T, Skinner JS, Wilmore JH, Gagnon J, Pérusse L, Leon AS, Rao DC (1999) Familial aggregation of V˙; O2max response to exercise training: results from the HERITAGE family study. J Appl Physiol 87:1003–1008

Breen L, Stokes KA, Churchward-Venne TY, Moore DR, Baker SK, Smith K, Atherton PJ, Phillips SM (2013) Two weeks of reduced activity decreases leg lean mass and induces "anabolic resistance" of myofibrillar protein synthesis in healthy elderly. J Clin Endocrinol Metab 98:2604–2612

Brook MS, Wilkinson DJ, Mitchell WK, Lund JN, Szewczyk NJ, Greenhaff PL, Smith K, Atherton PJ (2015) Skeletal muscle hypertrophy adaptations predominate in the early stages of resistance exercise training, matching deuterium oxide-derived measures of muscle protein synthesis and mechanistic target of rapamycin complex 1 signaling. FASEB 29:4485–4496

Burd NA, Holwerda AM, Selby KC, West DW, Staples AW, Cain NE, Cashaback JG, Potvin JR, Baker SK, Phillips SM (2010) Resistance exercise volume affects myofibrillar protein synthesis and anabolic signalling molecule phosphorylation in young men. J Physiol (London) 588:3119–3130

Burd NA, Andrews RJ, West DW, Little JP, Cochran AJ, Hector AJ, Cashaback JG, Gibala MJ, Potvin JR, Baker SK, Phillips SM (2011a) Muscle time under tension during resistance exercise stimulates differential muscle protein sub-fractional synthetic responses in men. J Physiol (London) 590:351–362

Burd NA, West DW, Moore DR, Atherton PJ, Staples AW, Prior T, Tang JE, Rennie MJ, Baker SK, Phillips SM (2011b) Enhanced amino acid sensitivity of myofibrillar protein synthesis persists for up to 24 h after resistance exercise in young men. J Nutr 141:568–573

Burke RE, Levine DN, Tsairis P, Zajac FE 3rd (1973) Physiological types and histochemical profiles in motor units of the cat gastrocnemius. J Physiol (London) 234:723–748

Burkholder TJ, Lieber RL (2001) Sarcomere length operating range of vertebrate muscles during movement. J Exp Biol 204:1529–1536

Burr DB, Milgrom C, Fyhrie D et al (1996) In vivo measurement of human tibial strains during vigorous activity. Bone 18:405–410

Camera DM, West DW, Burd NA, Phillips SM, Garnham AP, Hawley JA, Coffey VG (2012) Low muscle glycogen concentration does not suppress the anabolic response to resistance exercise. J Appl Physiol 113:206–214

Campbell WW, Haub MD, Wolfe RR, Ferrando AA, Sullivan DH, Apolzan JW, Iglay HB (2009) Resistance training preserves fat-free mass without impacting changes in protein metabolism after weight loss in older women. Obesity 17:1332–1339

Carolan B, Cafarelli E (1992) Adaptations in coactivation after isometric resistance training. J Appl Physiol 73:911–917

Cavanaugh DJ, Cann CE (1988) Brisk walking does not stop bone loss in postmenopausal women. Bone 9:201–204

Cermak NM, Res PT, de Groot LC, Saris WH, van Loon LJ (2012) Protein supplementation augments the adaptive response of skeletal muscle to resistance-type exercise training: a meta-analysis. Am J Clin Nutr 96:1454–1464

Christen P, Ito K, Ellouz R, Boutroy S, Sornay-Rendu E, Chapurlat RD, van Rietbergen B (2014) Bone remodeling in humans is load-driven but not lazy. Nat Commun 5:4855. https://doi.org/10.1038/ncomms5855

Christova P, Kossev A (2000) Human motor unit activity during concentric and eccentric movements. Electromyogr Clin Neurophysiol 40:331–338

Churchward-Venne TA, Pinckaers PJ, van Loon JJ, van Loon LJ (2017) Consideration of insects as a source of dietary protein for human consumption. Nutr Rev 75:1035–1045

Clauss W, Clauss C (2009) Humanbiologie. Spektrum, Heidelberg

Cormie P, McGuigan MR, Newton RU (2011) Developing maximal neuromuscular power: part 1-biological basis of maximal power production. Sports Med 41:17–31

Cribb PJ, Hayes A (2006) Effects of supplement timing and resistance exercise on skeletal muscle hypertrophy. Med Sci Sports Exerc 38:1918–1925

Cuthbertson D, Smith K, Babraj J, Leese G, Waddell T, Atherton P, Wackerhage H, Taylor PM, Rennie MJ (2005) Anabolic signaling deficits underlie amino acid resistance of wasting, aging muscle. FASEB J 19:422–424

Cuthbertson DJ, Babraj J, Smith K, Wilkes E, Fedele MJ, Esser K, Rennie M (2006) Anabolic signaling and protein synthesis in human skeletal muscle after dynamic shortening or lengthening exercise. Am J Physiol Endocrinol Metab 290:E731–E738

Da Boit M, Sibson R, Sivasubramaniam S, Meakin JR, Greig CA, Aspden RM, Thies F, Jeromson S, Hamilton DL, Speakman JR, Hambly C, Mangoni AA, Preston T, Gray SR (2017) Sex differences in the effect of fish-oil supplementation on the adaptive response to resistance exercise training in older people: a randomized controlled trial. Am J Clin Nutr 105:151–158

Dangin M, Boirie Y, Garcia-Rodenas C, Gachon P, Fauquant J, Callier P, Ballèvre O, Beaufrère B (2001) The digestion rate of protein is an independent regulating factor of postprandial protein retention. Am J Physiol Endocrinol Metab 280:E340–E348

De Luca CJ, Contessa P (2012) Hierarchical control of motor units in voluntary contractions. J Neurophysiol 107:178–195

DeFronzo RA, Jacot E, Jequier E, Maeder E, Wahren J, Felber JP (1981) The effect of insulin on the disposal of intravenous glucose. Results from indirect calorimetry and hepatic and femoral venous catheterization. Diabetes 30:1000–1007

Denny-Brown D, Pennybacker JB (1938) Fibrillation and fasciculation in voluntary muscle. Brain 61:311–344

Desmedt JE, Godaux E (1977) Ballistic contractions in man: characteristic recruitment pattern of single motor units of the tibialis anterior muscle. J Physiol (London) 264:673–693

Desmedt JE, Godaux E (1979) Voluntary motor commands in human ballistic movements. Ann Neurol 5:415–421

Desmedt JE, Godaux E (1981) Spinal motoneuron recruitment in man: rank deordering with direction but not with speed of voluntary movement. Science 214:933–936

Deutz NE, Wolfe RR (2013) Is there a maximal anabolic response to protein intake with a meal? Clin Nutr 32:309–313

Dobelli R (2011) Die Kunst des klaren Denkens: 52 Denkfehler, die Sie besser anderen überlassen. Hanser, München

Dreyer HC, Fujita S, Cadenas JG, Chinkes DL, Volpi E, Rasmussen BB (2006) Resistance exercise increases AMPK activity and reduces 4E-BP1 phosphorylation and protein synthesis in human skeletal muscle. J Physiol (London) 576:613–624

Enoka RM, Pearson KG (2013) The motor unit and muscle action. In: Kandel ER, Schwartz JH, Jessell TM, Siegelbaum SA, Hudspeth AJ (Hrsg) Principles of neural science, 5. Aufl. McGraw-Hill, New York, S 775

Eriksson A, Kadi F, Malm C, Thornell LE (2005) Skeletal muscle morphology in powerlifters with and without anabolic steroids. Histochem Cell Biol 124:167–175

EFSA Europäische Behörde für Lebensmittelsicherheit (2012). http://www.efsa.europa.eu/de/press/news/120727.htm. Accessed: 31. Juli 2014

Földhazy Z, Arndt A, Milgrom C et al (2005) Exercise-induced strain and strain rate in the distal radius. J Bone Joint Surg Br 87:261–266

Fouillet H, Mariotti F, Gaudichon C, Bos C, Tomé D (2002) Peripheral and splanchnic metabolism of dietary nitrogen are differently affected by the protein source in humans as assessed by compartmental modeling. J Nutr 132:125–133

Frost HM (1987) The mechanostat: a proposed pathogenic mechanism of osteoporoses and the bone mass effects of mechanical and nonmechanical agents. Bone Miner 2:73–85

Fujita S, Dreyer HC, Drummond MJ, Glynn EL, Volpi E, Rasmussen BB (2009) Essential amino acid and carbohydrate ingestion before resistance exercise does not enhance postexercise muscle protein synthesis. J Appl Physiol 106:1730–1739

Fuller B (1961) Tensegrity. Portfolio Artnews Annual 4:112–127

Garnett RA, O'Donovan MJ, Stephens JA, Taylor A (1979) Motor unit organization of human medial gastrocnemius. J Physiol (London) 287:33–43

Glynn EL, Fry CS, Drummond MJ, Dreyer HC, Dhanani S, Volpi E, Rasmussen BB (2010) Muscle protein breakdown has a minor role in the protein anabolic response to essential amino acid and carbohydrate intake following resistance exercise. Am J Physiol Regul Integr Comp Physiol 299:R533–R540

Greenhaff PL, Karagounis LG, Peirce N, Simpson EJ, Hazell M, Layfield R, Wackerhage H, Smith K, Atherton P, Selby A, Rennie MJ (2008) Disassociation between the effects of amino acids and insulin on signaling, ubiquitin ligases, and protein turnover in human muscle. Am J Physiol Endocrinol Metab 295:E595–E604

Hansen M, Langberg H, Holm L, Miller BF, Petersen SG, Doessing S, Skovgaard D, Trappe T, Kjaer M (2011) Effect of administration of oral contraceptives on the synthesis and breakdown of myofibrillar proteins in young women. Scand J Med Sci Sports 21:62–72

Heckman CJ, Enoka RM (2012) Motor unit. Compr Physiol 2:2629–2682

Henneman E (1957) Relation between size of neurons and their susceptibility to discharge. Science 26:1345–1347

Herbert RD, de Noronha M, Kamper SJ (2011) Stretching to prevent or reduce muscle soreness after exercise. Cochrane Database Syst Rev. https://doi.org/10.1002/14651858.CD004577.pub3

Hickson RC (1980) Interference of strength development by simultaneously training for strength and endurance. Eur J Appl Physiol 45:255–263

Hill AV (1922) The maximum work and mechanical efficiency of human muscles, and their most economical speed. J Physiol (London) 56:19–41

Hubal MJ, Gordish-Dressman H, Thompson PD, Price TB, Hoffman EP, Angelopoulos TJ, Gordon PM, Moyna NM, Pescatello LS, Visich PS, Zoeller RF, Seip RL, Clarkson PM (2005) Variability in muscle size and strength gains after unilateral resistance training. Med Sci Sports Exerc 37:964–972

Hubbard AW, Stetson RH (1938) An experimental analysis of human locomotion. J Physiol (London) 124:300–313

Ingber DE (2003a) Tensegrity I. Cell structure and hierarchical systems biology. J Cell Sci 116:1157–1173

Ingber DE (2003b) Tensegrity II. How structural networks influence cellular information processing networks. J Cell Sci 116:1397–1408

Item F, Denkinger J, Fontana P, Weber M, Boutellier U, Toigo M (2011) Combined effects of whole-body vibration, resistance exercise, and vascular occlusion on skeletal muscle and performance. Int J Sports Med 32:781–787

Item F, Nocito A, Thöny S, Bächler T, Boutellier U, Wenger R, Toigo M (2013) Combined whole-body vibration, resistance exercise, and vascular occlusion increases PGC-1a and VEGF mRNA abundances. Eur J Appl Physiol 113:1081–1090

Janssen I, Ross R (2005) Linking age-related changes in skeletal muscle mass and composition with metabolism and disease. J Nutr Health Aging 9:408–419

Janssen I, Baumgartner RN, Ross R, Rosenberg IH, Roubenoff R (2004) Skeletal muscle cutpoints associated with elevated physical disability risk in older men and women. Am J Epidemiol 159:413–421

Käser L, Mannion AF, Rhyner A, Weber E, Dvorak J, Müntener M (2001) Active therapy for chronic low back pain part 2 effects on paraspinal muscle cross-sectional area, fiber type size, and distribution. Spine 26:909–919

Katsanos C, Chinkes D, Paddon-Jones D, Zhang X, Aarsland A, Wolfe RR (2008) Whey protein ingestion in elderly persons results in greater muscle protein accrual than ingestion of its constituent essential amino acid content. Nutr Res 28:651–658

Katz B (1939) The relation between force and speed in muscular contraction. J Physiol (London) 96:45–64

Kelley G (1996) Mechanical overload and skeletal muscle fiber hyperplasia: a meta-analysis. J Appl Physiol 81:1584–1588

Kim IY, Schutzler S, Schrader A, Spencer H, Kortebein P, Deutz NE, Wolfe RR, Ferrando AA (2015) Quantity of dietary protein intake, but not pattern of intake, affects net protein balance primarily through differences in protein synthesis in older adults. Am J Physiol Endocrinol Metab 308:E21–E28

Kim IY, Schutzler S, Schrader A, Spencer HJ, Azhar G, Ferrando AA, Wolfe RR (2016) The anabolic response to a meal containing different amounts of protein is not limited by the maximal stimulation of protein synthesis in healthy young adults. Am J Physiol Endocrinol Metab 310:E73–E80

Kim IY, Schutzler S, Schrader A, Spencer HJ, Azhar G, Wolfe RR, Ferrando AA (2018) Protein intake distribution pattern does not affect anabolic response, lean body mass, muscle strength or function over 8 weeks in older adults: a randomized-controlled trial. Clin Nutr 37:488–493

Klass M, Baudry S, Duchateau J (2008) Age-related decline in rate of torque development is accompanied by lower maximal motor unit discharge frequency during fast contractions. J Appl Physiol 104:739–746

Kline JC, De Luca CJ (2016) Synchronization of motor unit firings: an epiphenomenon of firing rate characteristics not common inputs. J Neurophysiol 115:178–192

Koh TJ, Herzog W (1998) Excursion is important in regulating sarcomere number in the growing rabbit tibialis anterior. J Physiol (London) 508:267–280

Korhonen MT, Cristea A, Alén M, Häkkinen K, Sipilä S, Mero A, Viitasalo JT, Larsson L, Suominen H (2006) Aging, muscle fiber type, and contractile function in sprint-trained athletes. J Appl Physiol 101:906–917

Kosek DJ, Kim JS, Petrella JK, Cross JM, Bamman MM (2006) Efficacy of 3 days/week resistance training on myofiber hypertrophy and myogenic mechanisms in young vs. older adults. J Appl Physiol 101:531–544

Kumar V, Atherton P, Smith K, Rennie MJ (2009a) Human muscle protein synthesis and breakdown during and after exercise. J Appl Physiol 106:2026–2039

Kumar V, Selby A, Rankin D, Patel R, Atherton P, Hildebrandt W, Williams J, Smith K, Seynnes O, Hiscock N, Rennie MJ (2009b) Age-related differences in the dose-response relationship of muscle protein synthesis to resistance exercise in young and old men. J Physiol (London) 587:211–217

Lederman E (2010) The myth of core stability. J Bodywork Movement Therap 14:84–98

Lidegaard O, Schiodt AV, Poulsen EF (2001) Oral contraceptives: general aspects. Ugeskr Laeger 163:4544–4546

Lieber RL, Boakes JL (1988a) Muscle force and moment arm contributions to torque production in frog hindlimb. Am J Physiol 254:C769–C772

Lieber RL, Boakes JL (1988b) Sarcomere length and joint kinematics during torque production in frog hindlimb. Am J Physiol 254:C759–C768

Lynn R, Morgan DL (1994) Decline running produces more sarcomeres in rat vastus intermedius muscle fibers than does incline running. J Appl Physiol 77:1439–1444

Lynn R, Talbot JA, Morgen DL (1998) Differences in rat skeletal muscles after incline and decline running. J Appl Physiol 85:98–104

MacNaughton LS, Wardle SL, Witard OC, McGlory C, Hamilton DL, Jeromson S, Lawrence CE, Wallis GA, Tipton KD (2016) The response of muscle protein synthesis following whole-body resistance exercise is greater following 40 g than 20 g of ingested whey protein. Physiol Rep 4:e12893

Mamerow MM, Mettler JA, English KL, Casperson SL, Arentson-Lantz E, Sheffield-Moore M, Layman DK, Paddon-Jones D (2014) Dietary protein distribution positively influences 24-h muscle protein synthesis in healthy adults. J Nutr 144:876–880

Mannion AF, Junge A, Taimela S, Müntener M, Käser L, Dvorak J (2001a) Active therapy for chronic low back pain part 1 factors influencing self-rated disability and its change following therapy. Spine 26:920–929

Mannion AF, Taimela S, Müntener M, Dvorak J (2001b) Active therapy for chronic low back pain part 1 effects on back muscle activation, fatigability, and strength. Spine 26:897–908

Mathai JK, Liu Y, Stein HH (2017) Values for digestible indispensable amino acid scores (DIAAS) for some dairy and plant proteins may better describe protein quality than values calculated using the concept for protein digestibility-corrected amino acid scores (PDCAAS). Br J Nutr 117:490–499

Mauro A (1961) Satellite cell of skeletal muscle fibers. J Biophys Biochem Cytol 9:493–495

Milgrom C, Finestone A, Simkin A, Ekenman I, Mendelson S, Millgram M, Nyska M, Larsson E, Burr D (2000a) In vivo strain measurements to evaluate the strengthening potential of exercises on the tibial bone. J Bone Joint Surg Br 82:591–594

Milgrom C, Simkin A, Eldad A, Nyska M, Finestone A (2000b) Using bone's adaptation ability to lower the incidence of stress fractures. Am J Sports Med 28:245–251

Miller SL, Tipton KD, Chinkes DL, Wolf SE, Wolfe RR (2003) Independent and combined effects of amino acids and glucose after resistance exercise. Med Sci Sports Exerc 35:449–455

Miller BF, Olesen JL, Hansen M, Dossing S, Crameri RM, Welling RJ, Langberg H, Flyvbjerg A, Kjar M, Babraj JA, Smith K, Rennie MJ (2005) Coordinated collagen and muscle protein synthesis in human patella tendon and quadriceps muscle after exercise. J Physiol (London) 567:1021–1033

Miller BF, Hansen M, Olesen JL, Flyvbjerg A, Schwarz P, Babraj JA, Smith K, Rennie MJ, Kjaer M (2006) No effect of menstrual cycle on myofibrillar and connective tissue protein synthesis in contracting skeletal muscle. Am J Physiol Endocrinol Metab 290:E163–E168

Milner-Brown HS, Stein RB, Yemm R (1973) The orderly recruitment of human motor units during voluntary isometric contractions. J Physiol (London) 230:359–370

Mitchell CJ, Churchward-Venne TA, Parise G, Bellamy L, Baker SK, Smith K, Atherton PJ, Phillips SM (2014) Acute post-exercise myofibrillar protein synthesis is not correlated with resistance training-induced muscle hypertrophy in young men. PLoS ONE 9:e89431

Moore DR, Robinson MJ, Fry JL, Tang JE, Glover EI, Wilkinson SB, Prior T, Tarnopolsky MA, Phillips SM (2009) Ingested protein dose response of muscle and albumin protein synthesis after resistance exercise in young men. Am J Clin Nutr 89:161–168

Moore DR, Areta JL, Coffey VG, Stellingwerff T, Phillips SM, Burke LM, Cléroux M, Godin JP, Hawley JA (2012a) Daytime pattern of post-exercise protein intake affects whole-body protein turnover in resistance-trained males. Nutr Metab (London) 9:91. https://doi.org/10.1186/1743-7075-9-91

Moore DR, Young M, Phillips SM (2012b) Similar increases in muscle size and strength in young men after training with maximal shortening or lengthening contractions when matched for total work. Eur J Appl Physiol 112:1587–1592

Moore DR, Churchward-Venne TA, Witard O, Breen L, Burd NA, Tipton KD, Phillips SM (2015) Protein ingestion to stimulate myofibrillar protein synthesis requires greater relative protein intakes in healthy older versus younger men. J Gerontol A Biol Sci Med Sci 70:57–62

Morgan DL (1990) New insights into the behavior of muscle during active lengthening. Biophys J 57:209–221

Moro T, Brightwell CR, Deer RR, Graber TG, Galvan E, Fry CS, Volpi E, Rasmussen BB (2018) Muscle protein anabolic resistance to essential amino acids does not occur in healthy older adults before or after resistance exercise training. J Nutr 148:900–909

Morton RW, Murphy KT, McKellar SR, Schoenfeld BJ, Henselmans M, Helms E, Aragon AA, Devries MC, Banfield L, Krieger JW, Phillips SM (2018) A systematic review, meta-analysis and meta-regression of the effect of protein supplementation on resistance training-induced gains in muscle mass and strength in healthy adults. Br J Sports Med 52:376–384

Mouly V, Aamiri A, Bigot A, Cooper RN, Di Donna S, Furling D, Gidaro T, Jacquemin V, Mamchaoui K, Negroni E, Périé S, Renault V, Silva-Barbosa SD, Butler-Browne GS (2005) The mitotic clock in skeletal muscle regeneration, disease and cell mediated gene therapy. Acta Physiol Scand 184:3–15

Mudd LM, Owe KM, Mottola MF, Pivarnik JM (2013) Health benefits of physical activity during pregnancy: an international perspective. Med Sci Sports Exerc 45:268–277

Mueller SM, Aguayo D, Ruoss S, Lunardi F, Boutellier U, Frese S, Petersen J, Jung H, Toigo M (2014) High-load resistance exercise with superimposed vibration and vascular occlusion increases critical power, capillaries and lean mass in endurance-trained men. Eur J Appl Physiol 114:123–133

Nardone A, Schieppati M (1988) Shift of activity from slow to fast muscle during voluntary lengthening contractions of the triceps surae muscles in humans. J Physiol (London) 395:363–381

Nardone A, Romano C, Schieppati M (1989) Selective recruitment of high-threshold human motor units during voluntary isotonic lengthening of active muscle. J Physiol (London) 409:451–471

Nelson ME, Fisher EC, Dilmanian FA, Dallal GE, Evans WJ (1991) A 1-y walking program and increased dietary calcium in postmenopausal women: effects on bone. Am J Clin Nutr 53:1304–1311

Nissen S, Sharp R, Ray M, Rathmacher JA, Rice D, Fuller JC, Connelly AS, Abumrad N (1996) Effect of leucine metabolite β-hydroxy-β-methylbutyrate on muscle metabolism during resistance-exercise training. J Appl Physiol 81:2095–2104

Paddon-Jones D, Sheffield-Moore M, Katsanos C, Zhang XJ, Wolfe RR (2006) Differential stimulation of muscle protein synthesis in elderly humans following isocaloric ingestion of amino acids or whey protein. Exp Gerontol 41:215–219

Paul AC, Rosenthal N (2002) Different modes of hypertrophy in skeletal muscle fibers. J Cell Biol 156:751–760

Pencharz PB, Elango R, Wolfe RR (2016) Recent developments in understanding protein needs – How much and what kind should we eat? Appl Physiol Nutr Metab 41:577–580

Pérusse L, Lortie G, Leblanc C, Tremblay A, Theriault G, Bouchard C (1987) Genetic and environmental sources of variation in physical fitness. Ann Hum Biol 14:425–434

Phillips SM, Tipton KD, Aarsland A, Wolf SE, Wolfe RR (1997) Mixed muscle protein synthesis and breakdown after resistance exercise in humans. Am J Physiol 273:E99–E107

Pontzer H (2015) Constrained total energy expenditure and the evolutionary biology of energy balance. Exerc Sport Sci Rev 43:110–116

Reeves ND, Narici MV, Maganaris CN (2004) In vivo human muscle structure and function: adaptations to resistance training in old age. Exp Physiol 89:675–689

Reidy PT, Rasmussen BB (2016) Role of ingested amino acids and protein in the promotion of resistance exercise-induced muscle protein anabolism. J Nutr 146:155–183

Reisman S, Walsh LD, Proske U (2005) Warm-up stretches reduce sensations of stiffness and soreness after eccentric exercise. Med Sci Sports Exerc 37:929–936

Reitelseder S, Agergaard J, Doessing S, Helmark IC, Lund P, Kristensen NB, Frystyk J, Flyvbjerg A, Schjerling P, van Hall G, Kjaer M, Holm L (2011) Whey and casein labeled with L-[1–13C]leucine and muscle protein synthesis: effect of resistance exercise and protein ingestion. Am J Physiol Endocrinol Metab 300:E231–E242

Res PT, Groen B, Pennings B, Beelen M, Wallis GA, Gijsen AP, Senden JM, VAN Loon LJ (2012) Protein ingestion before sleep improves postexercise overnight recovery. Med Sci Sports Exerc 44:1560–1569

Roig M, O'Brien K, Kirk G, Murray R, McKinnon P, Shadgan B, Reid WD (2009) The effects of eccentric versus concentric resistance training on muscle strength and mass in healthy adults: a systematic review with meta-analyses. Br J Sports Med 43:556–568

Roth SM, Ivey FM, Martel GF, Lemmer JT, Hurlbut DE, Siegel EL, Metter EJ, Fleg JL, Fozard JL, Kostek MC, Wernick DM, Hurley BF (2001) Muscle size responses to strength training in young and older men and women. J Am Geriatr Soc 49:1428–1433

Rudroff T, Justice JN, Holmes MR, Matthews SD, Enoka RM (2011) Muscle activity and time to task failure differ with load compliance and target force for elbow flexor muscles. J Appl Physiol 110:126–136

Rutherfurd SM, Fanning AC, Miller BJ, Moughan PJ (2015) Protein digestibility-corrected amino acid scores and digestible indispensable amino acid scores differentially describe protein quality in growing male rats. J Nutr 145:372–379

Ryan AM, Reynolds JV, Healy L, Byrne M, Moore J, Brannelly N, McHugh A, McCormack D, Flood P (2009) Enteral nutrition enriched with eicosapentaenoic acid (EPA) preserves lean body mass following esophageal cancer surgery: results of a double-blinded randomized controlled trial. Ann Surg 249:355–363

Sanchez-Martinez J, Santos-Lozano A, Garcia-Hermoso A, Sadarangani KP, Cristi-Montero C (2017) Effects of beta-hydroxy-beta-methylbutyrate supplementation on strength and body composition in trained and competitive athletes: a meta-analysis of randomized controlled trials. J Sci Med Sport. https://doi.org/10.1016/j.jsams.2017.11.003

Saragiotto BT, Maher CG, Yamato TP, Costa LO, Menezes Costa LC, Ostelo RW, Macedo LG (2016) Motor control exercise for nonspecific low back pain. Spine 41:1284–1295

Schiessl H, Frost HM, Jee WS (1998) Estrogen and bone-muscle strength and mass relationships. Bone 22:1–6

Schoenau E, Werhahn E, Schiedermaier U, Mokow E, Schiessl H, Scheidhauer K, Michalk D (1996) Influence of muscle strength on bone strength during childhood and adolescence. Horm Res 45:63–66

Searle A, Spink M, Ho A, Chuter V (2015) Exercise interventions for the treatment of chronic low back pain: a systematic review and meta analysis of randomized controlled trials. Clin Rehabil 29:1155–1167

Seynnes OR, de Boer M, Narici MV (2007) Early skeletal muscle hypertrophy and architectural changes in response to high-intensity resistance training. J Appl Physiol 102:368–373

Simoneau JA, Bouchard C (1989) Human variation in skeletal muscle fiber-type proportion and enzyme activities. Am J Physiol 257:E567–E572

Simoneau JA, Bouchard C (1995) Genetic determinism of fiber type proportion in human skeletal muscle. FASEB J 9:1091–1095

Slater G, Phillips SM (2011) Nutrition guidelines for strength sports: sprinting, weightlifting, throwing events, and bodybuilding. J Sports Sci 29:S67–S77

Smalls LK, Hicks M, Passeretti D, Gersin K, Kitzmiller WJ, Bakhsh A, Wickett RR, Whitestone J, Visscher MO (2006) Effect of weight loss on cellulite: gynoid lypodystrophy. Plast Reconstr Surg 118:510–516

Smith GI, Atherton PJ, Reeds DN, Mohammed BS, Rankin D, Rennie MJ, Mittendorfer B (2010) Dietary omega-3 fatty acid supplementation increases the rate of muscle protein synthesis in older adults: a randomized controlled trial. Am J Clin Nutr 93:402–412

Snijders T, Res PT, Smeets JS, van Vliet S, van Kranenburg J, Maase K, Kies AK, Verdijk LB, van Loon LJC (2015) Protein ingestion before sleep increases muscle mass and strength gains during prolonged resistance-type exercise training in healthy young men. J Nutr 145:1178–1184

Spector SA, Simard CP, Fournier M, Sternlicht E, Edgerton V (1982) Architectural alterations of rat hind-limb skeletal muscles immobilized at different lengths. Exp Neurol 76:94–110

Staples AW, Burd NA, West DW, Currie KD, Atherton PJ, Moore DR, Rennie MJ, MacDonald MJ, Baker SK, Phillips SM (2011) Carbohydrate does not augment exercise-induced protein accretion versus protein alone. Med Sci Sports Exerc 43:1154–1161

Stotz PJ, Bawa P (2001) Motor unit recruitment during lengthening contractions of human wrist flexors. Muscle Nerve 24:1535–1541

Street SF (1983) Lateral transmission of tension in frog myofibers: a myofibrillar network and transverse cytoskeletal connections are possible transmitters. J Cell Physiol 114:346–364

Suetta C, Hvid LG, Justesen L, Christensen U, Neergaard K, Imonsen L, Ortenblad N, Magnusson SP, Kjaer M, Aagaard P (2009) Effects of aging on human skeletal muscle after immobilization and retraining. J Appl Physiol 107:1172–1180

Tabary JC, Tabary C, Tardieu C, Tardieu G, Goldspink G (1972) Physiological and structural changes in the cat's soleus muscle due to immobilization at different lengths by plaster casts. J Physiol (London) 224:231–244

Tang JE, Moore DR, Kujbida GW, Tarnopolsky MA, Phillips SM (2009) Ingestion of whey hydrolysate, casein, or soy protein isolate: effects on mixed muscle protein synthesis at rest and following resistance exercise. J Appl Physiol 107:987–992

Tax AA, van der Gon Denier JJ, Gielen CC, van den Tempel CM (1989) Differences in the activation of m. biceps brachii in the control of slow isotonic movements and isometric contractions. Exp Brain Res 76:55–63

ter Haar Romeny BM, van der Gon Denier, Gielen CC (1984) Relation between location of a motor unit in the human biceps brachii and its critical firing levels for different tasks. Exp Neurol 85:631–650

The International Fish Oil Standards Program (IFOS) (2013). http://www.nutrasource.ca/ifos. Accessed: 31. Juli 2014

Thompson D (1917) On Growth and Form. Cambridge University Press, Cambridge (abridged edition 1961)

Thomson WM, Poulton R, Hancox RJ, Ryan KM, Al-Kubaisy S (2007) Changes in medication use from age 26 to 32 in a representative birth cohort. Intern Med J 37:543–549

Toigo M (2006a) Trainingsrelevante Determinanten der molekularen und zellulären Skelettmuskeladaptation, Teil 1: Einleitung und Längenadaptation. Schweiz Zschr Sportmed Sporttraumatol 54:101–106

Toigo M (2006b) Trainingsrelevante Determinanten der molekularen und zellulären Skelettmuskeladaptation, Teil 2: Adaptation von Querschnitt und Fasertypusmodulen. Schweiz Zschr Sportmed Sporttraumatol 54:121–132

Toigo M (2013) Funktionelle Interaktion zwischen Muskeln und Knochen: Theorie und potenzielle klinische Relevanz. J Für Gynäkol Endokrinol 7:14–20

Toigo M, Boutellier U (2006) New fundamental resistance exercise determinants of molecular and cellular muscle adaptations. Eur J Appl Physiol 97:643–663

Van Cutsem M, Duchateau J, Hainaut K (1998) Changes in single motor unit behavior contribute to the increase in contraction speed after dynamic training in humans. J Physiol (London) 513:295–305 van Vliet S, Burd NA, van Loon LJ (2015) The skeletal muscle anabolic response to plantversus animal-based protein consumption. J Nutr 145:1981–1991

van Wijck K, Pennings B, van Bijnen AA, Senden JM, Buurman WA, Dejong CH, van Loon LJ, Lenaerts K (2013) Dietary protein digestion and absorption are impaired during acute postexercise recovery in young men. Am J Physiol Regul Integr Comp Physiol 304:R356–R361

Villareal DT, Smith GI, Shah K, Mittendorfer B (2012) Effect of weight loss on the rate of muscle protein synthesis during fasted and fed conditions in obese older adults. Obesity 20:1780–1786

Wallimann T (2008) Kreatin – warum, wann und für wen? Schweizer Zeitschrift für Ernährungsmedizin 5:29–39

Wallimann T, Tokarska-Schlattner M, Schlattner U (2011) The creatine kinase system and pleiotropic effects of creatine. Amino Acids 40:1271–1296

Walts CT, Hanson ED, Delmonico MJ, Yao L, Wang MQ, Hurley BF (2008) Do sex or race differences influence strength training effects on muscle or fat? Med Sci Sports Exerc 40:669–676

Wernbom M, Augustsson J, Thomeé R (2007) The influence of frequency, intensity, volume and mode of strength training on whole muscle cross-sectional area in humans. Sports Med 37:225–264

West DW, Kujbida GW, Moore DR, Atherton P, Burd NA, Padzik JP, De Lisio M, Tang JE, Parise G, Rennie MJ, Baker SK, Phillips SM (2009) Resistance exercise-induced increases in putative anabolic hormones do not enhance muscle protein synthesis or intracellular signalling in young men. J Physiol (London) 587:5239–5247

West DW, Burd NA, Churchward-Venne TY, Camera DM, Mitchell CJ, Baker SK, Hawley JA, Coffey VG, Phillips SM (2012) Sex-based comparisons of myofibrillar protein synthesis after resistance exercise in the fed state. J Appl Physiol 112:1805–1813

Wilkinson SB, Phillips SM, Atherton PJ, Patel R, Yarasheski KE, Tarnopolsky MA, Rennie MJ (2008) Differential effects of resistance and endurance exercise in the fed state on signalling molecule phosphorylation and protein synthesis in human muscle. J Physiol (London) 586:3701–3717

Wilkinson DJ, Hossain T, Hill DS, Phillips BE, Crossland H, Williams J, Loughna P, Churchward-Venne TA, Breen L, Phillips SM, Etheridge T, Rathmacher JA, Smith K, Szewczyk NJ, Atherton PJ (2013) Effects of leucine and its metabolite β-hydroxyβ-methylbutyrate on human skeletal muscle protein metabolism. J Physiol (London) 591:2911–2923

Wilkinson DJ, Hossain T, Limb MC, Philips BE, Lund J, Williams JP, Brook MS, Cegielski J, Philp A, Ashcroft S, Rathmacher JA, Szewczyk NJ, Smith K, Atherton PJ (2017) Impact of the calcium form of β-hydroxy-β-methylbutyrate upon human skeletal muscle protein metabolism. Clin Nutr. https://doi.org/10.1016/j.clnu.2017.09.024

Williams PE (1988) Effect of intermittent stretch on immobilised muscle. Ann Rheum Dis 47:1014–1016

Williams PE, Goldspink G (1971) Longitudinal growth of striated muscle fibres. J Cell Sci 9:751–767

Williams PE, Goldspink G (1973) The effect of immobilization on the longitudinal growth of striated muscle fibres. J Anat 116:45–55

Williams PE, Watt P, Bicik V, Goldspink G (1986) Effect of stretch combined with electrical stimulation on the type of sarcomeres produced at the ends of muscle fibers. Exp Neurol 93:500–509

Witard OC, Jackman SR, Breen L, Smith K, Selby A, Tipton KD (2014) Myofibrillar muscle protein synthesis rates subsequent to a meal in response to increasing doses of whey protein at rest and after resistance exercise. Am J Clin Nutr 99:86–95

Yang Y, Breen L, Burn NA, Hector AJ, Churchward-Venne TA, Josse AR, Tarnopolsky MA, Phillips SM (2012) Resistance exercise enhances myofibrillar protein synthesis with graded intakes of whey protein in older men. Br J Nutr 28:1780–1788

Zanchetta JR, Plotkin H, Alvarez Filgueira ML (1995) Bone mass in children: normative values for the 2–20-year-old population. Bone 16:393S–399S

# Index

**A**

Acetyl-coenzyme A (acetyl-CoA), 70–72
Actin, 22, 23, 25, 26, 30, 52, 53, 65, 139
Action potential (AP), 21, 23, 24, 41, 43, 45, 47, 51, 77, 98, 100, 102–110, 119, 226, 298
Activity, physical, 9, 153, 269, 274, 304
Adenosine diphosphate (ADP), 52, 53, 59, 64–67, 72, 74, 75, 77, 78, 317
Adenosine monophosphate (AMP), 66, 74, 75, 186–187, 196, 226
Adenosine triphosphate (ATP), 13, 51–54, 59, 60, 63–78, 184, 186–187, 196, 209, 226, 227, 256, 266, 317
Adenylate kinase (AK), 65, 66, 74
Adipocyte, 279
ADP, *see* Adenosine diphosphate (ADP)
Age, 56, 86, 91, 132, 136, 137, 149, 153, 155, 166, 173, 176, 177, 213–215, 217, 220, 238, 246, 248, 249, 257, 262–270, 280, 285, 287, 289–291, 300, 311, 312, 316, 321

Agonist
  inter-muscular coordination, 298, 299
All-or-nothing principle, 47
Amino acid
  availability, 155, 168, 173, 206, 208, 221, 265
  essential, 150, 154, 157–159, 161–163, 165, 174, 175, 202, 206, 208, 221, 255, 263, 314, 320
Amino acid profile, 163, 175
Amino acid scoring pattern (AASP), 158, 159, 162, 174
AMP/ATP ratio, 186–187, 196
Antagonist, 2, 12, 100, 258, 297–299, 309
ATP, *see* Adenosine triphosphate (ATP)
Axon, 23, 41, 44, 45, 47–50, 91, 100, 102–104, 107

**B**

Back problems, 302
Bag full hypothesis, 168
Birth control pill, 247–248
Bodybuilding, 192, 219, 240

Body composition, 272–274
Body fat percentage, 73, 259
Body mass, 10, 21, 58, 73, 153, 167, 168, 170, 173, 176, 207, 210, 211, 213, 215–222, 230, 255, 262, 271–272, 274, 281, 285, 287, 294, 316, 318, 319
Body mass index (BMI), 219, 271, 272, 281
Bone deformation, 258–262, 269
Bone geometry, 258
Bone mass, 213, 248, 258, 259, 269, 272, 300
Bone strength, 257–261, 300, 301

C

Calcium, 23–25, 43, 51, 63, 81, 109, 226, 313, 315
Cam disc, eccentric, 26, 30
Capacity
   metabolic, 74, 157
   transcriptional, 83, 89, 92, 212
Carbohydrate
   recording, 210
Cardiac output, 73, 231–233
Carnitine, 71
Casein, 157, 161–163, 165, 171, 172, 208
Cellulite
   cause, 281
   severity, 281
Central nervous system, 43, 44, 46, 78, 91, 98, 99, 105, 107, 116, 129, 301, 302
Change, statistically significant (LSC), 273, 274, 285
Chronotype, 285
Citrate cycle, 68, 71–73
Coactivation, 297, 298, 309
Combination exercise, 9, 178, 203, 213, 216, 220, 286

Compartment, neuromuscular, 117, 118, 126, 178, 212
Contraceptives, 247–248
Coordination
   intramuscular, 99, 190
Costamer, 122
Creatine, 65, 88, 317–319
Creatine kinase (CK), 65–67, 74, 317
Cross bridge cycle, 23–25, 52–54, 63, 65, 78
Cross-bridging, 23, 25, 52, 54, 63–65, 79
Cycling, 14, 16, 59, 72, 231, 232, 251, 252, 260, 268
Cytokines, 124, 257, 258, 280
Cytoskeleton, 78, 122–124

D

Degeneration, 81–83, 87, 90, 196, 227
Denervation, 91
Deoxyribonucleic acid (DNA), 82–86, 88, 89, 95, 129, 290, 291
Depolarization, 21, 24, 43
Detraining, 60, 91
Diet, 57, 153, 175, 210, 219, 221, 222, 249, 259, 268, 277, 279, 281, 282, 318
Digestibility, ileal, 158, 159, 161, 162, 174, 176
Digestible indispensable amino acid reference ratio (DIAARR), 155, 159, 161–162
Digestible indispensable amino acid score (DIAAS), 155, 158–163, 174, 175
DNA, *see* Deoxyribonucleic acid (DNA)
Domain, myonuclear, 87, 89, 95
Duchenne muscular dystrophy, 91
Dysbalances, 28, 31

## E

End plate, motorized, 41
Endplate strips, 45, 46
Endurance training (ET), 68, 71, 82, 155, 220, 225–236, 247, 252, 253, 265, 268, 285–287, 289
Energy, 12, 24, 51, 63, 157, 186, 226, 239, 252, 256, 271, 288, 312
Energy balance
  negative, 219, 220, 274
Energy consumption, 52, 63, 65, 211, 227
Energy release
  aerobic, 14
  anaerobic, 14
Energy storage, 6, 318
Energy stress, 186–187, 206, 226–227, 235, 252
Energy turnover
  musculoskeletal (MSE), 275
  total daily energy expenditure (TDEE), 275
Enzyme, 13, 54, 59, 63, 65, 67, 68, 73, 97, 184, 283, 317
Epigenetics, 291
Estradiol, 247, 248, 280
Excitation-contraction coupling, 41, 51, 77
Excitatory postsynaptic potential (EPSP), 23, 104–106, 116, 125, 126
Exerceuticals, 252–254, 285, 290, 292, 293
Exercise mimetics, 197
Exercise skills, motor skills, 32, 91, 299
Exhaustion, 16, 20, 114, 115, 120, 143, 144, 181–184, 186–187, 190, 191, 193, 198, 201, 253, 276
Explosivity, 14, 58, 60, 62, 107–109, 112, 115, 120, 140, 194

## F

Fascicle
  length, 5, 45, 133, 135, 136, 138–141, 143–145
Fat
  accumulation, 280
  mobilization, 71, 239
Fat cell, 71, 74, 239, 279, 280, 286
Fatigue, neuromuscular, 77
Fat loss, 220, 272, 274–275, 286
Fatty acid, 24, 59, 66, 70, 71, 73, 85, 239, 279, 280, 316, 317, 320
Fatty acid oxidation, 71
FF (fast fatigable), motor unit
  recruitment time integral, 184, 185, 189, 191, 193, 198, 201
Fiber force, 25, 30, 33, 34, 36, 43, 61, 69, 90, 104, 122, 252, 253, 285
Fibre, intrafusal, 92
Firing frequency, 99–100
Food protein, 85, 154
Force, 1–17, 19–39, 41–45, 47–52, 54, 58, 60–62, 65, 74, 76–82, 85, 87, 91, 98–116, 119–126, 131, 133, 134, 137–145, 170, 175, 178–183, 185–187, 189–195, 197–199, 201, 206, 208, 209, 226, 227, 233, 239, 243, 246, 247, 253, 257–263, 267, 269, 285, 287, 288, 290, 292, 295, 297–310, 312, 313, 318–320
  maximum voluntary, 20, 21, 259
Force curve, 27–31, 112, 308
Force drop, 199
Force target (force task), 301, 302
Frequency coding
  frequency, 43, 44, 99, 298
FR (fast fatigue resistant), motor unit, 50
Full body workout, 203, 237, 238, 243

## G

Gene doping, 197
Gluconeogenesis, 67, 69, 157, 255
Glucose, 24, 59, 66–69, 72, 85, 157, 158, 239, 255, 257, 265
Gluteofemoral region, 280
Glycogen, 24, 66–68, 74, 173, 197, 209–211, 239, 274
Glycogenolysis, 66–68, 74
Glycolysis
　aerobic, 70, 71
　anaerobic, 69–71, 75, 76, 184
Gravity, 10, 19, 123, 230, 259, 275
Ground reaction force, 19–21, 259
Gynecomastia, 248

## H

Henneman's recruitment principle, see Recruitment, size principle
High-intensity interval training (HIIT), 232–235, 252
High responder, 189, 223, 288, 289
Hormone
　anabolic, 172, 238–240, 242, 246
　catabolic, 242, 246
Hybrid fiber, 54, 59, 61, 97
Hyperactivation, 101
Hyperaminoacidemia, 154
Hyperglycemia, 257
Hyperinsulinemia, 157, 257
Hyperpolarization, 116
Hypoaminoacidemia, 154, 158
Hypohydration, 219

## I

Imitation illusion, 293
Impulse, 15, 43, 48, 306
Inflammation, 259, 263
Inflammatory process, chronic, 265, 281, 317
Innervation, 45, 47
Innervation number, 47, 103, 116, 117
Input current, synaptic, 104–106, 115, 125
Insulin
　resistance, 263, 265, 316
Integrity, tensional, 122–124
Interference effect, 225–227, 233–236, 252, 265
Intermediate filament, 122, 123
Isolation exercise, 27

## J

Jet lag, 284

## K

Kinetic chain exercise, 26
Klinefelter syndrome, 248

## L

Lactate
　dehydrogenase (LDH), 68
Latency, 168, 196, 206, 207
Law of Inertia, 10
Lean mass, 19, 163, 166, 167, 170, 171, 214–216, 219, 221, 222, 249, 253, 268, 274, 288, 314–316
Length-force relation, 28–31, 36, 39, 61, 79, 121, 133, 134, 136
Leucine
　threshold, 161
Lever arm, 3, 11, 20, 21, 27, 30, 52, 112, 195
Low responder, 223, 288, 289

## M

Machine training, 294, 304
Man, 73, 242, 246, 256
Master athlete, 266

Matrix, extracellular, 4, 13, 86, 122, 124
Maximum force, 20–21, 34, 261, 300, 309, 310
Measurement accuracy, 272
Mechanostat theory, 258, 259
Membrane potential, 52, 63, 103–105
Menstrual cycle, 238, 247
Messenger RNA (mRNA), 84, 85, 94, 148, 149, 197
Metabolite, 13, 66, 77–78, 197
Microtrauma, 45, 78–81, 86, 87, 123, 124, 134, 142, 196, 227
Mitochondria, 59, 65–76, 83, 90, 123, 284, 317
Modeling, 59, 118, 122, 134, 140, 159, 182, 197, 266, 293, 294, 314, 316
Moment arm, 11, 20, 21, 28–30, 110
Motoneuron, 23, 41–47, 91, 97, 100, 102, 104, 105, 107–109, 115, 116, 119, 125, 298, 308
Motoneuron axon, 41, 45
Movement phase
　miometric, 182, 193
　pliometric, 182, 193
Ms., 306, 308
Multi-set training, 293
Muscle activation, 21, 182, 302, 304
Muscle activity
　isometric, 4, 9, 297
　miometric, 9
　pliometric, 9, 195
Muscle afference, 78, 92, 302
Muscle architecture
　multipennate, 37
　spindle-shaped, 36
　unipennate, 37
Muscle atrophy, 91, 132, 146, 291
Muscle biopsy, 94, 215, 304
Muscle-bone unit, 258–260
Muscle cell, 24, 67, 84–86, 92, 95, 109, 122, 130, 145, 238, 257, 284, 314, 319
Muscle contraction
　eccentric, 4, 6, 16, 79
　concentric, 4, 6, 16
Muscle cross-sectional area, 36–38, 144, 145, 195, 212, 215, 218, 267, 272, 287, 288, 290, 292, 297, 299, 300, 308, 309, 317
Muscle fiber
　atrophy, 92, 146
　classification, 55, 129
　energy consumption, 52, 63, 65
　hyperplasia, 90, 146
　hypertrophy, 46, 87–90, 92, 94, 129, 130, 139, 142–144, 146, 168, 193, 212, 228, 229, 253, 268
　intrafascicular, 45, 46, 91, 123
　regeneration, 64, 83, 85
　repair, 86, 212, 265
Muscle fiber length, 30, 31, 33, 36, 80, 132, 134, 135, 143
Muscle fiber splitting, 91
Muscle fiber type, distribution, 55–59, 267, 300, 304
Muscle-full effect, 168, 169, 206, 241
Muscle injury, 78, 265
Muscle length, 5, 29–31, 33–38, 80, 90, 92, 131–133, 135, 137, 138, 140, 141, 143, 144, 189, 199
Muscle mass, 10, 19, 32, 38, 56–58, 85, 90–92, 98, 100, 109, 120, 129, 146, 147, 149, 153, 157, 158, 166, 167, 171, 178, 183, 192, 197, 202, 211, 213, 215, 217, 219, 220, 222, 225, 227, 229, 230, 233, 235, 239, 241, 245–249, 255–259, 263, 264, 269–275, 282, 286, 290–292, 294, 295, 298, 300, 309, 312, 313, 316–321
Muscle memory, 91, 92
Muscle pH, 78

Muscle power, internal, 19–20, 28, 30, 34, 111, 112, 189
Muscle protein breakdown rate (MPB), 147–150, 154, 157, 158, 166, 168, 170–174, 176, 177, 179, 201, 204, 209–211, 213, 220, 227, 241, 245–247, 255–258, 264, 269, 314–316, 320
Muscle protein metabolism, 153–154, 175, 247, 256, 316
Muscle protein synthesis (MPS), 88, 94, 109, 114, 147–150, 154, 157, 158, 160–184, 186–187, 189–191, 193, 195, 196, 198, 201–213, 217, 219–221, 226–227, 241–243, 245–247, 251–253, 256, 258, 263, 264, 269, 312, 314–316, 320
Muscle protein synthesis rate (MPS) increase, 149, 165, 166, 176, 178–180, 196, 204, 207, 211, 246, 252, 253, 256
Muscle shortening, 2, 3, 5, 8, 17, 34
Muscle soreness, 69, 78–82, 125
Muscle spindle, 92, 302
Muscle stem cell, 86, 95
Muscle-tendon unit, 4–6, 11, 12, 78, 115, 130–132, 138, 141, 142, 144, 193, 231, 301, 308
Muscular atrophy, 91, 92, 132, 146, 291
Musculature, striated, 25, 139
MyHC isoform, 54, 55, 58, 60, 63, 64, 74, 97, 108, 139
Myoblast, 86
Myofibrils, 22, 25, 67, 73, 79, 90, 130, 145, 146
Myofilament, 23–25, 43
Myoglobin, 51, 72
Myokin, 257, 262
Myosin
    heavy and light chains, 53, 55, 228

Myostatin, 290, 291
Myotubulus, 86, 91

N

Necrosis, 83
Negative training, 8, 16, 17, 83, 144, 194, 195, 262
Nerve, 3, 32, 41, 42, 44, 45, 78, 93, 117, 131, 196, 319, 320
Nerve impulse, 43
Net muscle protein balance (NBIL), 147–150, 158, 160–164, 166, 169–173, 175, 176, 178, 179, 189, 191, 198, 201, 202, 204, 207, 213, 222, 264, 269, 316
Neurotransmitter, 105, 157
Newton, I., 10, 14
Nutrition, 161, 164, 214, 216, 217, 222, 268, 271, 276, 278, 285, 286, 293, 295, 321
Nutritional supplements, 293

O

Obesity, 256, 257, 271, 276
Omega-3 fatty acid, 317
One-repeat maximum (1RM), 180–184, 189, 190, 210–212, 214–216, 219, 225, 226, 228, 251, 253, 268, 284, 287–289, 315
Orange peel skin, see Cellulite
Osteoblasts, 258
Osteoclasts, 258
Osteocytes, 258
Osteoporosis, 257, 263, 311
Overtraining, 227, 278
Overweight, 219, 256, 257, 271, 274
Oxygen
Oxygen species, reactive, 77, 78

## P

Peak power, 230, 252
Pennation angle, 37–39, 308, 309
Periodization, 227–229
Phosphate, inorganic, 52, 65
Phosphocreatine (PCr), 65
Phosphorylation, oxidative, 65, 72, 76
Polymorphism, genetic, 290
Popping sarcomere theory, 79, 134, 142
Position drop, 302
Position target (position task), 302
Power
   critical, 230
   mechanical, 13, 14, 16, 68, 70, 76, 182, 230, 232, 263, 298, 299, 318
   metabolic, 14, 64, 65, 70, 76, 239
Power production
   miometric, 6, 8, 11, 82, 111, 115, 137, 140, 141, 189, 191
   pliometric, 6, 8, 21, 61, 79, 80, 82, 115, 116, 137, 138, 140, 142, 189, 299
Pregnancy, 154, 262
Propagation effect, 124, 237, 242
Progenitor cell, myogenic (MPC), 86, 87, 159, 162
Progesterone, 247
Progestin, 247, 249
Protein, 13, 51, 63, 78, 81, 105, 129, 147, 153, 177, 201, 226, 241, 245, 251, 255, 271, 290, 314
Protein amounts, 166, 170, 218
Protein content, 60, 90, 129, 147, 160, 161, 164, 175, 176
Protein degradation, 85, 91, 139, 149
Protein digestion, 208–209
Protein intake, 91, 145, 154, 161–163, 166, 168–172, 174, 177, 178, 201–223, 241, 245, 256, 264, 268, 274, 313
Protein metabolism, 153–154, 162, 163, 169, 172, 175, 241, 315
Protein quality, 155, 158–165, 174, 176, 217, 218
Protein requirement, 217, 255
Protein shake, 167, 168, 171–173, 176, 211, 218, 220, 222
Protein source, 158–165, 167, 174–176, 218, 221, 222
Protein supplementation, 163, 203, 213–221
Protein synthesis
   splanchnical, 163
Proteolysis, 81
Pyruvate
   dehydrogenase, 68, 70

## R

Range of motion (ROM), 20, 26–28, 30, 32, 111, 132–134, 139–144, 180–182, 193, 195, 253, 288, 304
Reaction matrix, 222, 285, 287, 290, 292
Recruitment, size principle, 106, 109, 125
Recruitment threshold, 50, 100–102, 107–113, 115, 125, 191, 210
Refractory period, 43
Refractory phase, 202, 204
Regeneration, 64–76, 81–83, 85–87, 90, 184, 196, 209, 210, 227, 317
Repetitions, number of, 143, 180, 182, 191, 193–195, 198, 212, 306
Reserve, autonomous, 100–101
Resistance, anabolic, 166, 176, 177, 203, 263–266, 269, 312
Respiration, mitochondrial, 64, 66, 72–75, 317
Reticulum, sarcoplasmic, 23, 24, 43, 53, 63, 67, 73, 77, 81, 123

Retraining, 91, 92
Rhythm, circadian, 282–284
Ribonucleic acid (RNA), 83, 84
Ribosome, 84, 94
RNA, *see* Ribonucleic acid (RNA)
Rotational resistance, 27

S

Sarcolemma, 21, 23, 24, 41, 43, 51, 67, 69, 77, 81–83, 86, 319
Sarcomere
 connected in parallel, 25, 36, 43, 145, 299
 serial, 30, 33, 131–139, 144, 145
Sarcopenia, 263, 265, 312
Satellite cell, 86–90, 95, 124, 129, 130, 132, 241, 265, 266
Secretom, 259
Shortening speed, 7, 34, 52, 54, 107, 134
Signal (transduction) cascade, 124, 197
Signal transmission, paracrine, 124
Single twitch, 48–50
S (slow), motor unit, 48–50, 97, 106, 109, 114, 185–187
Soy protein, 159, 161–163
Speed
 of the force development, 263
 of the movement, 7, 35, 120
Speed, critical (critical velocity), 230
Speed-force relation, 61
Split training, 237–238, 294
Steroid, anabolic, 91, 220, 240
Strength endurance, 15, 16
Strength training, sport-specific, 120
Stretching, 7, 8, 21, 79, 80, 82, 130–134, 136, 137, 139, 140, 142–144, 304
Stretch-shorten cycle, 5, 6
Summation of the force, 43
Supercompensation, 197–198

Suprachiasmatic nucleus (SCN), 283, 284
Synapse, 23, 41, 45, 46
System
 glycolytic, 67
 phosphagenes, 65–68, 74, 317
*Système International d'Unités* (SI), 9, 20, 43, 66

T

Task, motor, 99, 100, 102, 107, 110, 111, 114, 116, 120, 121, 178, 181, 189, 298, 301, 309
Testosterone, 57, 238–242, 246, 248, 249, 280
Test-retest reliability, 272, 273
Thermogenesis, 14
Titin, 139
Torque, 1, 11, 12, 19, 20, 27–29, 31, 35, 77, 110, 112–114, 116, 120, 138–140, 144, 190, 195, 197, 213, 242, 243, 253, 263, 267, 287, 288, 292, 298, 304, 317
Torso musculature, 29, 110
Total daily energy expenditure (TDEE), *see* Energy expenditure
Training
 ballistic, 107, 110, 120
 explosive, 14, 60, 62, 107, 194
 plyometric, 7
Training adaptation, specificity, 225, 251–254, 305
Training machine, 294, 304
Training volume, 184, 228, 229, 278
Transcription, 83–85, 129
Translation, 84, 85, 94–96, 129, 130, 142, 148, 149, 285
Trigger zone, 41, 47, 103, 105, 107, 108, 119
Triglycerides, 24, 74
Tropomyosin, 23, 24, 53

Troponin, 23, 53, 78
Trunk stabilization training, 303, 305, 309, 310
Type 2 diabetes, 74, 257, 263

### U
Unit, motor
  activity, 307, 309
  derecruitment, 111, 116
  FF type, 48–49, 54, 97, 114, 185–187, 190, 201
  FR type, 48–49, 97, 185, 186
  recruitment, 98, 102–106, 109, 111, 114–117, 120, 125, 126, 179, 186–187, 190, 198, 201
  S-type, 48–50, 54, 97, 185

### V
Variability, interindividual, 211, 287–289, 291, 293
VibroX, 253
Vitamin D, 311–314, 319

Voltage duration
  effective time under tension, 114, 115, 120, 183, 185–187, 190, 193

### W
Watt, J., 13
Weight
  free, 27
Weight force, 8, 11, 12, 21, 27, 301
Weight-gainer, 211
Weight training, 27, 170, 192, 209, 247
Whey protein, 159, 162–163, 165–167, 169, 171–176, 201–203, 205–207, 220, 245
Work, mechanical, 12–14, 17, 76, 180–182, 184, 191, 195, 292

### Z
Z-disk, 26, 78, 122, 139

GPSR Compliance

The European Union's (EU) General Product Safety Regulation (GPSR) is a set of rules that requires consumer products to be safe and our obligations to ensure this.

If you have any concerns about our products, you can contact us on

ProductSafety@springernature.com

In case Publisher is established outside the EU, the EU authorized representative is:

Springer Nature Customer Service Center GmbH
Europaplatz 3
69115 Heidelberg, Germany